D0193056

Praise for Ann Louise Gittleman's Work

I deeply respect and honor the work of Ann Louise Gittleman, whom I consider as a teacher, as well as what she has done to bring intelligence to the world of nutrition.
—**Mark Hyman**, MD, author of *Eat Fat, Get Thin*

I always admired her passion for healing for all, her desire to look deeper, and her healing wisdom.
—**Dr. Raphael Kellman**, Kellman Center for Functional & Integrative Medicine

A powerful "Force of Nature" in the healing community, Ann Louise is used to being on the cutting edge. Want to see what the experts will be saying in 25 years? Simply see what she is saying NOW!
—**Jacob Teitelbaum**, MD, author of *The Complete Guide to Beating Sugar Addiction*

A longtime guiding light in the world of nutritional medicine, Ann Louise continues to be The First Lady of Nutrition and someone I can always count on for the best information for my patients, my readers, and me. Not only is she knowledgeable and a pioneer in the field, but she is a truly caring person who is dedicated to changing the world, one body at a time. I'm proud to call her my friend.
—**Hyla Cass**, MD, author of *Supplement Your Prescription*

Ann Louise's Fat Flush Plan is dietary common sense for all the right reasons—it's balanced, it's a program you can safely stay on for life, and it works.
—**Dr. Barry Sears**, author of *The Zone*

If nutrition has glamour, she's got it!
—The late **Robert C. Atkins**, MD, author of *Dr. Atkins' New Diet Revolution*

Ann Louise Gittleman has demonstrated extraordinary leadership when it comes to reporting on the fundamental causes of illness and disease. Whether it's parasites in *Guess What Came to Dinner?* or environmental toxins in *The Fat Flush Plan* or toxic EMF or RF in *Zapped*, she reaches the hearts of the public by not only demonstrating what causes illness, but she also offers solutions on how to fix them! I'm proud to be one of her colleagues.
—**Stephen Sinatra**, MD, FACC, integrative cardiologist and coauthor of *Health Revelations from Heaven and Earth*

I have been privileged to know Ann Louise Gittleman for a number of decades and respect her dedication in assisting others to achieve vibrant health with nutrition and natural therapies. She is truly at the top of her field, deserving designation as "The First Lady of Nutrition."

—**Jonathan V. Wright**, MD, Medical Director,
Tahoma Clinic, Tukwila, Washington

Ann Louise Gittleman is a dynamic pioneer and leading authority in nutrition, health, and wellness. She is a beacon of light and inspiration for millions of people who seek advanced healing information that genuinely transforms their lives.

—**Anthony William**, author of *Medical Medium:*
Mystery & Chronic Illness

Ann Louise Gittleman is to be commended for getting the detox message out to mainstream Americans. I couldn't agree more with her message and her methods.

—**Elson M. Haas**, MD, author of *Staying Healthy*
with New Medicine

Ann Louise Gittleman has been one of my closest "sisterfriends" for years. Not only do we enjoy a warm personal relationship but I have been a huge professional fan of hers for decades. We share a mutual passion as "nutrition detectives" to find underlying root causes of disease and disharmony and a healthy respect for the emerging field of energy medicine.

—**Nan Kathryn Fuchs**, PhD, nutrition expert and author

Over the years, Ann Louise has always been at the forefront when it comes to nutrition for optimal health and weight loss. As a guest on my radio show, she frequently and generously shared her knowledge and cutting-edge advice with my listeners, answering their questions and discussing all aspects of healthy eating for both general health and healthy weight loss. I incorporated her Fat Flush Plan into my popular Fit Camps with successful results and was honored to coauthor *The Fat Flush Fitness Plan*. In a world where advice can be so questionable, Ann Louise continues to offer sound advice.

—**Joanie Greggains**, original star of TV's *Morning Stretch*;
health and fitness educator

Ann Louise has always been one of my favorite go-to nutritionists. Her Fat Flush Plan and other programs, supplements, and test kits have paved the way for a whole new generation of health and environmentally like-minded advocates and activists. She is STILL a superstar in our changing world and we are all very grateful for her tireless efforts to bring the most cutting-edge wisdom to a world that desperately needs it.

—**Donna Gates**, author and creator of *Body Ecology*

When it comes to wellness through nutrition, Ann Louise Gittleman not only pioneered the field; she continues to be ahead of her time and on top of the game. At *First for Women*, we rely on Gittleman to alert us to the newest scientific studies with the most urgent relevance for our readers—and she always delivers.

—**Carol Brooks**, editor in chief of *First for Women* magazine

the
NEW

Fat
Flush
Plan

Also by Ann Louise Gittleman, PhD, CNS

Fat Flush for Life

The Complete Fat Flush Program

The Fat Flush Cookbook

The Fat Flush Journal and Shopping Guide

The Fat Flush Fitness Plan

Zapped

The Gut Flush Plan

The Fast Track Detox Diet

Hot Times

The Fat Flush Foods

Ann Louise Gittleman's Guide to the 40/30/30 Phenomenon

Eat Fat, Lose Weight Cookbook

The Living Beauty Detox Program

Why Am I Always So Tired?

Super Nutrition for Men

How to Stay Young and Healthy in a Toxic World

Eat Fat, Lose Weight

Overcoming Parasites

Super Nutrition for Menopause

Beyond Probiotics

The 40/30/30 Phenomenon

Before the Change

Your Body Knows Best

Get the Salt Out

Get the Sugar Out

Guess What Came to Dinner? Parasites and Your Health

Super Nutrition for Women

Beyond Pritikin

Eat Fat, Lose Weight for Kindle

The Fat Flush App for iPhone and iPad

the NEW Fat Flush Plan

ANN LOUISE GITTLEMAN, PHD, CNS

Mc
Graw
Hill
Education

New York Chicago San Francisco Athens
London Madrid Mexico City Milan New Delhi
Singapore Sydney Toronto

Fat Flush, and all variations thereof, is a registered trademark exclusively owned by First Lady of Nutrition, Inc., including but not limited to the accompanying trade dress, symbols, designs and goodwill associated therewith.

Copyright © 2017 by Ann Louise Gittlemen. All rights reserved. Printed in the United States of America. Except as permitted under the United States Copyright Act of 1976, no part of this publication may be reproduced or distributed in any form or by any means, or stored in a database or retrieval system, without the prior written permission of the publisher.

1 2 3 4 5 6 7 8 9   LWI   21 20 19 18 17 16

ISBN   978-1-259-86113-0
MHID   1-259-86113-9

e-ISBN   978-1-260-01111-1
e-MHID   1-260-01111-9

This book is for educational purposes. It is not intended as a substitute for medical advice. Please consult a qualified healthcare professional for individual health and medical advice. Neither McGraw-Hill Education nor the author shall have any responsibility for any adverse effects arising directly or indirectly as a result of the information provided in this book.

Throughout this book, trademarked names are used. Rather than put a trademark symbol after every occurrence of a trademarked name, we use names in an editorial fashion only, and to the benefit of the trademark owner, with no intention of infringement of the trademark. Where such designations appear in this book, they have been printed with initial caps.

Library of Congress Cataloging-in-Publication Data
Names: Gittleman, Ann Louise, author.
Title: The new fat flush plan / Ann Louise Gittleman.
Other titles: Fat flush plan
Description: Second edition. | New York : McGraw-Hill Education, [2017] |
    Originally published: Fat flush plan. c2002.
Identifiers: LCCN 2016040689 (print) | LCCN 2016041461 (ebook) | ISBN
    9781259861130 (hardback) | ISBN 1259861139 (hardback) | ISBN 9781260011111
    () | ISBN 1260011119
Subjects: LCSH: Weight loss. | Reducing diets—Recipes. | BISAC: HEALTH &
    FITNESS / Diets.
Classification: LCC RM222.2 .G5373 2017 (print) | LCC RM222.2 (ebook) | DDC
    613.2/5—dc23
LC record available at https://na01.safelinks.protection.outlook.com/?url=https%3a
    %2f%2flccn.loc.gov%2f2016040689&data=01%7c01%7ckari.black%40mheducation
    .com%7c9a53c8498e1d4fa42ab008d3d8302451%7cf919b1efc0c347358fca0928ec39d8d
    5%7c1&sdata=DI4agHcBY3kkEXxajUHVNxs6dqDp01HfciAqPT4%2bvnc%3d

McGraw-Hill Education books are available at special quantity discounts to use as premiums and sales promotions or for use in corporate training programs. To contact a representative, please visit the Contact Us pages at www.mhprofessional.com.

To my longtime agent and friend, the late Mike Cohn
—this one's STILL for you!

Contents

The Fat Flush Phenomenon

This updated and revised edition is right on time. In light of the game-changing health ideas that *Fat Flush* first championed over 15 years ago that are trending today, this edition couldn't come any sooner. Like its pioneering predecessor, *The New Fat Flush Plan* offers evidence-based detox and diet strategies for weight loss, for improvement of the hormonal and metabolic impact of foods, and for liver cleansing and overall wellness. It features a heightened emphasis on the forgotten importance of bile—a focus that the earliest health pioneers of the twentieth century wrote about prolifically. Today we recognize that the bile connection is linked to a myriad of conditions that the Fat Flush Plan targets, including inadequate fat metabolism, gallbladder issues, constipation, poor estrogen metabolism, and hypothyroidism.

As many of my fans have told me, the first edition of *Fat Flush* was the "first" in many arenas: it was the first to declare that calories don't count, that food sensitivities—including gluten—and chemical toxins can make us fat, that prescription meds can be fattening, and that too little sleep and stress are major fat promoters thanks to fluctuating cortisol levels. With emerging trends and promising research currently focused on higher-fat diets (like paleo and ketogenic) and fasting-cleansing (think green drinks), the Fat Flush Plan continues to evolve and focus on lifestyle medicine that is easy and doable.

We all know there are no quick fixes—but the Fat Flush Plan comes close. As an integrative functional medicine advocate always on the lookout to identify and correct metabolic and nutritional imbalance, I have unrelentingly searched beyond the conventional answers to uncover the root causes of unexplained weight gain. Thankfully, my investigative nature has paid off. Years of hands-on experience and avidly following the latest research studies and diet trends led me to insights into lasting weight control that I am excited to share with you in this book.

The Fat Flush phenomenon really began in the year 2000. That year marked not only the beginning of the new millennium but also the birth of the expanded and complete Fat Flush Plan—a quick and easy way to feel fit and strong while erasing those pockets of fat that bother us the most. Previously, Fat Flush appeared as a chapter in my first book, *Beyond Pritikin*, which came out over 10 years prior.

The year 2000 was also when iVillage, the most popular women's health site on the Internet at that time, approached me to be a guest expert on its

Diet and Fitness channel. The iVillage online Fat Flush community received so many positive reviews within the first four months after release, along with over 400,000 hits monthly, that it soon became one of the leading traffic drivers of the Diet and Fitness channel.

The media picked it up and dubbed this initial diet blueprint the Internet Miracle Diet. Since then, the Fat Flush Message Board on iVillage has become one of the most popular diet and fitness boards in the history of the website—a fact that truly amazed me. Magazines followed suit, featuring my rapid weight loss diet. *Woman's World* made Fat Flush its cover story in the early spring of 2000 as well as in January and February of 2001. *First for Women* also featured an adaptation of my diet on the cover, and the magazine included my own testimonial inside.

All of this unexpected national attention, however, did more than just spotlight this burgeoning diet plan. It was the catalyst for its development into a full-fledged book.

When *Fat Flush* was launched in the bookstores in 2002, it quickly climbed onto bestseller lists in publications nationwide including the *New York Times*, *Wall Street Journal*, *USA Today*, and *Publishers Weekly*. I remember my agent calling me at six o'clock in the morning when the book first hit the *New York Times* bestseller list, wanting to know what I had done to generate sales. He said the publisher was also curious, as the book's success was an unexpected surprise to all of them—but not me. I knew that dieting was not just about calories in and calories out. There was a whole slew of underlying factors that needed to be reckoned with for optimal health.

The concept of fat flushing was beginning to revolutionize weight loss and change the way Americans ate by introducing the principles of clean eating, detox with targeted liver and lymphatic support, and lifestyle modifications (journaling, movement, and stress reduction) on a daily basis. The Fat Flush Plan became the basic template behind a myriad of other diets, cleanses, juicing fasts, and detox regimens out there—which today is commonplace, but back then, it was revolutionary!

Soon a tsunami of Fat Flush interviews, spin-off diets, and critiques not only hit the airwaves, in shows such as *Dr. Oz* and *The View*, but also graced the pages of major national media, including *Time* magazine, *O Magazine*, *Self*, and the *New York Times*, among many others. The growing interest in my Fat Flush concepts led to seven "Cruise to Lose" cruises to Alaska, the Caribbean, and the Mexican Riviera. Fat Flushers learned how to adapt the diet and exercise program to real-life challenges. One of our cruisers lost a record 13 pounds in 8 days!

The Fat Flush phenomenon also led to the creation of an in-house detox, diet, and exercise residential program at one of the finest women's spas in the country in the early 2000s—the Greenhouse Spa, a five-star destination spa in Arlington, Texas. This was accompanied by a family of Fat Flush books including the *Fat Flush Cookbook, Fat Flush Journal and Shopping Guide, Fat Flush Foods, Fat Flush Fitness Plan*, and *Fat Flush for Life*, which was named "one of the Top 10 Diet Books" by *Time* magazine. The book takes a seasonal approach to well-being with a more detailed fitness program and advanced wellness treatments for the whole body.

However, what I probably valued the most throughout the years was the online community spirit that Fat Flush spawned. For a period of close to 15 years, a number of dedicated and devoted veteran Fat Flushers manned messaging boards and forums 24/7 to answer a myriad of daily questions and concerns ranging from protocol clarifications, to day-to-day detox symptoms, to challenges of the "working mom." These groups encouraged me to examine every aspect of the plan under a huge magnifying glass to learn why Fat Flush was supporting them on so many levels: body, mind, and spirit.

I soon realized that Fat Flush was way more than just a diet program. It was also a journey into self-care.

Simply put, you deserve to put self-nurturing at the top of your to-do list. Sometimes repressed emotions and self-sabotaging patterns become embedded in the cells. They trigger all types of behavior that can impede your best weight loss efforts, not to mention overall health. Researchers have suggested that the most prevalent reason women fail at their diets is due to a lack of support. The right kind of support can empower individuals to cope with the emotional, social, and even spiritual issues commonly associated with foods. Maybe that's why one of our online community members once wrote, "I would have never in my wildest imagination conceived that I could be so fed, so fortified, so supported, so connected to an online community."

TEND AND BEFRIEND

A landmark study from UCLA proves something that my online community members have already suspected: a unique friendship forms between women. Your circle of friends makes life so much brighter and the tough times not so dark. The researchers at UCLA have demonstrated that women who are under stress produce brain chemicals that open them up to making and maintaining friendships with other women. One of the study's leading researchers, Laura Cousin Klein, PhD, explains that before this study, it was generally assumed that when a person experienced stress, the hormones released created a fight-or-flight response, but women have a distinct response to stress.

"In fact," says Dr. Klein, "it seems that when the hormone oxytocin is released as part of the stress responses in a woman, it buffers the 'fight-or-flight' response and encourages her to tend children and gather women instead." Men do not have this response because of the high amounts of testosterone they produce when they are under stress. So when men are stressed, they tend to go off by themselves, and when women are stressed, they gather other women around them.

While women may especially need community in times of stress, isolation in itself is an innately stressful experience for both genders. As you will read, nothing sabotages weight loss efforts like excess stress. Humans are pack animals and are therefore programmed to feel more comfortable and be more successful in a community setting. Not feeling that sense of community is paramount to fighting a bear with your bare hands: it can be done, but it's exponentially harder than if you had the aid of even the most basic of weapons. Psychological research has proved over and over again that social support aids in weight loss. For both men and woman, going through this health-seeking process with even one other person who has the same goal as you and who will hold you accountable can be the difference between creating a new way of living and letting this journey turn into another failed diet.

There is simply no reason to go it alone anymore. In addition to the guidance you will have from my book, my online Facebook community (Fat Flush Community) is nurturing, supportive, and nonjudgmental. We also have the Fat Flush App to connect you to resources and make healthy choices. I invite you to check it out!

WHAT'S NEW?

As the past 10 years have flown by since my first mini-update of the plan in 2006, I have heard from people across the globe, and they have requested "more." Specifically, they asked for more healthy fats, more food options, more snacks, more recipes, more vegan substitutes, and more exercise variations.

What distinguishes this book from the earlier version is that this edition presents a whole array of breakthroughs. Among them: an accelerated Three-Day Ultra Fat Flush Tune-Up as a jump-start to the phase 1 two-week program. There is a brand-new Fat Flush bone broth that is a supercharged side and snack and can be tweaked for specific health concerns. Popular slimming fats are introduced much earlier in the program, such as metabolism-revving coconut oil, appetite-taming avocado, and chia and hemp seeds, which are now a "legal" exchange for phytohormone-rich flax seed. There is a new vegan protein powder made from GMO-free pea and rice as well as expanded natural sweetening options beyond stevia, such as a monk fruit–erythritol blend and chicory root syrup. A large, updated recipe section includes more family-friendly meals, and there's a shopping list that mentions brand names.

As alluded to earlier, a key innovative concept that this version showcases is how bile—the body's ignored but key method of breaking down fats and eliminating toxins—can be linked to stubborn fat deposits and a host of seemingly unrelated symptoms. While the original Fat Flush introduced the importance of the liver as an unrecognized fat-burning organ, the updated program takes this many steps further by explaining the importance of bile, especially for those without a gallbladder—and those with a gallbladder still intact!

WHAT'S IN STORE?

The first part of the book introduces you to the progression of the Fat Flush concept and expands upon the hidden weight gain factors to include five more than the original. Not only will you read the science behind each one, but you'll learn all about how each facet of the Fat Flush protocol addresses each factor. And I know you will feel encouraged by reading some of the fresh testimonials, observations, and stories from Fat Flushers everywhere.

Then we move on to the easy Fat Flush game plan. You'll gain a practical understanding of the principles behind each phase of the plan and see how simple it is to put them into action as you graduate from one level to the next. There are details about the fat-burning supplements needed for each phase, with helpful tips and words of wisdom from Fat Flushers who have been there. And you'll discover the power of ritual in your life in supporting your weight loss goals. You'll learn how to keep a daily journal, tracking your progress, eating patterns, and emotional triggers. You will also discover how to sculpt a healthy and strong body—without strenuous exercises. And you will see how to boost your body's immune system, physical repair, and even fat-burning ability while you experience the "art" and science of proper sleep and rest.

You will also find a wealth of information at your fingertips, including the updated Master Shopping List with brand names (like the best-tasting flaxseed oils and bone broths) and quick tips on food preparation and storage as well as useful health tips. You will also discover more than 50 quick and delicious recipes, as well as ideas on how to modify your favorite recipes and holiday delights the Fat Flush way. You'll learn smart, no-stress ways to take Fat Flush on the road, whether it's eating out at your favorite restaurant, attending a business luncheon, or celebrating that special occasion.

The last part of the book gives you straight answers to the more commonly asked questions about the plan itself as well as special concerns. You'll also find a comprehensive "Resources and Support" chapter of helpful products, educational resources, nutritional organizations, labs, magazines, newsletters, and pure food and clean water sources where you can purchase products and get more information about the items or ideas mentioned in this book.

As you embark on your Fat Flush experience, I'd like you to keep a few things in mind. You are an individual, and so is your rate of weight loss. Your body is unique, which means your weight loss challenges are not necessarily like your best friend's or even other family members'. This is probably the most frustrating concept for Fat Flushers to accept. You will discover your own roadblocks and learn how to remove them, one step at a time, at your own pace.

I've tried to make the plan as easy as possible for this reason. You will start slowly and gradually make a few dietary and lifestyle changes, one at a time, even before you start. By easing into each progressive phase, you won't feel overwhelmed.

And take things one day at a time. Remember, Fat Flush is a journey toward your weight loss destination. Be kind to and supportive of yourself. It's important to learn how to recognize and applaud even your smallest accomplishments of the day. And even if you slip sometimes—as we all do— that's okay. It's called being human.

But most of all, you can accomplish your weight, health, hormonal, and fitness goals because I will be there with you to help guide the way. I also have been there. You and I will do this together. Be patient with yourself and let your most radiant and authentic self emerge.

Let your journey begin . . .

Ann Louise Gittleman

Acknowledgments

The updated and revised Fat Flush Plan was a bittersweet labor of love. It brought back many fond memories of the original book that was written in my hometown of West Hartford, Connecticut, at my parents' home during the spring and early summer of 2001. It was a magical time for me, where I hung out with my mother and father after long days (and nights) of nonstop writing to meet my deadline. And just like when I was in high school, my parents would stay up late with me and would make sure I was eating three square meals a day and snacks—but this time in Fat Flush style. My mother lost 10 pounds that summer!

My parents have since passed—and these days "the presence of their absence" (by Rabbi David Small) is always with me . . .

This time around, the words have flowed much more easily with more than a decade of firsthand experience and research. I owe much of this to the continual support and love of my staff, researchers, and moderators who selflessly man my online communities day and night. How can I ever thank you?

So, heartfelt thanks first and foremost to my intern, Emily Carmichael, who provided the millennial perspective with an extraordinary grasp of the science—far beyond her years. Her creative assistance with the foundation of the program shines through and through. In equal measure, I must recognize my brand manager, Ally Mortensen, who kept us all on track and orchestrated various generations of the manuscript. Stuart Gittleman, my significant brother, provided his research expertise in numerous ways with references and resources.

My marketing team headed by the very talented Carol Templeton Volanski has been a godsend to me. Chris Todd and Shae Janda are blessed with talents and know-how that constantly amaze me.

My IT department headed by the brilliant Matt Carnegey is always ready to assist—morning, noon, and night!

My sincere appreciation goes out to my moderators past and present: Linda Leekley, Linda Mitchell, Linda Shapiro, Charli Sorenson, Nina Moreau, Janine Forbes, Terri White, Carol Ackerman, Sue Durand, Michelle O'Reardon, Cathy Gorbenko, Elisa Bieg, Linda Pankhurst, Kathy Jensen, Lisa Nectoux, Kathleen Sullivan, Jackie Scott, Mary Dodge, Barbara Anderson, Chris Patterson, and Priscilla Underwood.

Without the oversight and encouragement of my agent, Coleen O'Shea—this edition would not have been possible. Coleen has been in my literary life since my first book nearly three decades ago. I must also thank the remarkable Nancy Hancock, who was the first to understand my vision and was the original editor who made the book such a success. Thanks also to the team at McGraw-Hill Education, especially publisher Chris Brown, Cheryl Ringer, Donya Dickerson, Ann Pryor, and Chelsea Van Der Gaag. Major kudos extended to Patty Wallenburg—who was an absolute doll to work with. My deepfelt thanks are also extended to Judy Duguid, Alison Shurtz, and Claire Splan.

I have been very blessed to have had continual coverage in many of the top women's magazines in this country, especially *First for Women*. I owe a huge dept of gratitude to the Bauer Publishing Company CEO Hubert Boehle, Bauer Media Sales President and Publisher Ian Scott, Editor in Chief Carol Brooks, Deputy Editor in Chief Maggie Jaqua, as well as their wonderful staff: Melissa Gotthardt, Melissa Sorrells, Rebecca Haynes, Lisa Maxbauer, Julie Relevant, Brenda Kearns, and Jennifer Joseph.

On the home front, I am surrounded by many helping hands. These devoted souls include Bonnie Cerillo, Cheryl Siroshton, Dave Stetzelberger, Liz Patton, Sierra Hamm, Rhonda Watts, Jeff Legg, Jan Cramer, and Kea Fisher. And I would be most remiss if I didn't recognize my personal chef, Teresa Pfaff, who transformed my kitchen into a Fat Flush testing station.

And as always, to JWT—wouldn't want to spend forever with anybody but you.

1 Someone Like You . . .

He who controls others may be powerful, but he who has mastered himself is mightier still.

—LAO-TZU

It's downright frustrating. Hormonal weight gain, cravings, bloating, and those stubborn fat deposits on your belly, hips, and thighs. And that's just what you can see. There's also exhaustion, anxiety, depression, leaky gut, and more, all associated with the dietary choices you make. But you're not alone. There are more than 100 million of us currently fighting the infamous battle of the bulge. For most of us, it's challenging combat at best, trying one diet plan after another. Some regimens are simply too restrictive to follow, whereas others lack any real variety or satiety. In the end, we usually wind up back where we started—unhappy and overweight once again.

Over the years, I've had my own ups and down with weight gain. Right from the start, I had to deal with a stacked deck, genetically speaking. Part of my body shape—the proverbial pear—I inherited from my mother and her side of the family, judging from the pictures of my maternal grandmother, aunts, and female cousins that graced our den wall when I was growing up. And like me, all the women on my mother's side were always on a diet, trying to lose those infamous last 10 to 20 pounds that seemed to stockpile below the waist.

On my father's side, my family history of diabetes didn't help matters any. From as early as I can remember in both junior high and high school, I suffered from low blood sugar, or "reactive hypoglycemia." I was always craving something sweet (such as cookies, candy, cake, or ice cream) to raise my blood sugar, which piled on the pounds. I simply couldn't find the time to eat on schedule. Back then (much like today), I was too busy being responsible and a caretaker for everyone else—writing as a high school correspondent for the *Hartford Courant* newspaper, serving as the president of the Service Club, and teaching religious school after regular school—to pay attention to my own body. So it's no wonder that I was always going up and down on the weight scale.

My use of food as a drug to offset the stress of a competitive college environment during my freshman and sophomore years only compounded the matter. I would drift into one eating hall for lunch and then into another one for yet another meal. In fact, men used to love to take me out because I didn't drink, but had a hearty appetite. The truth is that I could eat anyone under the table. In addition, my body never seemed to firm up the way some women's do when they exercise. I had to literally force myself to exercise anyway.

THE FAT FLUSH GENESIS

I spent my junior year abroad in London. There I started to frequent health food restaurants. Vegan eating and drugless healing fascinated me. My whole life took an about-face once I began a program of cleansing and detoxification (which, by the way, helped me lose fat from those stubborn hips of mine rather effortlessly!). For the first time, I realized that whole foods (like fruits and vegetables), herbs, and dietary supplements could become a path not just to healing and wholeness but also to weight loss.

Back in the United States, after I graduated from college, I decided to enroll in the New York Institute of Dietetics as part of the Dietetic Technician Program. Later I received a master's degree in nutrition education from Teachers College at Columbia University. I went on to become a certified nutrition specialist (CNS) with accreditation from the American College of Nutrition.

It was a classroom experience at Columbia, however, that foreshadowed the nature of my professional journey and eventual Fat Flush discovery. While I was a student there, I heard the "lamppost story," which continues to this day to motivate me. It goes something like this:

> A gentleman goes out for a walk on an extremely dark evening and arrives at his destination, only to find that he has lost his wallet along the way. He immediately retraces his steps and starts looking for the wallet under the lamppost, where there is light. But he is unable to find his wallet because he had really lost it in the dark, where the light didn't reach. The moral of the story is that the answers are out there somewhere; you just have to look in the right places that have yet to come to light.

Inspired by this to search for answers outside the box, I was convinced that the real answers to weight gain, cellulite, and bloating were out there somewhere. I believed that we had yet to search in the right places, evidenced by the enormous number of unsuccessful diet plans. So, I embarked on a quest to find the missing links to weight loss. In my heart, I knew that the solution wouldn't be like any other diet plan. It had to be a program that authentically addressed the true sources of weight gain and also embodied sound nutritional guidelines.

Today, while many women in their twenties, thirties, forties, and fifties are concerned about their changing bodies, I've been able to keep my body fit and fat resistant for nearly three decades now. And that's despite my genes. I learned that "biology is not your biography." Once I had discovered an entirely new approach to managing my weight, it no longer mattered how the genetic cards were stacked. And now, thanks to the emerging science of epigenetics, we know that heredity is not a death sentence and that DNA can be controlled most effectively by diet, exercise, lifestyle, and even our thoughts and beliefs.

Optimizing genetic expression—tuning up the good genes and turning down the bad ones—is the basic approach of my Fat Flush Plan, a program based on a unique diet model using smart and healthy fats, balanced proteins, fiber-filled seeds, colorful carbohydrates, special spices, and a positive lifestyle. It is also designed to address and correct the 10 most prevalent underlying causes of weight gain. These unseen root causes have little to do with your genes. Instead they reflect toxic overload or simple body chemistry imbalances that you probably never suspected. I call them the 10 hidden weight gain factors, which are the key to just about all of our overweight and obesity issues. You'll find that most diet plans typically target only one or two of these factors, which may explain why they don't work in the long term and why they cause recurring weight gain.

Ignored, overlooked, or simply not taken seriously enough, the 10 hidden weight gain factors include the following: an overworked liver, a unique take on "when fat is not fat," lack of fat-burning fats, insulin resistance and inflammation, the stress-fat cycle, microbiome matters, a poor quality bile, thyroid dysfunction, parasites, and magnesium deficiency. These factors are mainly caused by a stagnant lymph system, sneaky food allergies, prescription drugs like birth control and hormone replacement therapy, chemicals in the environment, poor food choices, and a lack of the proper digestive juices. You will learn all about these problematic factors and how to solve them in the next two chapters, along with the scientific developments behind each factor that have reached a critical mass.

To tell you the truth, the development of my Fat Flush Plan didn't happen overnight. It progressed naturally out of every area of my life, from my personal weight control quest and my work alongside my nutrition mentors, to a wide variety of professional experiences spanning my entire career in counseling, consulting, and researching.

Early in my career, I had the privilege of working beside such nutrition pioneers as Hazel Parcells, PhD, Nathan Pritikin, and Robert Atkins, MD. Their contributions helped me on my own weight control journey, which in turn enabled me to assist thousands of my own clients in their weight control efforts. In fact, when my first book, *Beyond Pritikin*, came out, my private practice in California grew, and soon my message that essential fats were absolutely necessary for rapid weight loss, longevity, and good health resonated with people everywhere. For years I had a thriving practice that included professional athletes like Don Meredith, the beloved "Dandy Don" of *Monday Night Football* fame, movie stars, fashion designers, producers, and members of the Joffrey Ballet. In this way, I was helping others, who in turn were helping me fine-tune my program and stay on track myself as the messenger of a new weight loss approach.

Insight: The Liver, Your Major Fat-Burning Organ, and the Lymph, Your Major Fat-Processing System

Over 35 years ago, a health-conscious friend shared an ad with me about the Parcells School of Scientific Nutrition in Albuquerque, New Mexico. The ad promised "five days that would change your life." Nothing could have been more true. After meeting Hazel Parcells, PhD, DC, ND, my life was changed forever. She inspired me to become a nutritionist with a foot in both clinical and integrative nutrition. Dr. Parcells was 84 years old when I met her—and lived to the incredible age of 106 with all her senses fully intact. A true pioneer in natural medicine, she was a woman far ahead of her time.

Under Dr. Parcells's masterful tutelage, I first became acquainted with several innovative concepts that nobody was talking about back in the day—many of which later became the foundation of my Fat Flush Plan. The first revelation was the surprising connection between weight loss and the liver. I recognized early on what researchers are only now beginning to understand: not only is the liver the main organ for detoxifying pollutants, hormones, and chemicals in the body, but this vital organ also is a hidden key to effortless weight loss.

Based on simple biochemistry and the charts from *Gray's Anatomy*, I learned quite early and firsthand that one of the best-kept secrets to weight loss and lasting weight control is keeping the liver, the key organ for fat metabolism, in tip-top shape. For example, bile, which is synthesized and secreted by the liver and stored in the gallbladder, helps the liver break down fats. Bile cannot do its job, however, if it is lacking certain nutrients that make up the bile salts, or if it is congested or thickened with chemicals, toxins, excess sex hormones, drugs, or heavy metals. Bile deficits for individuals who have had their gallbladders removed are rampant, and even for those fortunate enough to still have their gallbladder, issues like bile-related constipation, dry skin, sciatica-like pains, and sleeplessness are all too common.

So I researched all the "liver-loving" and, later on, bile-impacting foods and nutrients that would enable the body to produce quality bile and aid in decongesting the liver. Since one of the primary ingredients of bile is lecithin—a highly effective emulsifier with a detergent-like ability to break up fats—I decided to add non-GMO soy lecithin to the signature Fat Flush Smoothie recipe. For those who are suffering from gallbladder pain and possibly stones, I made lecithin-rich eggs an optional component of the diet because of the strong allergy link to eggs and gallbladder issues. Fresh lemon juice and water—a well-known bile thinner—was later added. When I implemented these measures into my own life, not only did my own liver enzymes come down, but my LDL cholesterol was reduced (a good 20 points to be exact), and so was my weight.

Today, light is finally being shed on the liver—a vitally important organ. The liver performs over 500 tasks and utilizes not just one but three methods of detoxification of the myriad of chemicals, metabolic wastes, viruses, bacteria, heavy metals, medications, and hormones your body comes in contact with daily. The first detox method is the filtering of the blood. The second is the cytochrome P-450 phase I and phase II detoxification enzymes.

The liver's two cytochrome P-450 detoxification pathways are responsible for breaking down, eliminating, and neutralizing toxins. In this petrochemical world of ours, the sheer number of toxins we ingest from medications, drugs, pollutants, and pesticides can overwhelm the liver's ability to break them down and deactivate them. In addition, the detoxification pathways can become drained of the antioxidants, enzymes, and other nutrients necessary for detoxification because of the overload. The resulting metabolic by-products of incomplete detoxification are often more poisonous to the body than the original toxins.

The glutathione conjugation pathway in phase II is far and away the most important detox pathway in the cytochrome P-450 process, and it governs almost 60 percent of toxins carried into the bile, which is yet another of the liver's main detox methods. The bottom line is that with so many toxins being dumped into the bile, its storage, concentration, production, and ability to do its primary job of digesting fats are seriously impaired.

Another valuable insight I learned from Dr. Parcells was that cellulite— that dimpled accumulation of stored fat on our thighs and buttocks—was just as much connected to a sluggish lymphatic system as it was to poor muscle tone or weakened connective tissues. The lymphatic system, a relatively unknown secondary circulatory system underneath the skin, rids the body of toxic wastes, bacteria, heavy metals, dead cells, trapped protein, and fat globules. In essence, the lymphatic system is the liver's partner in toxic waste removal.

Thanks to Dr. Parcells, I was given a head start decades ago in learning about the importance of cleansing both the liver and the lymphatic system for effective weight loss and cellulite control.

Insight: The Role of Fat-Burning Fats

Another major piece of the weight loss puzzle fell into place during my tenure as director of nutrition at the Pritikin Longevity Center in Santa Monica, California. In the early 1980s, the Pritikin diet was widely credited with being the model for the low-fat, high-carbohydrate diet prescription. At the center, as well as later in private practice, I found that many women following this type of program were complaining about distressful premenstrual syndrome (PMS) symptoms and other health ailments. I began to study their diet and health histories, hoping to find some underlying patterns.

For the most part as early as the 1980s I found that they were loading up on unlimited fat-free complex carbohydrates such as pasta, bread, crackers, cereal, and potatoes. I discovered that the more they overate wheat-based carbohydrates (in particular, pasta, bread, cereal, and crackers), the more they craved them—and the more they seemed to become depressed with lower thyroid function. And these high amounts of grains were somehow contributing to their bloating—along with all that fat-free milk and yogurt they used with cereal. The unlimited use of fat-free but yeast-related seasonings such as soy sauce, tamari, tomato sauce, and oil-free vinegar dressings of every persuasion added insult to injury. Of course, the reason they were overusing these kinds of seasonings was that their zero-fat meals lacked any real flavor.

As it turned out, these same women were the ones complaining about retaining fluid, feeling tired and cold, and having allergies and recurring yeast infections, in addition to severe PMS. Therefore, I recommended a highly touted supplement used widely by European doctors for hormone-related problems known as evening primrose oil. Evening primrose oil is rich with a fatty acid called gamma-linolenic acid (GLA). And this is when the unexpected happened. Besides eradicating symptoms of inflammation, lack of energy, and bloating, these women also experienced a welcomed side benefit—weight loss!

The GLA Fat-Fighting Connection. Although generations have used the evening primrose plant for its many medicinal and healing properties, the oil in the seeds—containing the powerful GLA—was making a splash in the weight loss arena. In fact, it was through research conducted by David Horrobin, MD, at the University of Montreal, and M. A. Mir, MD, a senior researcher and consultant physician at the Welsh National School of Medicine in Cardiff, Wales, that helped me realize how the right kind of fat stimulates the body's metabolic ability to burn fat. Their work demonstrated that evening primrose oil was most effective for those who were overweight by at least 10 percent.

The key to this calorie-burning mechanism appeared to be the way the GLA-rich evening primrose oil worked via the prostaglandin pathways, a network of hormones that control virtually all body functions at the cellular level.

The GLA found in evening primrose oil mobilizes the metabolically active fat known as brown adipose tissue (BAT). This special form of fat, if available in sufficient amounts, can burn off extra calories and boost energy. BAT is a particular insulating kind of fat found deep within the human body that surrounds your vital organs such as the kidneys, heart, and adrenal glands. It cushions your spinal column as well as the neck and major thoracic blood vessels.

The series I prostaglandins created from GLA are believed to regulate many aspects of metabolism. GLA-induced prostaglandins regulate BAT by acting as a catalyst to either turn BAT on to trigger calorie burning or turn it off to trigger calorie conservation. Prostaglandins are also connected to a metabolic process referred to as ATPase. ATPase is also known as the sodium pump, a biochemical process necessary to keep the right amount of potassium inside cell walls and too much sodium out. It is this balance between sodium and potassium that allows your neurons to fire and send messages throughout your body. GLA-rich substances such as evening primrose oil, by means of prostaglandin activity, control the sodium pump, which in turn revs up metabolism.

Taking into account mounting evidence that essential fatty acids were important to overall health—from studies that started to appear in such prestigious medical journals as the *New England Journal of Medicine* in the mid-1980s—I published my first book, *Beyond Pritikin*.

Years before the current spate of "eat fat to get thin," "smart fat," and "big fat surprise" books hit the market, I extolled the virtues of "skinny" fats—to the horror of traditional dietitians and doctors. When *Beyond Pritikin* was released in 1988, the book became a bestseller and boldly defied the conventional dietary wisdom of the day; it featured a chapter entitled "The Two-Week Fat Flush" that, as I look back, was really the origin of today's Fat Flush Plan. I inserted this program in my book as an antidote to the high-carbohydrate, high-grain-based, yeast-rich, fat-free diets of the era. It contained a one-day sample menu and touched on liver cleansing for more efficient fat metabolism. The diet featured the GLA supplements I had worked with in my private practice.

Insight: Insulin Resistance, Inflammation, and Fat Storage

A fat-free diet, low in proteins but high in pro-inflammatory, fast-acting, or high-glycemic carbohydrates (starches and simple sugars), keeps insulin levels elevated, which promotes fat accumulation. Since insulin is a fat storage hormone, and excess fat is a strong producer of pro-inflammatory molecules, a vicious cycle is triggered. It is now believed that inflammation, like insulin, is one of the underlying factors of weight gain, loss of muscle mass, and aging. Abnormal inflammation has been tied to a variety of diseases including heart disease, cancer, and autoimmune challenges such as type 2 diabetes, systemic lupus, and multiple sclerosis.

Thankfully, insulin awareness has ushered in a brand-new era of balanced nutrition and has legitimized the return of insulin-lowering fats and proteins to America's dining tables. The Fat Flush formula of healthy fats, lean proteins, fiber-rich seeds, and flavor-filled spices, with slow-acting carbohydrates, is right on the low-insulin track.

Insight: Ignored Hidden Weight Gain Factors

I learned about the remaining weight loss stumbling blocks through my most dependable sources—you (my readers) and clients. Time and time again I was finding that even when some of my clients were doing everything else right, they still couldn't lose weight. Thanks to the nutritional assessment questionnaire, food diary record sheets, and travel and environmental history I had every client fill out, a pattern began to emerge. I discovered that many of those who were resistant to weight loss had a history of long-term use of birth control pills, hormone replacement therapy, antidepressants, and other medications as well as hidden food allergies. In Chapter 2 you will learn that this kind of weight gain is really not fat per se, but rather severely waterlogged tissues masquerading as fat, or "false fat"—a term coined by my friend and holistic doctor extraordinaire, Dr. Elson Haas.

In addition, I noted from my clients' assessment forms that those who had the hardest time losing weight were also those who were the most stressed out. They were living on caffeine (from two to four cups of coffee daily), juggling home and career, definitely not getting enough rest (four to six hours daily), feeling "on edge" most of the time, and reporting an increase in food cravings and fat storage, particularly in the abdominal area. I suspected that the adrenal glands—our "fight-or-flight" glands that produce hormones, including cortisol, in response to stress—were intimately connected to the stress-fat cycle. And I had a very strong hunch that I could disrupt this cycle with some simple changes in lifestyle habits.

So I honed the Fat Flush Plan to include more sleep and stress-relieving protocols (such as exercise and journal keeping) that would zap the stress trigger and accelerate weight loss. Probably the most vigorous stress-busting dietary suggestion was to increase protein—at least eight ounces or more of poultry, fish, lean meat, or a vegan substitute—because the body has higher protein needs when it is under stress. Clients were elated by the results. Just by adding another couple of ounces of protein to lunch and dinner, they were dropping two pants sizes in two weeks—at last!

The other overlooked hidden weight gain factors like low thyroid, poor quality bile, magnesium deficiency, out-of-whack GI flora, and parasites can all throw the body into a "metabolic slowdown," which I will touch on shortly in the next chapters.

DESTINATION: A NEW BODY AND A NEW YOU

In Chapters 2 and 3, I will briefly explain how *all* the hidden weight gain factors can sabotage your weight loss goals. There are real reasons you can't drop your weight. It's not just a lack of willpower, and science can now verify this. For over a decade I have been collecting the latest studies, research, and books (which are listed in the References at the end of the book) that have helped to substantiate my Fat Flush discoveries so many years ago.

Finally, there is an answer for someone like you, like me, like all of us.

My name is Linda Shapiro, and I am a 14-year veteran of the Fat Flush Plan. I'm ecstatic to share that over the years I have lost 45 POUNDS and multiple inches, including several from my belly, which despite regular exercise wouldn't budge! For a "slow as a turtle" loser like me, this is truly magical. Plus, I'm wearing TWO dress sizes smaller and recently gave away almost an entire wardrobe of clothes.

And . . .

- *I no longer fit the profile for metabolic syndrome*
- *My thyroid is finally balanced again*
- *I no longer have PCOS or estrogen dominance*
- *My osteopenia has greatly improved*

I cannot tell you how wonderful it feels to share my success with others including my clients—who in turn are experiencing fantastic results! My Fat Flush journey has given me the unique ability to understand what those with frustrating issues causing an inability to lose weight (and keep it off) endure, allowing me to be an important partner in their quest for healthy and enduring weight loss. I am hoping my story inspires you to give this revolutionary eating lifestyle a try!

—LINDA SHAPIRO, OWNER OF MEALPLANNINGMAVEN.COM

2 Top 10 Hidden Weight Gain Factors #1 Through #5

All truths are easy to understand once they are discovered; the point is to discover them.

—GALILEO GALILEI

Spoiler Alert: It's not always your fault you're fat. Your struggles with weight are not the result of simply too much food and too little exercise. There's more to the metabolic math going on in your body than the equation Calories in + calories out = weight loss or gain. A myriad of unsuspected elements come into play. It's time to balance the weight loss equation, and Fat Flush is here to do it.

Before we look more closely at these, take this Quick Quiz to put your own lifestyle in focus.

QUICK QUIZ

	Yes	No
Do you drink caffeinated beverages daily?	——	——
Are you taking antidepressants or prescription or over-the-counter drugs?	——	——
Do you eat margarine or foods made with hydrogenated (solid or semisolid) fats?	——	——
Do you take birth control pills?	——	——
Are you on estrogen or hormone replacement therapy?	——	——
Did you take antibiotics two or more times during the past 12 months?	——	——
Do you avoid fat at all cost (e.g., by eating fat-free yogurt and fat-free cookies)?	——	——
Do you often crave sweets, bread, or other high-carbohydrate foods?	——	——

QUICK QUIZ (continued)

	Yes	No
Do you eat pasta, potatoes, bread, or other carbohydrates two or more times daily?	___	___
Does at least one meal a day contain processed or packaged foods (e.g., frozen entrées or lunch meats)?	___	___
Do you eat fewer than two servings of protein (e.g., meat, eggs, or fish) daily?	___	___
Do you regularly sleep fewer than eight hours a night?	___	___
Do you lead a high-stress life?	___	___
Do you frequently skip a meal because you are "too busy to eat"?	___	___
Would you describe your lifestyle as sedentary?	___	___
Do you have depression, anxiety, or mood swings?	___	___
Did you have your gallbladder removed?	___	___
Do you avoid trans fat but see no problem with canola oil, sunflower oil, and safflower oil?	___	___
Do you experience occasional constipation regardless of how much fiber you eat?	___	___
Did you travel outside the country in the past year?	___	___
Do you have pets?	___	___
Do you frequently eat wheat and dairy?	___	___

If you answered yes to any of these questions, reading this and the next chapter will help you understand what is really weighing you down.

If you are like most people, the Fat Flush Plan is not your first attempt at weight loss. You've exercised, counted calories, and cut out fat, then protein, and now even carbohydrates. Perhaps you peeled off the pounds; perhaps not. Chances are you've regained most, if not all, of whatever you lost.

For thousands of individuals, the Fat Flush Plan has been different. They've lost pounds and inches and kept them off, as well as embraced a healthier, more wholesome way to live. I believe this is so because the plan, unlike any other weight loss program, targets the 10 hidden factors that bring on unwanted pounds:

✓ Tired, toxic liver
✓ False fat
✓ Fear of eating fat
✓ Insulin resistance and inflammation
✓ Stress as a fat maker
✓ Messy microbiome
✓ Poor quality bile
✓ Tuckered-out thyroid
✓ Hidden hitchhikers—parasites
✓ Missing magnesium

How do these factors really affect your weight? Over the past 15 years, I have followed the research, and, in some cases, the work of the nutritional pioneers who spearheaded the breakthroughs, to answer this question. If you are like most of the Fat Flushers who have been my followers, then you will understand some of the no-nonsense reasoning and the science behind the plan. You'll have the knowledge and insights to make smart choices for your body and forge confidently toward your best body yet.

As you begin your journey, I want you to remember that fully restored health won't be achieved on a short-term diet; it's a way of living. While the Three-Day Ultra Tune-Up and the Two-Week Fat Flush may appear to make the program look like a fad diet, the complete Fat Flush Plan is a full-fledged lifestyle plan, helping to reset and detoxify your body while you learn how to take care of yourself in the long run. That's why I named the third and final phase of Fat Flush "The *Lifestyle* Maintenance Plan"—because Fat Flush is for life.

Each of these hidden factors affects not only your weight but also your overall health. As you slim down with the Fat Flush plan, you will simultaneously balance your hormones and optimize your bodily functions from your toenails to your brain and everywhere in between. You will feel better *physically, mentally, and emotionally too.*

Let's get started!

HIDDEN FACTOR #1: YOUR TIRED, TOXIC LIVER

Poets and songwriters may wax poetic about the heart, but your liver is by far the most versatile organ in your body and one of the most important. Weighing between 2.5 and 4 pounds in adults, the liver is the largest internal organ as well. Between 3 and 4 pints of blood flow through it every minute.

The Vital Liver

Researchers now estimate that the liver performs nearly 500 different jobs. It functions as a living filter to cleanse the system of toxins, metabolize proteins, control hormonal balance, and produce immune-boosting factors. Many of these functions not only are essential to your overall health but have a direct bearing on your weight loss efforts. These functions are the focus of the Fat Flush Plan.

A Fat-Burning Machine. Each day your liver produces about a quart of a yellowish-green liquid called bile that carries toxins out of the body and emulsifies and absorbs fats in the small intestine. It is the real key to the liver's ability to digest and assimilate fats. Bile is so important, in fact, that I have made it one of my hidden weight loss factors. More about this in the next chapter. For now, know that the worse the quality of the bile, the less fat your body can break down, the less your body can use fat and the vital nutrients in it, and the more fat your body stores as extra pounds.

If you have a roll of fat at your waistline, you may have what is common-ly called a "fatty liver." Your liver has stopped processing fat and begun stor-ing it, for reasons I'll explain in a moment. *Only when you bring your liver back to full function will you lose this fat.* This truth, and Fat Flush's excellent job of addressing it, is the cornerstone of Fat Flush's success.

An Efficient Metabolizer. The liver metabolizes not only fats but also car-bohydrates and proteins for use in your body. Carbohydrates are the number one source of glucose, one of the body's basic energy molecules. The organ has a triple role in carbohydrate metabolism:

1. The liver converts glucose and galactose into glycogen, a storable version of these energy molecules.
2. When your blood sugar level drops and no new carbohydrates are avail-able for your body to use as energy, the liver converts stored glycogen back into glucose and releases it into your bloodstream.
3. If your diet is regularly low in carbohydrates, the liver will convert fat or protein into glucose to maintain your blood sugar levels.

In protein metabolism, the liver converts amino acids from food into various proteins that may have a direct or indirect impact on your weight. For example, many proteins transport hormones through the bloodstream, and the balance of these hormones is crucial to avoid water retention, bloat-ing, and cravings, as well as other health problems. As you read, you will see over and over again how essential hormonal communication is to regulating your weight. Proteins also play an important role part in the detox process helping transport wastes to the liver for detoxification and elimination through the kidneys.

A Potent Detoxifier. Perhaps the liver's most important function, and the one that puts it at greatest risk for damage, is to detoxify the myriad toxins that assault our bodies daily. A toxin is really any substance that irritates or creates harmful effects in the body. Some toxins, called endotoxins, are the natural by-products of bodily processes. Other toxins you consume by choice, such as alcohol, sugar (especially fructose), caffeine, and prescription drugs (more about these later). Still others are the thousands of toxic chem-icals we breathe, consume, or touch in our environment: pesticides, car exhaust, secondhand smoke, chemical food additives, and indoor pollutants from paint, carpets, and cleaners, among others.

Working with your lungs, skin, kidneys, and intestines, a healthy liver detoxifies many harmful substances and eliminates them without contami-nating the bloodstream. Under ordinary circumstances, your body handles toxins by:

1. Neutralizing them with antioxidants, like the body's premier antioxidant glutathione
2. Transforming them from fat-soluble chemicals to water-soluble ones
3. Eliminating them through urine, feces, sweat, mucus, and breath

When the Liver Is Overloaded

Your liver is a workhorse that can even regenerate its own damaged cells. However, it is not invincible. When it lacks essential nutrients or when it is overwhelmed by toxins, it no longer performs as it should. Hormone imbalances may develop. Fat may accumulate in the liver and then just under the skin or in other organs. Toxins build up and get into your bloodstream. Among the signs of "toxic liver" are:

✓ Weight gain, especially around the abdomen
✓ Cellulite
✓ Abdominal bloating
✓ Indigestion
✓ High blood pressure
✓ Elevated cholesterol
✓ Fatigue
✓ Mood swings
✓ Depression
✓ Skin rashes

When your liver is sluggish, every organ in your body is affected, and your weight loss efforts are blocked. Blood vessels enlarge, and blood flow becomes restricted. A toxic liver is unable to break down the adrenal hormone aldosterone, which accumulates to retain sodium (and water) and suppress potassium. This can also raise your blood pressure. If the liver fails to detoxify the components of estrogen for excretion, symptoms of estrogen dominance arise. Unable to carry out its activities to control glucose, a toxic liver can lead to hypoglycemia, which can produce sugar cravings, weight gain, and candida overgrowth. A toxic liver is unable to process toxins, enabling them to escape into your bloodstream and set off an inflammatory immune response. With repeated assaults from escaped toxins, your immune system becomes overworked. Fluid accumulates, and you may develop one or more autoimmune diseases such as lupus or arthritis. A liver overloaded with pollutants and metabolic waste cannot efficiently burn body fat. All these things work in concert to sabotage your weight loss efforts from almost every angle. By the end of Chapter 3, you will clearly see how this works.

Liver Stressors

Probably nothing you do to control your weight is as important as keeping your liver healthy. This means avoiding as many of the damaging elements (like alcohol) as possible while embracing liver boosters. Among the lesser-known compromisers of liver function are sugar, trans fats, caffeine, medications, and inadequate fiber.

Fructose and Other Sugars. Annually, Americans consume approximately 150 pounds of sugar and artificial sweeteners per person (although this number is controversial). You may not even know when you're consuming sugar. Food producers don't use it just for sweetening. Sugar helps retain color in foods like ketchup, gives a brown crust to breads and rolls, and adds body to soft drinks. Cigarettes, toothpaste, aspirin—even hairspray and postage stamps—contain sugar.

Sugar, a simple carbohydrate, comes in many forms, not all of which you may recognize in an ingredients list:

✓ Glucose
✓ Fructose
✓ Sucrose
✓ Maltose
✓ Lactose
✓ Raw sugar, brown sugar, powdered sugar
✓ Molasses, maple sugar, honey, corn syrup, erythritol, high-fructose corn syrup
✓ Sugar alcohols: sorbitol, mannitol, and xylitol
✓ Cane syrup

In the process of being metabolized, these sugars rob your body of valuable nutrients; some of these, such as zinc, are essential for liver function. Sugar also inhibits your liver's production of the enzymes needed in the detoxification process. Your liver must go into overdrive to convert the sugar into fats such as cholesterol and triglycerides. Unfortunately, once the liver has made this heroic effort, the fats may pile up in your liver and other organs, or these fats may accumulate in the most typical fat storage areas of your body—thighs, buttocks, and abdomen.

Speaking of fat deposition, one sugar in particular poses a unique danger to your liver: fructose. Found primarily in fruit, fructose was previously thought of as "better" sugar because it does not trigger insulin release and comes from a natural, whole food source. However, instead of insulin metabolizing the fructose, it goes straight to the liver, which cannot efficiently metabolize it. The liver converts the fructose into triglycerides, which can eventually turn into another source of excess body fat and lead to nonalcoholic fatty liver disease. In fact, nonalcoholic fatty liver disease has seen a skyrocketing number of cases.

Sugar is also a favorite food of candida, a yeast that can overgrow and not only bring on bloating and water retention but also stress your liver. The yeast causes sugar to ferment and form acetaldehyde, a neurotoxin that increases ammonia levels in your bloodstream and can damage the liver. In addition, your liver must work overtime to detoxify the toxins produced by the fungal form of flourishing candida, compromising the organ's fat-burning ability.

Trans Fats. As I indicated in Chapter 1, I introduced to the public the concept of adding the right fats back into the diet way back in 1988. I was labeled a "nutritional heretic" at the time, but now scientists caught up because the concept is definitely mainstream today, decades after I came onto the scene as the lone advocate of fat. Of course, I didn't and don't promote just any type of fat, but the really smart fats that have shown themselves to be both healthful and helpful in weight loss and beyond.

What I have been urging my readers to avoid for years are *trans fats*, also called *trans fatty acids*.

Trans fats are created when liquid vegetable oils are hydrogenated. This process produces solid or semisolid fats widely used in commercial baked goods, other processed foods, and the food in fast-food restaurants. By adding hydrogen and metals, under high heat, processors create a very stable oil that won't easily go rancid, but in the process the oil molecules have been altered. Trans fats impede your liver's ability to burn fat. They retard detox-ification, increase fatty deposits within the liver, and thicken the bile, thus impeding bile flow. You'll find trans fats in margarine (not butter), hydro-genated and partially hydrogenated vegetable oils, and shortening, as well as in processed foods made with these ingredients. As a general rule, the less refined, softer, or more fluid the oil, the fewer trans fats it contains.

Medications. As with food, the medications you take must be processed before they can be used by your body. Once again, your liver plays an impor-tant role. Some drugs, however, cause the liver to work harder and can also pack on pounds. Hormone replacement therapy, for example, causes the liver to make more clotting factors, and the organ must work harder to break down the drug's hormones. Other drugs may produce waste products that can accumulate in the liver. Acetaminophen, the active ingredient in the popular pain reliever Tylenol, is one such drug. Studies by researchers at the University of Texas Southwestern Medical Center found that 38 percent of more than 300 cases of liver failure and 35 percent of 307 cases of severe liver injury were associated with excessive acetaminophen use. The common antidepressants Zoloft and Paxil can typically add 10 to 20 pounds of weight gain, while a Depo Provera birth control shot can be responsible for as much as 30 pounds of extra weight.

Drugs that can potentially harm your liver or may cause weight gain include:

✓ Nonsteroidal anti-inflammatory drugs (NSAIDs)
✓ Cholesterol-lowering drugs
✓ Antidiabetic drugs
✓ Triglyceride-lowering drugs
✓ Anticonvulsants
✓ Hormones (e.g., estrogen and tamoxifen)
✓ Antidepressants
✓ Antihistamines
✓ Beta-blockers and other blood pressure medications
✓ Corticosteroids
✓ Antiestrogens
✓ Sleeping pills and tranquilizers

Do note that anywhere between one-third to one-half of people have a mutation in their MTHFR (methylenetetrahydrofolate reductase) gene. This mutation impairs their body's ability to break down toxins. Because of their impaired metabolism, people with a MTHFR mutation cannot metabolize drugs properly and therefore cannot receive the full benefit of medications they might take. When taking medications like the ones listed above, people with the MTHFR mutation get a double whammy of distress. Not only do they get less of a benefit from the medication than the majority of people, but their liver is also more heavily taxed as it tries to keep detoxifying substances it is not genetically equipped to metabolize in the first place.

If you are currently taking any medications and have concerns about their effects on your liver, do *not* stop taking the drugs before you consult your physician. Liver function tests are available. You may be able to take an alternative drug with less potential for liver damage. Many drugs, for example, are available in lower doses or in different forms (e.g., patch, pill, or injection), or a natural form may replace a synthetic product. These alternatives may provide the treatment that you need without the added weight and liver dysfunction that you don't need. Know and weigh the benefits of the medication versus weight gain and any other side effects you're experiencing.

Inadequate Fiber. If you are like most Americans, you eat only about 10 to 12 grams of fiber a day when experts believe that more like 35 grams is ideal for long-term health. Among fiber's healthful benefits is its role in moving toxins out of your body. Insoluble fibers, from flaxseed, for example, absorb water in your digestive tract. This speeds up transit time (the time it takes materials to move through your intestine) to move waste products out of your body. Without adequate fiber, up to 90 percent of cholesterol and bile acids will be reabsorbed and recirculated to the liver. This taxes your liver and reduces its fat-burning abilities. No matter what the cause, a sluggish, overworked liver does a poor job metabolizing fat, and you gain weight.

Caffeine. Interestingly, the latest studies suggest that coffee ranks high in antioxidants. Japanese researchers in the *Journal of the National Cancer Institute* have even reported that people who drank coffee daily had half the liver cancer of those who never drank it and that the protective effect occurred in people who drank one to two cups per day and increased at three to four cups. But what these studies neglect to report is how the caffeine in coffee is a powerful diuretic, doubling the rate at which calcium leaves your body in urine. The excretion of calcium stimulates the parathyroid gland to secrete the hormone responsible for drawing more calcium from the bone to replace it in the bloodstream. In addition, coffee contains about 30 different acids, which draw even more calcium from the bone to act as a neutralizer.

Excessive consumption of coffee, as well as other foods containing caffeine like tea, regular soft drinks, and chocolate, will increase your risk of osteoporosis by reducing blood calcium levels, triggering calcium to be pulled from bone, thus weakening the bones and flushing needed calcium out of your body. And it doesn't take much to be excessive. A mere three cups of black coffee a day can result in a 45-mg calcium loss. Unfortunately, women between the ages of 36 and 50, who often need calcium the most, drink more coffee than people in any other age group.

You may be thinking, "I only drink one or two cups of coffee a day." However, you may be unknowingly consuming much more caffeine, from chocolate, cocoa, tea, some soft drinks, kola nut and guaraná root supplements, and a host of over-the-counter medications, including Excedrin, Anacin, Vanquish, Midol, Cope, Premens, Vivarin, NoDoz, and Dexatrim.

What the Fat Flush Plan Does for Your Tired, Toxic Liver

Detoxifying Drink. We start with the plan's cran-water, which is composed of diluted cranberry juice and water. This Fat Flush water is a potent source of phytonutrients such as anthocyanins, catechins, luteins, and quercetin. These powerful phytonutrients act as antioxidants, providing nutritional support and cofactors for the liver's cytochrome P-450 phase I and phase II detoxification pathways. These nutrients also seem to help digest fatty globules in the lymph thereby reducing cellulite deposits. The plan's cran-water elixir will assist your liver in diluting and expelling the increased body wastes from the two-phase detoxification process. Water helps empty stubborn fat stores because your liver is more efficient at using stored fat for energy when your body is well hydrated.

If you are missing lots of coffee, you will find satisfying fat-flushing alternatives such as dandelion root tea, ginger tea, and fennel tea that keep your liver happy. While all of these promote liver health, ginger and fennel teas add an extra metabolism boost, with ginger capable of boosting metabolism up to 20 percent. Dandelion root tea, my personal favorite, is especially supportive of liver function while still giving you an energy boost. It promotes bile health as an herbal bitter and lowers elevated liver enzymes for those who have overdone alcohol, sugar, trans fats, and medications.

Protein. Daily protein is important to your liver's health and function. Only protein can raise metabolism by 25 percent and activate the production of enzymes needed during detoxification to break down toxins into water-soluble substances for excretion. Your liver needs protein to produce the bile that is essential for absorbing fat-soluble nutrients. Protein also provides amino acids, such as cysteine, that your body needs to produce the antioxidant glutathione. This enzyme is one of several that overcome the damaging free radicals (toxins) produced in your liver (and elsewhere) during detoxification.

Red meats such as lean beef and lamb are high in L-carnitine, which plays a vital role in both the normalization of liver enzymes in the blood and the liver's use and metabolism of fatty acids. This nutrient carries fat to the mitochondria in your cells, where the fat is converted to energy. L-carnitine also helps clear waste products from the mitochondria to avoid free-radical accumulation (and damage). In animal studies, L-carnitine has been shown to protect the liver from powerful toxins. To ensure that you get enough of this fat-burning nutrient, the plan includes not only dietary sources but also a supplement. You'll get 1 gram or more of L-carnitine per day, which at least one study has shown is enough to burn off 10 extra pounds in 12 weeks when combined with a Fat Flush–type diet and light exercise.

Plant Products. By including flax, coconut, and MCT (medium-chain triglyceride) oil, the plan takes advantage of the metabolism-raising action of these oils and their ability to attract and bind to the oil-soluble poisons that are lodged in the liver and carry them out of the system for elimination. The essential fatty acids in flaxseed oil also stimulate bile production, which is crucial to the breakdown of fats.

Plants have protein, too! For vegans and vegetarians, and also those who don't have access to organic, pasture-raised meat or those who simply want to vary their diet, the plan includes non-GMO pea and rice protein powder, beans, and legumes. These options provide a good source of protein without the allergens associated with eggs, soy, milk, and tree nuts, as well as none of the environmental and ethical concerns associated with animal products. Pea protein powder, in particular, isolates the protein found in peas, but all the carbohydrates have been removed so you get a pure protein punch.

You'll find lots of cruciferous vegetables in the menus. Broccoli, brussels sprouts, and kale are very high in sulforaphane, a substance your liver uses in converting toxins into nontoxic waste for elimination.

Many of the herbs and spices featured in the Fat Flush Plan were selected for their liver-supporting and fat-metabolizing properties. Garlic and onion encourage bile secretion and aid liver function. Gingerroot boosts metabolism, helps reduce toxic buildup in fat cells, and supports bile flow.

Supplements. Supplements are an integral part of the plan, including the lipotropic herbs dandelion root, milk thistle, turmeric, and Oregon grape root. Lipotropic substances decrease the fat storage rate in liver cells and accelerate fat metabolism. Dandelion root, which contains moderate levels of vitamin A and other nutrients, has been shown to aid the liver and fat metabolism in two ways. As a bitter herb, dandelion stimulates the liver to produce more bile to send to the gallbladder, while at the same time causing the gallbladder to contract and release its stored bile, thus assisting in fat metabolism.

Milk thistle, in use for over 2000 years, increases liver enzyme production, helps repair damaged liver tissue, and blocks the effects of some toxins. Over 100 research reports have been published on the liver-supporting properties of its active ingredient, silymarin.

Turmeric, a relative of gingerroot, is the highest known source of beta-carotene, one of the powerful antioxidants that help protect the liver from damage by free radicals. Oregon grape root helps stimulate the liver by helping to control bile production.

Among the other lipotropic factors featured in the plan's supplements are the B-complex vitamins phosphatidylcholine and inositol, the amino acid methionine, and the fat-digesting enzyme lipase. They help prevent excess fat buildup and thin or emulsify fat for easy movement through the bloodstream.

A bile builder supplement is highly recommended. It is useful for those with and without a gallbladder. For those without a gallbladder, a bile builder simply supplements the missing bile salts as a replacement therapy and helps to provide the missing bile when fat is consumed during a meal or snack. For those with a gallbladder, a bile building supplement helps to promote complete digestion of fats, detoxification, regularity, and supports healthy thyroid function. Ideally, a bile building formula should also contain choline, taurine, beet root, and pancreatic lipase.

Many individuals seek a glutathione-promoting formula to assist the liver in its massive detox functions. While the whey protein on the plan provides the precursor amino acids to make glutathione, there are a number of glutathione formulas currently on the market that can help with detoxification and overall Fat Flush success. One in particular that has caught my eye is known as ASEA, which is a redox signaling product that can elevate glutathione production by 350 percent. (See Chapter 15.)

Toxic Turnover. Just as important as what is included is what is excluded. Among the missing are caffeine; sugar; alcohol; yeast-based foods such as bread and soy sauce; most vinegars (except the anti-candida apple cider vinegar and coconut vinegar); and trans fats from fried foods, margarine, vegetable shortenings, and commercial vegetable oils. These seriously disrupt liver function by clogging the detoxification pathways or increasing candida production. The yeast-related poison acetaldehyde is extremely toxic to the liver and inhibits fat burning.

You also won't find several herbs popularized for their thermogenic qualities. Most widely known is ephedra, or ma huang. Ephedra acts as a stimulant to the adrenal glands, which are responsible for your body's stress response and for maintaining blood sugar levels. Prolonged use of ephedra can create adrenal exhaustion. The herb also can constrict blood vessels, elevate blood pressure, and raise the heart rate. These can be serious side effects, especially for individuals with diabetes, heart disease, hypertension, or kidney disease. Kola nut, guaraná, and mate ontain caffeine, and the fifth thermogenic, white willow bark (from which aspirin is derived), is high in salicylate, which can have unwanted blood-thinning effects.

HIDDEN FACTOR #2: FALSE FAT

On a "good" day, your body is 60 to 70 percent water by weight. About two-thirds of the water is in your cells; the rest is in blood, body fluids, and spaces between cells. This water is essential. It flushes toxins, moistens your respiratory system, and is part of every metabolic process. Cells take the water they need from capillaries, which in turn carry waste products and excess water to the kidneys.

However, many individuals carry an extra 10 to 15 pounds of water trapped in their tissues. This water contributes to abdominal bloating, cellulite, and face and eye puffiness. It is what my esteemed colleague Elson Haas, MD, calls "false fat"—or when fat is really not fat. That is, the weight is not the result of additional adipose tissue, or true body fat, but of excess water. Waterlogged tissues result from various causes, including:

✓ Consumption of too little water and protein
✓ Food sensitivities
✓ Hormonal fluctuations
✓ Certain medications

Deficiencies and Water Retention

It's ironic, but consuming too little water can cause your body to retain water. Your kidneys must have adequate water to flush waste from your body. When your fluid intake is low, the kidneys hoard water.

Insufficient fluid also slows the lymphatic system. This system of organs, tissues, and tiny channels filters cellular waste and other foreign particles, propelling this debris along lymph vessels. Some researchers spectulate that when a sluggish lymphatic system fails to carry wastes away in a timely fashion, the waste accumulates in fat cells and causes cellulite. At least one study, conducted at Brussels University in Belgium and cited by Elisabeth Dancey, MD, in *The Cellulite Solution*, has found that women with cellulite showed lymphatic system deficiencies.

Protein plays a crucial role in tissue growth and healing, strengthening the immune system and burning fat. But it is its hydrophilic—literally, "water loving"—properties that have an impact on water retention. Proteins that circulate in your blood control water levels between and within cells and within your arteries and veins by attracting water molecules. As the blood circulates through your kidneys, this excess water is removed and eliminated. When your body is deficient in protein, however, fluid leaks from the vascular spaces into the spaces between the cells. It becomes trapped there, resulting in cellulite, water retention, bloating, and water weight gain.

When You React to Food

An estimated 60 to 80 percent of people are sensitive to one or more foods. Unlike true allergies, sensitivities often cause delayed, rather than immediate, reactions after you eat the offending food. This delay can make it difficult for you to tie your symptoms to the food you eat. Among the vast array of food sensitivity symptoms are:

✓ Headache
✓ Coughing
✓ Blurred vision
✓ Rapid heartbeat
✓ Indigestion

✓ Skin rashes
✓ Fatigue
✓ Joint swelling
✓ Mood swings

Food sensitivities are also one of the most common causes of weight gain through fluid retention and through overeating brought on by cravings.

The Response to Reactive Foods. Your body's immune system releases antibodies in response to signals from foreign substances. In the case of food sensitivities, the antibody is immunoglobulin G (IgG), found only in the bloodstream. The "foreign substance" is food macromolecules that have left the digestive tract and entered the bloodstream. When IgG meets a macro-molecule, the entire immune response is kicked off. Histamines and other chemicals are released, and the area is flooded with extra fluid to wash away the reactive food particle. Your body holds onto this water as long as such molecules remain in your tissues.

At the same time, your body produces hormones, including cortisol and aldosterone, which increase sodium intake. This sodium attracts more water to the cells and tissues. In your gastrointestinal system, reactive foods can stimulate production of the gut hormones cholecystokinin and somatostatin, which cause water retention in gut tissues.

The production of histamine and other chemicals causes blood vessels to expand and contract, leaking fluids into tissues and setting off a secondary inflammatory response and swelling. This leaking fluid often carries protein with it, and the protein attracts sodium and still more fluid.

To compound the false fat weight gain from waterlogged tissues, food sensitivities also trigger weight gain from adipose tissue. This results from either heightened cravings for reactive foods or disruption of your metabolism.

The same immune response that pumps excess fluid into your tissues also triggers your body's distress mechanisms, centered on various natural chemicals and hormones. First, endorphins hit your system. These natural opiates give you a pleasant feeling of relief—but only for a few minutes to several hours. As your supply of endorphins dwindles, you are uncomfort-able and seek to re-create the pleasant feelings with more of the reactive food. Cravings strike!

Second, your adrenal glands release epinephrine, norepinephrine, and cortisol (take special note of the latter because I will be discussing it quite a bit), which give you a burst of energy and a mood lift. When these hormones are depleted, fatigue and irritability set in. Once again, you crave the reactive food to bring back your energy level.

Third, your insulin levels become destabilized, which lowers your blood sugar levels. Cells are starved for this energy booster, and you are weak and starved for food, especially carbohydrates. Destabilized insulin dramatically promotes an increase in fat storage, as you will see in the section "Hidden Factor #4: Insulin Resistance and Inflammation."

Finally, as if all this weren't enough, your levels of the neurotransmitter serotonin drop. This chemical is produced in the gut and the hypothalamus, the part of the brain that controls hunger, and is carried primarily by white blood cells. When you eat nonreactive foods, serotonin helps signal that you are full and shuts off your hunger. However, when your immune system goes into high gear in response to a reactive food, your white blood cells are too busy fighting the "invader food" to carry serotonin. The result is a craving for high-carbohydrate foods to help move serotonin to the brain. Low serotonin levels are also the biological basis for depression and other mental health issues.

Not surprisingly, these disruptions in hormone and chemical levels severely affect your metabolism and make putting on pounds oh-so easy. Metabolism is slowed when your epinephrine levels are depleted, causing increased fat storage, or when your thyroid gland doesn't function properly because signal hormones are imbalanced. Some food reactions also interfere with your body's ability to absorb the fat-burning essential fatty acids—such as the gamma-linolenic acid (GLA) that I mentioned in Chapter 1.

Food Triggers. What foods are most likely to trigger this destructive immune response? Elson Haas, MD, Jacqueline Crohn, MD, and others have identified the most commonly reactive foods. Among them are:

✓ Wheat
✓ Dairy products
✓ Sugar
✓ Yeast

These account for up to 80 percent of food reactions, although almost any food can be reactive. Reactions to these foods develop primarily because of poor digestion, which results in partially digested food macromolecules entering the bloodstream and setting off the immune response. Reasons for poor digestion vary from eating too fast to eating too little fiber to eating the same foods repeatedly, or simply from the foods themselves.

Excessive consumption of processed foods, loaded with corn syrup, monosodium glutamate, and gluten, is particularly disastrous. Surprisingly, celiac disease (an autoimmune disease triggered by the protein-containing gluten in wheat, rye, and barley) is more common than people usually suspect. Celiac is found in 1 in every 167 healthy children in the United States and 1 in every 111 healthy adults. Gluten sensitivity arises most commonly with wheat, used in practically everything from breads and pastas to piecrust, muffins, bagels, and cakes. Gluten can damage the intestinal lining, create inflammation, and disrupt nutrient absorption, especially of the precious B vitamins. Consequently, if gluten-containing foods are your triggers, you may experience not only bloating but also eczema, fatigue, intestinal gas, and anemia.

William Davis, MD, author of *Wheat Belly*, showed the world the nutritional hazards of wheat. He points the finger at the entire grain, not only the gluten it contains. Wheat contains things like gliaden, glutenin, amy-lopectin A, and wheat germ agglutinin that Davis says cause blood sugar imbalance, leptin resistance, brain fog, impulsivity, anxiety, and appetite stimulation. He even implicates wheat in arthritis, obesity, asthma, irritable bowel syndrome, and psychiatric disorders such as schizophrenia. I will go more in depth on the perils of wheat when I discuss Hidden Factor #4, below. For now, know that whether it's the gluten or the grain it's in, this food trigger has got to go!

A Woman's Hormones: Natural and Synthetic

From puberty, women's bodies are subject to the effects of an estrogen-progesterone balance. At ovulation, estrogen secretion increases fat produc-tion by inhibiting thermogenesis (fat burning). In turn, fat stimulates more estrogen production, which prompts more fat deposition. At the same time, progesterone levels decrease, which is thought to stimulate production of an antidiuretic hormone, so less progesterone means more water retention. This balance of estrogen and progesterone is a crucial component in your body's preparation for pregnancy, which requires increased body fluids and fat.

When Balance Is Lost. For too many women, however, this natural cycle is disrupted, and weight gain—from both actual fat and water retention—becomes permanent. Estrogen levels remain high, resulting in a condition known as estrogen dominance. Among the symptoms of estrogen domi-nance are:

✓ Fat gain (especially around your abdomen, hips, and thighs)
✓ Sluggish metabolism
✓ Bloating
✓ Water retention
✓ Depression
✓ Mood swings
✓ Sugar cravings

Estrogen can promote sodium retention (and thereby more water reten-tion). The hormone changes the way your body metabolizes the amino acid tryptophan, which is necessary to produce serotonin. You'll remember that serotonin deficiency can lead to food cravings, weight gain, and depression. When you have much more estrogen than progesterone or are really defi-cient in progesterone levels, with estrogen more or less normal, you may develop hypothyroidism. A healthy thyroid gland secretes hormones that help signal the pancreas to produce insulin. With a sluggish thyroid, your body may produce too much insulin and trigger low blood sugar (hypo-glycemia), along with intense cravings for carbohydrates.

Fluctuating estrogen levels are only one-half of the equation, of course. Thanks to the pioneering research of Raymond Peat, PhD, and John Lee, we are becoming better informed about the role of progesterone. This hormone signals the hypothalamus to increase your core body temperature, thereby increasing your resting metabolism rate. Low levels of progesterone cause your body to burn 15,000 to 20,000 fewer calories per year and increase water retention. You may not produce enough progesterone because (1) you are deficient in zinc and vitamin B6, nutrient precursors of progesterone, (2) you are not ovulating regularly, or (3) your body is converting progesterone into other chemicals as a result of excessive stress.

High levels of progesterone, on the other hand, increase your appetite. They also slow down intestinal transit time to increase food absorption, which can increase insulin levels. The resulting additional blood glucose is absorbed by fat cells to add pounds of true fat.

Causes of Imbalance. Estrogen replacement therapy (ERT) and hormone replacement therapy (HRT) are common causes of estrogen-progesterone imbalances, with millions of American women currently on HRT. Research into the effects of these therapies on weight has found conflicting results. For example, when researchers gave monkeys estrogen with synthetic progestin (a form of progesterone), their weight increased, fat tended to accumulate around their abdomens, and they secreted excess insulin. On the other hand, monkeys given estrogen with natural progesterone did not experience these effects.

In 2002, the directors of the Women's Health Initiative, a major, long-term study analyzing the effects of HRT, abruptly brought the study to a halt. They realized that the risks associated with HRT far overshadowed the benefits. Those risks included a 26 percent greater chance of breast cancer; 41 percent higher rate of stroke; 29 percent greater risk of heart disease; and double the rate of blood clots in the legs and lungs. While there are still specific circumstances under which HRT is necessary, in general, I advise against it, unless you are monitored with bioidentical hormone replacement therapy. Following the Fat Flush diet will balance hormones and help mitigate and correct the effects of estrogen-related problems.

However, since the Women's Health Initiative, we have learned about a period of time in a woman's life called the "estrogen window" during which she can receive the most benefit from ERT with the least amount of risk. This window typically opens right after the onset of menopause and closes 5 to 10 years later. Using estrogen in this window can help relieve menopausal symptoms and, contrary to the results of the Women's Health Initiative, lower the risk for breast cancer, heart disease, and type 2 diabetes. But outside of the estrogen window, the findings of the Women's Health Initiative still hold true. I encourage you to use discretion when considering HRT or ERT. I would have a candid conversation with your doctor taking into consideration the potential risks and side effects.

If you are among the millions of women taking birth control pills to prevent pregnancy, regulate your menstrual cycle, or treat acne, an unwanted side effect may be weight gain. Contraceptives can create a state of anovulation, and the absence of ovulation can lead to progesterone deficiency, slowing metabolism and encouraging water retention. Birth control pills also aggravate problems with insulin regulation and resulting carbohydrate cravings, as well as encourage candidiasis.

Unbound copper is also closely associated with estrogen dominance. Think of copper and zinc as the mineral mirrors of estrogen and progesterone. Copper and estrogen seem to vary together, as do zinc and progesterone. On top of the relationship to estrogen dominance, high copper and low zinc levels can lead to osteoporosis, acne, eczema, sensitive skin, sunburn, frontal headaches, white spots on the fingernails, food cravings, mood swings, menstrual irregularities, fatigue, constipation, depression, weight gain, and yeast infections.

Many people are unaware of the amount of copper they are actually exposed to on a daily basis. Using copper cooking ware, copper IUDs, drinking water from copper pipes, and prenatal and birth control pills can all contribute to high copper levels. Even a healthy diet can sneak an abundance of copper into the system. Common foods like chocolate, nuts (especially cashews), seeds (especially sunflower), soy, shellfish, and black teas are all high in copper.

Do note that vegetarians, people who experience chronic stress, and people who eat a diet high in refined carbohydrates and sugar are more likely to have high copper levels because their lifestyles zap the zinc from their system. While stress seems to have a super power to drain your body of nutrients, the other two categories result largely from dietary choices. The foods with the most plentiful amount of zinc tend to be high-protein foods such as zinc-rich eggs, pumpkin seeds, grass-fed beef, oysters and other seafood, lamb, kelp, sunflower seeds, mushrooms, poultry, and beans. Without the fail-safe of animal products, vegetarians and people who eat a highly processed diet do not usually eat sufficient quantities of these foods to maintain appropriate zinc levels. This leads to a zinc deficiency, which in turn leads to excess copper in the body.

Unequalized Ecosystem

Our urban environment is the main cause of exposure to petrochemical molecules and other pollutants in our air, water, food, and more. Many of us would cringe at the prospect of drinking jet fuel; yet depending upon your location, your water supply can overflow with invisible poisons like lead, chloramine (which has replaced chlorine as the major disinfectant in municipal water systems), pharmaceutical drugs, Teflonlike chemicals (PFOA), gasoline additives, and, yes, even perchlorate, the chemical name for jet fuel. These are but a few of the potentially lethal petrochemicals and other impurities found today in water. And that's only the water.

Pollutants have disturbing endocrine-disrupting and waistline-expanding effects within our bodies. The Chinese government funded a study at Duke University that compared rats exposed to imported air from the notoriously polluted Beijing with a control group of rats exposed to filtered air that contained minimal pollution. After only eight weeks, the rats exposed to the polluted Beijing air showed increased lung and liver inflammation; had higher

LDL cholesterol, higher triglyceride levels, and higher overall cholesterol; developed insulin resistance (Hidden Factor #4); and *were significantly heavier* compared with the rats who breathed the purified air. The kicker: both groups of rats ate the exact same diet.

Up to 800 environmental pollutants can qualify as fat-mongering obesogens. Obesogens are foreign chemicals in your body that disrupt your endocrine system and impact how your body handles fats. They can affect the fat cells themselves, or they can take a more indirect approach to weight gain and affect your metabolism. If you ever felt you gained weight simply by breathing, you aren't entirely wrong!

Allergies. Once rare, pollution and poor diet have drastically increased the occurrence of allergies in the global population. Today, according to the European Academy of Allergy and Clinical Immunology, over 1 billion people suffer from allergies. Symptoms include not only the typical runny nose but also stomachaches, insomnia, headaches, fatigue, brain fog, depression or anxiety, and, yes, weight gain.

Allergies and weight gain have a cyclical relationship. Allergies make fat cells larger, and fat cells in turn create a type of inflammation that intensifies allergic reactions. Both environmental and food allergies can cause this kind of inflammatory reaction that literally grows fat in the body.

Xenoestrogens. Many of these petrochemicals are estrogen-disrupting substances called xenoestrogens. Xenoestrogens have molecular structures that resemble that of estrogen closely enough to occupy the same receptors. Their effect in the body can vary from altering estrogen receptor sites, to disrupting the detoxification of estrogen, to interfering with the production of estrogen itself. Any of these creates an estrogen imbalance. Your well-being and your waistline pay the price.

Medication Bloat

Unfortunately, birth control pills, ERT, and HRT are not the only medications that cause water retention, bloating, and weight gain. Chances are that your medicine cabinet contains one or more other prescription drugs that are undermining your weight loss efforts. These are the same medications that affect your liver, as you read previously, and other parts of your body.

How these drugs stimulate weight gain varies with their mechanism of action. Statins and blood pressure meds interfere with exercise; beta-blockers slow fat burning; antibiotics and antacids alter the microbiome (Hidden Factor #6); and antidepressants and fibromyalgia drugs increase appetite. When the receptors are blocked, you gain weight. Prednisone, a corticosteroid, is five times more potent than the natural cortisol it's related to, with much the same action as the hormone (I will explain cortisol's fat-promoting action in Hidden Factor #5). Drugs also may cause weight gain indirectly. Side effects such as headaches, fatigue, and joint pain may keep you from exercising or from preparing healthful meals.

I will reiterate: if you are currently taking any medications—including birth control pills, ERT, HRT, and even drugs not listed in this chapter—do not stop taking them. If you suspect that they are causing weight gain, you must consult with your physician to explore potential alternatives.

And, of course, try the Fat Flush Plan. As I describe in the next section, various components of the plan are designed to target the weight you gain when fat's not fat. At the same time, with your hormones in balance, your insulin under control, and key nutrients and oils included, you may find that you no longer need the medication you're taking. Acne may clear up without birth control pills; depression and fatigue caused in part by food sensitivities may improve, decreasing your need for antidepressants.

What the Fat Flush Plan Does for False Fat

Cranberries and Water. The Fat Flush Plan targets water retention from the very first day. The Fat Flush Cran-Water beverage that you'll drink throughout the day in phase 1 is a powerful diuretic. Arbutin, an active ingredient of cranberries, pulls water out to be eliminated through your kidneys. At the same time, cranberry juice works on cellulite because the flavonoids in the fruit improve the strength and integrity of connective tissue and help keep your lymphatic system working smoothly.

Drinking 64 ounces of cran-water daily will ensure that your kidneys and lymphatic system have the fluid they need to work properly to remove wastes and fat. Ideally, water should be filtered and noncarbonated. Water helps rid the body of waste, keeps tissues moist and lubricated, and may even help burn calories.

The hot water with lemon juice you'll drink throughout the plan gives your kidneys another boost with lemon's diuretic action. And even the Fat Flush Plan exercise regimen, based on the mini-bouncer and brisk walking, has been designed to strengthen your lymphatic system and help rid your body of cellulite.

Additionally, the flaxseed and GLA components of the plan act as natural hormone therapy, from PMS to postmenopausal and beyond. They help to reduce hot flashes, level out mood swings, reduce sleep disturbances, and lubricate dry tissues without the side effects of fat-promoting synthetic estrogens and progestins. And for those Fat Flushers who are seeking even more individualized natural hormone therapy to replace their current drug prescriptions, there are pharmacies all over the country that specialize in compounding tailor-made natural hormones.

Fiber and Protein. Daily portions of selected fruits and unlimited quantities of selected crunchy vegetables ensure that you'll get additional dietary fiber. According to B. A. Stoll, a high-fiber diet reduces recirculating estrogen by binding to excess estrogen and carrying it out of the body. You'll also find that the plan's various fiber sources will help you feel full.

By including eight ounces or more of animal protein, rice and pea protein, and whey protein, the plan prevents protein deficiency that can slow

metabolism and cause cellulite and water retention. Without enough protein, your body loses muscle tissue, which slows metabolism. Pound for
pound, muscle burns five times as many calories as other tissue. You'll find
protein sources in the menus for all three daily meals because (1) your body
needs protein to rebuild tissue overnight, (2) protein helps you feel full, and
(3) it helps avoid midday fatigue that can lead to overeating.

Diuretic Don'ts. As you read through the recipes for phase 1, you'll notice
that they feature tasty herbs and spices, including sea salt. Commercial salt's
water-retaining properties are well known, but you may be less familiar with
the diuretic qualities of selected herbs. This is why the plan specifies parsley,
cilantro, fennel, and anise.

Phase 1 eliminates two of the most reactive food groups, grains and dairy
products. Following the two-week cleansing, phase 2 gradually reintroduces
hypoallergenic carbohydrates. By keeping a journal (see Chapter 7), you'll be
able to quickly identify any food reactions and make adjustments accordingly. In phase 3, "The Lifestyle Eating Plan," dairy and some grain-based foods
are part of the menu, and you are encouraged to continue to note your
body's responses, removing any reactive food permanently.

In phase 1, you'll not only avoid wheat and other grains, which can
cause gluten intolerance and candidiasis; you'll also skip other candida
boosters—starches, sugars, and fermented flavor enhancers such as soy
sauce. I have selected metabolism-boosting and diuretic herbs and spices
such as dry mustard, cayenne, garlic, mineral-rich apple cider vinegar, and
coconut vinegar to add flavor to my recipes without providing an environment for candida to flourish.

HIDDEN FACTOR #3: FEAR OF EATING FAT

In Chapter 1 I explained how I came to learn about the benefits of gamma-
linolenic acid for good health and weight loss. You read about your need for
essential fatty acids such as GLA. However, you still don't quite believe it, do
you? Eating fat to lose fat flies in the face of reason, of everything you've
heard about the dangers of fat.

You're not alone in your fear of eating fat. Many Americans have an
unhealthy fat intake, not because they eat too much fat, but because they
eat too much of the wrong types of fat, like trans fats, and too little of the
right types, like essential fatty acids (EFAs), particularly omega-3s. Well-
intentioned, but misinformed, dieters especially tend to avoid fat altogether, good and bad. This is unfortunate, because our bodies cannot make
EFAs. Yet, as precursors to hormonelike prostaglandins, EFAs regulate
every body function at the cellular level. This includes water retention,
sodium balance, and fat metabolism.

In your efforts at weight control, fat also:

✓ Carries fat-soluble vitamins A, D, E, and K through the bloodstream
✓ Activates the flow of bile (Hidden Factor #7)

✓ Helps your body conserve protein
✓ Slows the absorption of carbohydrates to balance blood sugar levels (Hidden Factor #4)
✓ Is a building block for production of estrogen, testosterone, and other hormones
✓ Is a precursor for serotonin, which controls cravings and elevates your mood

Every cell in your body is protected by a membrane that is composed largely of fat. Even your brain is 60 percent fat. Is it any wonder then that your body craves fat—any fat—when you eat a high-carbohydrate, low-fat diet?

Of course, the Fat Flush Plan does not suggest that you eat unlimited quantities of any fat. With the right fats, however, you'll end fat cravings, feel full, have more energy, and lose weight.

Fat Tames the Hunger Hormones

Many of our hunger and satiety cues are controlled by a group of four hormones called the "hunger hormones." The hunger hormones consist of leptin, ghrelin, cholecystokinin (CCK), and adiponectin. Just as diet can throw hormones such as insulin into disarray, how you eat greatly affects how your hunger hormones operate, too. The biggest dietary regulator of hunger hormones: fat.

CCK is the hormone responsible for the immediate sense of fullness that we have after a meal—and it is released by high-quality fats in our food (think the omega fats). Without this hormone that comes as a courtesy of fat, we will continue to feel hungry and dissatisfied after a meal. This explains why people who eat low-fat, high-carb diets often still feel hungry despite a big and hearty, high-carb dinner. To top it off, fat provides flavor to our food. So not only is your low-fat meal dissatisfying, but it doesn't taste all that great either!

In the opposite role of CCK, you have ghrelin. Ghrelin is a major appetite-stimulating hormone made by the pancreas and stomach. It triggers immediate hunger, especially cravings for salty and sweet foods that contain unhealthy fats. Levels are lower when you are thin and higher when you are fat. Typically, ghrelin should increase before meals and then decrease after eating. But these levels can get out of whack in response to things like stress, skipped meals (especially breakfast), restrictive dieting, and lack of sleep. Eating, you guessed it, good fats, especially omega-3s, helps to keep ghrelin levels balanced.

Leptin is a hormone that controls your hunger more in the big picture rather than in the existing moment. Think of it as a hallway monitor for fat. It is secreted by the fat cells and gives instructions on whether the body needs to pack on or shed the pounds based on the amount of fat it is carrying. Leptin levels are low in people at a healthy body weight and higher in those who are overweight or obese. Higher leptin levels decrease appetite and trigger the body to increase physical and immune system activity. Lower levels of leptin increase appetite. If you never feel quite satisfied after a meal, then you have low leptin levels to thank. With good fat, leptin can clearly communicate to the body whether it needs to eat more or less in order to, respectively, gain or lose weight. Without good fat, things don't go quite as smoothly. Like resistance to insulin, you can develop leptin resistance by eating too many refined carbs, causing the body to become insensitive to the appetite-decreasing effects of leptin. Obviously, leptin resistance results in weight gain.

Adiponectin has been referred to as the body's "fat-burning torch." It is also produced by fat cells in the body and circulates in the bloodstream. The more you have of it, the more fat you will burn for fuel, especially from the abdominal area. It's no surprise, then, that low levels of adiponectin have been linked with higher levels of obesity and insulin resistance. Monounsaturated fats boost adiponectin levels.

The Amazing Omegas

Two of the most important types of fat are the polyunsaturates omega-3 and omega-6. They make up the essential fatty acids, meaning your body cannot produce them on its own, and you must obtain them from your diet. When consumed in the correct balance, they are absolutely foundational for good health.

Omega-3 fats raise your metabolism, help flush water from your kidneys, and lower your triglyceride level. These fatty acids also increase the activity of L-carnitine to help your body better burn fat and to lower the risk of breast cancer. Studies in animals have shown that omega-3 fats even help prevent the development of excessive numbers of fat cells when the fatty acids are consumed early in life.

Alpha-linolenic acid (ALA) is one of the omega-3 fatty acids. It is found in flax seeds, hemp seeds, and walnuts. Under ideal circumstances, your body converts the ALA into eicosapentaenoic acid (EPA), then into docosahexaenoic acid (DHA), and then finally into prostaglandins. However, circumstances are seldom ideal. Excess sugar, a high intake of trans fats, stress, vitamin deficiencies, pollution, and viral infections are among the inhibitors of this transformation.

The omega-6 fat called linoleic acid (LA) can be found in *unheated, unprocessed* safflower, sunflower, and corn oil. Your body can convert the LA to GLA and arachidonic acid (AA) and then into prostaglandins. But as in the ALA conversion, many of the same saboteurs often interfere with this process. Thus, it is usually advisable to rely on the preformed GLA found in borage oil (24 percent GLA), evening primrose oil (8 to 10 percent GLA), or black currant seed oil (15 percent GLA). The omega-6 fatty acids stimulate your thyroid, raising your metabolism, and activate your brown adipose tissue (BAT) to burn fat, rather than storing it in your white adipose tissue. GLA also helps the skin maintain tone, firmness, and hydration during and after weight loss.

BAT is high-energy fat. It is dense in mitochondria, giving the tissue its darker color, and its only job is to burn calories for heat. When properly activated, BAT can become your own fat-burning machine. The key words are *properly activated.* In thinner people, according to researchers, BAT is quite active. However, overweight people tend to have more sluggish brown fat. Age appears to be a factor as well, with BAT activity slowing down as we get older. Thermogenic vitamins, minerals, herbs, and amino acids can help stimulate brown fat activity.

As I mentioned in Chapter 1, prostaglandins can augment the metabolic process called ATPase, which acts like a sodium-potassium pump to keep the right amounts of potassium in the cell and excess sodium out. The prostaglandins produced from GLA stimulate ATPase, causing this sodium-potassium pump to burn even more calories.

About 30 prostaglandins are known, and they are categorized into three families. For each prostaglandin performing one function, there is another performing the opposite function. The prostaglandins produced from the omega-3 and omega-6 essential fatty acids perform different functions and must be kept in balance for good health and effective weight loss. GLA becomes PGE1, an anti-inflammatory prostaglandin and diuretic. AA becomes PGE2, which causes inflammation, triggers the kidneys to retain salt, and encourages water retention. PGE3, produced from EPA, works with PGE1 to control inflammation, along with blood clot prevention and other functions. All three are needed at various times; for example, if you cut yourself, you'll need the inflammatory action of PGE2. However, to keep water retention under control, you need PGE1 and PGE3.

Omega-3 fats are burned off more quickly than other fatty acids, so when you diet, you lose omega-3s first—unless you include EFA supplements and food sources. This is just what the Fat Flush Plan does. Otherwise, if you lose weight at the expense of your omega-3 supplies, you'll find that you regain the weight easily and will have a hard time losing that regained weight. Your metabolism will have slowed because your body is less effective in using insulin when omega-3 fats are missing.

The New Fat Fighter

In the early 1980s, a research team headed by Michael Pariza, MD, of the University of Wisconsin isolated a form of linoleic acid called conjugated linoleic acid (CLA). This fatty acid is produced by cows and other grazing farm animals from linoleic acid in the grass they eat. It comes into our food supply via meat, whole milk, and full-fat dairy products.

More than 300 studies, mostly in animals, have been reported since CLA's initial discovery, highlighting its promise in cardiac, cancer, and diabetes therapy. However, it was CLA's special properties for weight control that were the subject of the first human studies.

Dr. Pariza and Ola Gudmundsen, PhD, of the Scandinavian Clinical Research Facility in Kjeller, Norway, were among the researchers reporting at the American Chemical Society meeting in 2000. The American study of 80 overweight people found that those who took CLA when they dieted, and who regained the weight when the diet ended, regained the weight as 50 percent muscle and 50 percent fat. Those who did not take CLA regained the weight as 75 percent fat and 25 percent muscle, the usual ratio of weight gain.

According to Dr. Pariza, whose team carried out the study, "CLA works by reducing the body's ability to store fat and promotes the use of stored fat for energy." CLA helps convert fat to lean muscle tissue, and muscle is one of your best metabolism enhancers.

The Norwegian study found that overweight people who did not diet but took CLA lost a small but significant amount of weight over a 12-week period. This study, also reported in the *Journal of Nutrition* in 2000, showed a stunning 20 percent decrease in body fat percentage, with an average loss of 7 pounds of fat in the group taking CLA without any diet changes.

The New Omega on the Block

While omega-3 and omega-6 tend to get all the glory, they are not the only omega fats that are mega fat burning. In fact, omega-7 is the most active fatty acid in regulating lipid (fat) metabolism. When observing omega-7 in a petri dish, researchers at Harvard found that it acts like a fat-burning signal to fat cells—which can become inactivated because of age, stress, or environmental toxins. Not only does omega-7 help you burn fat, but it helps keep you full, too. This fat elevates satiety hormones over 25 percent, helping people to feel satisfied with less food and significantly reducing their caloric intake by almost as much.

Omega-7 also improves heart health, insulin sensitivity (Hidden Factor #4), and cholesterol levels. It reduces levels of fat and triglycerides in the blood, which in turn leads to reduced fatty liver. And remember the inflammatory immune response that helped create false fat and is even part of Hidden Factor #4? Well, omega-7 is one of the most anti-inflammatory omega fatty acids. Studies have shown that omega-7 supplementation causes inflammation markers like C-reactive protein to fall by nearly 75 percent within 30 days.

Needless to say, omega-7 fatty acid may be the new omega on the block, but it has certainly made itself right at home as an essential part of the weight-regulating and health-promoting fat family. You find it most biologically available in anchovy oil and also in macadamia and macadamia nut oil.

Not So Crazy About Canola and Its Friends

I know this may seem confusing because I have just sung the praises of omega-6s and the vegetables oils they come from, but I was only referring to omega-6s from *unprocessed* fat, eaten in *balance* with omega-3s. The ubiquitous processed vegetable oils that have pumped our Western diet with a disproportionate amount of refined omega-6s are an entirely different story.

The most common vegetable oils like canola, corn, and soybean are almost always genetically modified and highly refined in food products. You will remember that refined or hydrogenated oils contain trans fats that sabotage the liver and make your body sick.

These oils are also polyunsaturated fats, which are not stable. This instability means the oils go rancid quickly, are more likely to denature in high-heat situations like the refining process, and oxidize quickly in the body. When a substance oxidizes, it creates free radicals—highly reactive molecules that damage DNA and cell membranes. Cellular damage caused by free radicals has been linked to aging, cancer, and other diseases.

Out of all the processed vegetables oils, canola oil has the worst offense record. While canola is high in omega-3s, not omega 6s, many of those omega-3s don't make it to your body. Because canola oil is a polyunsaturated fat and easily goes rancid, it must be deodorized to remove any rancid smell. The deodorization process transforms most of canola oil's omega-3s into trans fats. Studies have shown that canola oil blocks vitamin E in the body, which protects cells from free radicals and protects the heart. And for the cherry on top, canola plants do not actually exist in nature! Canola oil plants were fabricated in a laboratory, only coming to life out of the genetic modification of rapeseed.

As you now know, fake fat makes you fat. If the fat isn't real and has been synthesized or altered in some way, don't eat it!

Beyond the Fear

As I mentioned, your body converts EFAs from food into prostaglandins under ideal circumstances. However, circumstances often are far from ideal.

Our fear of fats, especially saturated fat, has driven us away from beef, dairy products, and butter. In their place, we've put refined vegetable oils, low-fat or no-fat dairy foods, and margarine. As a result, the balance between omega-3 and omega-6 fats is substantially skewed. We've also dangerously increased our consumption of trans fats, those damaged oil molecules produced when oils are heated or hydrogenated. Both results interfere with EFA conversion to prostaglandins. Other saboteurs include:

✓ High sugar consumption
✓ Chronic alcohol consumption
✓ Smoking
✓ Use of cortisone or excessive antibiotic use
✓ Stress
✓ Pollution
✓ Vitamin deficiencies

Another change over the past 20 to 30 years has had a whole range of unforeseen (and perhaps some as yet unknown) consequences, including several affecting our intake of EFAs and CLA. Almost without our noticing, farmers and commercial food producers converted from feeding cattle grass to feeding them grains. Few of us would suspect this relatively simple and straightforward change to have the potential for long-term health consequences, but this now appears to be the case. Grass-fed cows have three to five times more CLA than grain-fed cows.

What the Fat Flush Plan Does for Your Fear of Fat

Fat-Loving Food and Supplements. Your selections for your daily proteins on the plan can provide some of the EFAs and CLA you need. I've even included suppliers of grass-fed beef in Chapter 15. However, I know that getting the proper balance of omega-3s, omega-6s, and CLA is so important to your successful weight loss that I've made specific oils and supplements integral to the plan.

Daily servings of flaxseed oil ensure that you get adequate supplies of the omega-3 ALA. Adding flaxseed oil to foods creates a feeling of fullness and satisfaction following a meal. The EFAs in the oil cause your stomach to retain food for a longer period of time compared with no-fat or low-fat foods. The physiologic effect is a slow, sustained rise in blood sugar and then a prolonged plateau. The net result is a corresponding feeling of stamina, energy, and satisfaction with no immediate hunger pangs to lure you into overeating.

Throughout the plan you'll take a daily supplement of GLA, made from evening primrose, borage, or black currant seed oil, and in phase 3 you'll add a CLA supplement. To ensure that your body makes the best use of these oils and supplements, the plan also eliminates or minimizes many of the saboteurs, including sugar, alcohol, vitamin deficiencies, and stress.

Another delicious fat-filled option you'll enjoy is avocado. The avocado is a beautifully balanced fruit. These nutritional champions pack fiber, monounsaturated fat (including omega-9), and protein into a delicious green package. It promotes the hunger hormone adiponectin; and the abundance of omega-9, the most satiating omega fat, makes avocados especially filling. Its fiber content supports critically important liver functions and detoxification. All these factors combined give avocados an uncanny ability to fire up fat burning—to the tune of six pounds in two months.

HIDDEN FACTOR #4: INSULIN RESISTANCE AND INFLAMMATION

After reading this far, you must be marveling at just how complex and interrelated your body systems are. Too much or too little of a key component disrupts the natural balance, and you end up overweight and tired and a victim of any of a wide range of diseases. Such is the case with the intricate system for metabolizing carbohydrates.

Putting Carbohydrates to Work

When you eat carbohydrates or food high in sugar, glucose is released into your bloodstream. This signals the islets of Langerhans in the pancreas to produce the hormone insulin. Insulin takes some of the glucose to cells for immediate energy; it converts more glucose to a starchy version, glycogen. Glycogen is transported to the liver and muscle tissue for short-term storage, ready to be used quickly as blood sugar levels start to fall again. Short-term storage capacity is limited, however, so any remaining glucose is converted, again with the help of insulin, into triglycerides (body fat) for long-term storage. In short, insulin uses all the blood sugar it needs and stores the rest as fat.

When your blood sugar level drops, the islets produce the hormone glucagon. This hormone causes the glycogen stored in your liver to be released once again into your bloodstream and protein to be converted to glucose, all to restore your blood sugar level. Glucagon also releases fat from storage in your adipose tissue to be burned as fuel.

This process works very well when blood sugar is released slowly into the bloodstream, ensuring an equally controlled release of insulin. However, some carbohydrates are quickly converted to glucose, flooding your bloodstream and triggering an equally high level of insulin. The excess insulin causes your blood sugar level to drop sharply, bringing on fatigue and cravings for more carbohydrates. When this happens repeatedly, a series of events is set off.

✓ Insulin levels remain high.
✓ Insulin struggles to convert all the glucose for storage but succeeds only partially, and excess glucose is stored as fat; your body fat increases.
✓ Excess body fat is an active organ, producing proteins that prompt inflammation, which further inhibits insulin and energy usage.
✓ Cells no longer respond to insulin and refuse to store all the fat.
✓ Glucose that can't be converted to fat remains circulating in the bloodstream, wreaking havoc on your heart, kidneys, nerves, eyes, and blood vessels.

In the late 1980s, in a report in the journal *Diabetes*, Gerald Reaven, MD, professor emeritus of medicine at Stanford University, gave this sequence a name: insulin resistance. Robert C. Atkins, MD, author of *Dr. Atkins' Age-Defying Diet Revolution*, and others estimate that about 25 percent of apparently healthy, normal-weight individuals are affected by insulin resistance. If you're overweight, your chances are significantly higher. Possibly as many as 75 percent of overweight people are insulin resistant.

Inflammation Proliferation

One of the most dangerous and fat-fueling consequences of elevated insulin and blood sugar is the inflammation they create throughout the body. While inflammation itself serves as one of the immune system's primary weapons against pathogens, it causes a multitude of illnesses when it becomes chronic or misdirected. Insulin is an anabolic hormone, meaning it not only encourages cellular growth but also promotes fat retention and inflammation. In addition, excess glucose can be toxic, so your body responds to elevated blood sugar levels by triggering your immune system and creating inflammation.

Sugar also causes a process called *glycation*. In glycation, sugar attaches to proteins and specific fats, creating deformed molecules called *advanced glycation end products* (AGEs). AGEs do not function properly, and the body cannot recognize them, making the AGEs appear as foreign invaders to your immune system. The immune system responds to AGEs with yet another round of sugar-induced inflammation.

This is important because obesity is a disease of inflammation. Fat produces pro-inflammatory substances such as cytokines that rev up inflammation in the body. Not only does fat cause inflammation, but fat, visceral fat in particular, becomes inflamed itself. As the body cleanses itself of all the inflammatory substances produced by fat, the substances go straight to the liver, which responds by producing more inflammatory reactions and becoming tired and toxic. Inflammation is part of what makes obesity so dangerous, leading to many obesity-related illnesses such as diabetes. If you have too much excess fat, you are on inflammatory fire. When you calm inflammation, you calm your struggles with weight, too.

Not All Carbohydrates Are Created Equal

Carbohydrates—sugars, starches, and certain fibers—come primarily from plant foods, such as fruits, vegetables, grains, and beans. Milk products also contain some carbohydrates. Traditionally, nutritionists have categorized carbohydrates as either simple or complex based on their chemical structure. Sugars were simple and were thought to be digested quickly to release high levels of glucose. Starches were complex and released glucose slowly as they were digested.

However, it's not as simple as the difference between simple and complex carbohydrates. What matters is where the carbs come from. Different sources of carbohydrates have different impacts on blood sugar levels. Carbs from low-sugar, unprocessed, plant-based sources, like vegetables and beans, take longer for the body to process, so they can provide all the good nutrients that carbs have to offer while not causing dramatic changes in blood sugar levels. On the other hand, high-sugar, refined (processed) carbohydrates (think those foods in which grain has been processed into flour) are processed quickly by the body, creating erratic changes in blood sugar levels. As you now know, it is those drastic changes in blood sugar—the spikes and the drops—that destabilize your hormones, including insulin, leading to weight gain and insulin resistance.

Good Riddance, Grain

It's easy to spot some bad carbs. Cookies, candy bars, packaged breakfast pastries—they all obviously contain high levels of processed sugar that send your blood sugar and hormonal levels haywire. Others, like whole grain bread, are not quite as obvious.

When a grain is ground into flour, it behaves exactly like sugar in the body. Just two slices of whole wheat bread, high in the sugar-spiking carb found in wheat called amylopectin A, can raise blood sugar levels higher than most candy bars!

Wheat also contains a protein called wheat germ agglutinin that may block leptin receptors, which can lead to leptin resistance. Not only does grain send your blood sugar through the roof and mess with hormones like leptin, but it is particularly inflammatory as well. Inflammation, as you have been reading, contributes to weight gain, insulin resistance, and also leptin resistance.

Gluten. By now, almost everyone in the United States has heard of the infamous gluten. Gluten is a protein found in especially high concentrations in wheat and also in rye, barley, spelt, farina, faro, durum, emmer, semolina, couscous, triticale, kamut, and graham. Gluten free or gluten gluttony—it seems everyone has an opinion on whether or not gluten harms the body. Let me explain to you the science behind my thinking on the controversial grain protein.

Bottom line, gluten damages your health—and not only because of its inflammatory properties. I have already implicated wheat, and the gluten it contains, as a food trigger that causes false fat in Hidden Factor #2, but it is more dangerous than simply the waterlogged tissue it creates.

Today's genetically modified grain contains gluten that is high in gliadin, a protein that is foreign to our bodies. Gliadin is a shameless, druglike appetite trigger. In fact, gliadin is actually considered an opiate. The gliadin protein binds to the pleasure-producing opiate receptors in the brain, creating an addictive response in the body. Gliadin consumption leads to brain fog, impulsivity, anxiety, and, most commonly, appetite stimulation. People can consume nearly 400 extra calories per day when gluten is added to certain food products by manufacturers.

Furthermore, modern wheat contains 10 times more gluten than the wheat of 50 years ago. That's 10 times more of the inflammatory substance inundating your body every time you eat that piece of whole grain toast. Neurologist David Perlmutter, who has written extensively about the dangers of grain, points to grain-induced inflammation as a causal factors in various diseases such as leaky gut syndrome, autoimmunity, diabetes, Alzheimer's and dementia, depression, attention deficit hyperactivity disorder, digestive disorders like Crohn's and celiac disease, irritable bowel syndrome, and cancer.

When it comes to gluten, it's not only those with celiac disease or wheat allergy who suffer. Multiple studies have documented non-celiac gluten sensitivity (NCGS) in which people without celiac disease still experience symptoms such as diarrhea, abdominal pain, behavioral changes, foggy mind, and anemia. More research still needs to be done to determine the prevalence of NCGS, but researchers have noted its close relationship and substantial overlap with irritable bowel syndrome. One study estimates that 30 percent of people with symptoms of irritable bowel syndrome have wheat sensitivity or multiple food hypersensitivities.

I believe that whether officially diagnosed celiac, NCGS, or not, we all have some degree of gluten sensitivity. The trouble is that nearly 100 percent of gluten-intolerant individuals are unaware of it because gluten's negative reactions typically occur a good 12 to 24 hours after consumption. It's high time to get off our whole grain high horse and admit that glutenous grain in all its forms is not good for your health.

What the Fat Flush Plan Does for Insulin Resistance and Inflammation

In a single generation we Americans have made significant changes in our diet. Since 1977, the percentage of fat in our average daily calorie intake has dropped from 39.7 to 33.4 percent as of 2008. That equates to 10 grams less of fat per day. Unfortunately, this has been achieved largely by consuming low-fat, highly refined carbohydrates so obligingly created by food producers. To replace the fat, they filled their baked goods with sugar. We also eat much larger portions—mega-muffins and mega-bagels, giant plates of pasta—again in the mistaken belief that low fat equals low calorie.

The Rebalancing Diet. The Fat Flush Plan is designed to restore equilibrium to your diet and to control your insulin levels. About 30 percent of your daily calories come from natural healers in the form of highly colored vegetables and fruits. Many are also high in vitamin C, which researchers at Arizona State University have shown delays the insulin response to glucose, and in fiber, which slows the release of glucose into the bloodstream. What you won't find, however, are pro-inflammatory sugar, bread, white potatoes, and other high-glycemic carbohydrates.

Another 30 percent of your calories come from protein. Protein stimulates the pancreas to produce glucagon, the hormone that counteracts insulin and mobilizes fat from storage. Grass-fed beef, whey, butter and cream are also valuable food sources of CLA, which has been shown in animal studies to improve glucose tolerance.

Finally, up to 40 percent of your calories come from high-quality anti-inflammatory fats, in particular, flaxseed oil, coconut oil, MCT oil, and avocados. Their fatty acids have also been shown to rev up metabolism, satisfy hunger, and reduce insulin resistance significantly in people with diabetes, according to a report by Australian researchers published in the *New England Journal of Medicine*. These researchers also found that the more fatty acids from hydrogenated oils and high-fat meats found in a person's bloodstream, the more resistant that person is to insulin.

Inflammation-Quelling Condiments. Studies have shown that consuming apple cider vinegar or lemon juice with meals can lower blood sugar by as much as 30 percent. The acidity in these foods helps slow stomach emptying, which means that food takes longer to reach your small intestine and bloodstream. Carbohydrates are digested more slowly, and glucose levels are thus lower. Thus, the plan includes a daily drink of hot water and lemon juice and suggestions throughout the menus for using apple cider vinegar.

The plan also includes sesame seeds and sesame seed oil that help to curb the output of insulin, thereby slowing fat storage and preventing uncontrolled blood sugar swings that result in cravings and chronic fatigue. Sesame contains an amazing amount of antioxidants—like sesamol, sesamin, and sesamolin—which keep the oil stable despite its high linoleic acid omega-6 content. Coupled with a high vitamin E content, this unique antioxidant system also aids cellular sensitivity to insulin. This makes the inimitable sesame oil a wonderful seasoning agent and cooking oil for blood sugar regulation.

Speaking of flavorful additions to your meals, you'll find several anti-inflammatory herbs and spices regularly featured in the plan's recipes that boost your body's ability to metabolize sugar. Most prevalent is cinnamon. Researchers from the U.S. Department of Agriculture have shown that just ¼ to 1 teaspoonful of cinnamon with food metabolizes sugar up to 20 times better than turmeric, cloves, bay leaf, coriander, cayenne, dry mustard, and ginger, and lessens your risk of inflammation and excess insulin by speeding your metabolism or by lowering glucose levels.

However, the other Fat Flush herbs are far from living in cinnamon's shadow. Cayenne, ginger, and mustard can all boost metabolism between 20 and 25 percent. Turmeric aids fat digestion by decongesting the bile. The thermogenic cumin heightens metabolism so effectively that one study found that only a tablespoon can increase weight loss 50 percent.

The Fat Flush Plan may cut out sugar, but don't worry, I'm not asking you to forgo forever the taste of sweetness. In the plan, you will find sweet treats like low-fructose berries and natural sugar alternatives such as stevia and Lakanto, a type of sweetener that combines monk fruit and erythritol. While they may taste like sugar, these alternatives will not send you on that perilous blood glucose roller coaster. In fact, stevia is actually 30 times sweeter than sugar but with zero calories and zero carbohydrates. Lakanto is a whopping 300 times sweeter, has zero calories, and prevents tooth decay!

Supplements. Among the plan's supplements you'll find not only the EFAs mentioned earlier, but also several nutrients known to aid insulin action or regulate glucose. These include vitamins A, C, and E and magnesium, zinc, and chromium. Chromium is particularly important, and yet our diets are frequently deficient in it. It acts as a transport mechanism to enable insulin to work more quickly and efficiently. In turn, you store less fat and use more calories to build muscle. A 1998 study reported in *Current Therapeutic Research* found that individuals who took chromium supplements had an average weight loss of 6.2 pounds of body fat, whereas those taking a placebo lost 3.4 pounds. This weight loss represented a significant reduction in body fat for the chromium takers without their losing any lean body mass.

Once again, the plan's omission of pro-inflammatory saturated and trans fats, sugars, and refined carbohydrates will help its insulin-boosting components work at highest efficiency and effectiveness.

Even the exercise regimen, with the mini-trampoline, brisk walking, and, in phase 3, weight training, helps keep your insulin levels low. You'll have fewer cravings for sugary foods, feel more energetic, be more alert, and lose the weight you want—and keep it off. Exercise also helps another kind of resistance—leptin resistance!

HIDDEN FACTOR #5: STRESS AS A FAT MAKER

Living in this information age has most of us going nonstop at "cyberspeed." So it's no surprise to me, after assessing my own clients' stress levels for so many years, that in 2015 the American Psychological Association found 75 percent of Americans reported experiencing at least one symptom of stress in the past month—or that 33 percent of us admit to using food as our drug of choice to pacify our hectic lives by either overeating or eating unhealthy foods. The irony of the matter is that stress, as I suspected, is making the adrenals kick out certain hormones—such as cortisol—that can cause you to gain weight.

Stress is at the root of almost every disease. It impacts every part of the body, and especially the brain. Stress can disrupt our ability to think and feel clearly, even shrinking the brain with prolonged exposure to stressful experiences. This means the primary organ responsible for keeping you balanced and at a healthy weight cannot do its job properly.

It all starts when a part of our brain called the amygdala perceives a threat and alerts its neurological next-door neighbor, the hypothalamus, that the body is in danger. The hypothalamus controls our primal urges by using the endocrine system to send our body hormonal messages. Think of the primal urges as the four Fs: feeding, fighting, fleeing, and fornicating. You can already see stress's close relationship with food and weight—they are influenced by the same part of the brain. When stressed, the hypothalamus sends out a particularly important hormone for our purposes in this book: cortisol.

Stress and Cortisol

In the early 1990s, noted researcher Pamela Peeke, MD, spent three years at the National Institutes of Health examining the unsuspected side effect of stress: weight gain. Her work was published initially in 1995 in *The Annals of the New York Academy of Sciences*. Dr. Peeke discovered that stress makes you fat through a cycle of events that begins in the brain. The hypothalamus signals the nearby pituitary gland to release adrenocorticotropic hormone (ACTH). Then the adrenal gland, aware of ACTH in the blood, sends out stress hormones to handle things, including high levels of cortisol.

Cortisol's job is to release glucose and fatty acids so that muscles have energy. However, after the stress moment has passed, the cortisol level remains high, stimulating your appetite to replenish fuel your body has burned. A high consumption of sugary foods prompts more cortisol production and causes the body to store more fat than needed, usually in the abdominal area. Dr. Peeke's work also indicates that if stress remains a problem, cortisol levels in the bloodstream will continue to rise, in which case the stress-fat cycle goes on indefinitely—along with those extra pounds.

In earlier eras, that enhanced appetite would have worked to your advantage. You would have burned through a substantial amount of calories running from a wild animal while hunting and gathering. Today, however, the type of stress you have to contend with is usually emotional—being stuck in traffic, juggling job and family, dealing with a difficult employer, coping with computer crashes at critical moments, and so on. And as frustrating as all that is, it doesn't call for the same level of energy expenditure as earlier physical stresses, so now the calories you pile on are stored in your deep abdominal fat, ready for quick energy during the next crisis.

Psychology researcher Elissa S. Epel has confirmed and expanded on Dr. Peeke's findings, according to research published in the September–October 2000 edition of *Psycho-Somatic Medicine*. In Epel's research, 59 pre-menopausal women, over several days, experienced a series of stress-filled tasks, from puzzles and math to public speaking. Interestingly, the women who felt the most stress were those with central fat, poundage behind the abdominal muscles. Not only did they demonstrate a tendency toward more stress, but they also produced more cortisol than the slimmer-tummied participants.

Cortisol activates enzymes to store fat when it contacts fat cells—any fat cells. Central fat cells are deep abdominal visceral cells, which are a fast source of energy in times of stress. These central fat cells also happen to have four times more cortisol receptors than the fat cells found right beneath the skin. Consequently, cortisol is drawn to the central fat cells, which ultimately ups fat storage in that area. Thus, every time you're stressed, you're encouraging your body to have enough reserves of fat to handle the problem. This concept helps explain why chronic psychological stress, according to Epel, actually has an effect on body shape through fat distribution, creating what is commonly referred to as an "apple" body shape.

The cortisol-pumping stress response will only stop once the body relaxes and can shut off its reaction to the stressful circumstance.

Compounding Factors

Modern Mayhem. In his landmark book, *Why Zebra's Don't Get Ulcers*, Robert Sapolsky addresses the question his book's title poses. The answer: zebras use their stress response how it is meant to be used. Humans, on the other hand? Not so much.

A lion chasing a zebra on a savanna puts a zebra into an immediate, short-lived stressful situation that has only two outcomes: the lion catches the zebra, or the zebra escapes. This is the exact type of life-or-death stress the human fight-or-flight reaction evolved to handle. Surviving this stressful situation utilizes every measure of the fight-or-flight response to the full capacity, including all of that excess cortisol, in order to survive something that is about to kill or severely threaten the zebra.

In contrast, humans in modernized, civilian societies like that of the United States do not frequently face life-threatening danger. Instead, the "danger" we face is psychological. It's that unexpected traffic jam that makes us late to work, a fight with our spouse, a last-minute assignment from our overbearing boss, a snide comment from our teenage child. All these things elicit the exact same fight-or-flight response as that zebra has as she sprints for her life across the savanna. However, contrary to popular belief, our snarky kids probably won't kill us.

This leaves our body biologically prepared to take on a lion, but with no lion in sight. All our biological preparations go to waste, and if stress becomes chronic, they can end up hindering our survival instead of promoting it.

Today, we find ourselves anxious, depressed, tired, sick, and overweight, in no small part because the stress we face never ends. Unlike the zebra, which calms down after the encounter with the lion, we have psychological lions around every corner. Chronic stress means chronic cortisol production and increased accumulation of that infamous belly fat that puts people at risk for heart disease and type 2 diabetes.

Dangerous Distractions. Everyone handles stress differently. Some reach for a cigarette, some for a relaxing cocktail after work, and others for a hot cup of coffee. Interestingly, the more heavily a person smokes, the more visceral fat she or he has. About 30 minutes after a smoker puts out a cigarette, the person's cortisol level shoots up, and it remains high for at least another 30 minutes. In a study of 2,000 smokers over age 50 years, the individuals who smoked the least were the thinnest. Alcohol has similar effects, raising cortisol levels and upping the amount of central fat. One Swedish study reported that nondrinkers had 38 percent visceral fat, whereas alcoholic men had 49 percent.

Caffeine. Caffeine isn't much better. Just 15 ounces of your favorite coffee contains enough caffeine to raise your epinephrine (also called adrenaline) level by more than 200 percent. And that epinephrine pumps out more stress hormones, including cortisol. Chugging down around three cups of coffee a day could cause your serum cortisol to stay at high levels 18 out of every 24 hours, instead of just the couple of hours our bodies were designed to handle.

Caffeine also promotes norepinephrine production. This stress-involved hormone targets your nervous system and brain. Along with epinephrine, it increases your heart rate, raises your blood pressure, and stimulates your fight-or-flight stress response. In fact, caffeine actually reduces your threshold for stress, so that you aren't able to handle it as well. This might lead you to cope in different, counterproductive ways, including the oh-so-common eating of comfort foods (invariably loaded with sugar and other high-glycemic carbohydrates), which creates more metabolic stress and fat storage.

And remember, as I mentioned in the section on the liver toxicity factor, caffeine is in much more than coffee. It's found in over-the-counter medications (e.g., Anacin, Vivarin, and Vanquish), chocolate (e.g., baking chocolate, cocoa, and milk chocolate), sodas (e.g., Pepsi, Mountain Dew, Diet RC, and Coke Zero), and tea.

Sleep. Sleep and cortisol are entwined. Chronically high cortisol levels disturb moods and even sleep. Lack of sleep, in turn, keeps your body stressed out and your cortisol levels high. Sleep deprivation has reached epidemic proportions in the United States. Indeed, founder of the *Huffington Post* Arianna Huffington has declared we are in a sleep deprivation crisis in her book *The Sleep Revolution*. According to Huffington, sleep deprivation is the new smoking, glamorized in today's culture when it in reality is corroding our health. A national poll conducted by the National Sleep Foundation found 45 percent of Americans reported that poor or insufficient sleep affected their daily activities at least once in the past seven days. A study published in 2000 by the University of Chicago's Department of Medicine revealed that not only does sleep deprivation affect tiredness and immunity, but too little sleep impairs the way the body handles food, creating impaired glucose tolerance. This can result in insulin resistance and obesity. It is believed that a lack of quality sleep, known as rapid eye movement sleep, can impede surges of growth hormone, resulting in increased fat tissue and reduced muscle mass. Sleep deprivation, which causes lower body temperature and fatigue, usually leads to increased food consumption to boost energy and help you stay warm.

Insulin. I've highlighted the effects of excess insulin on your weight. In his book *Sweet & Dangerous*, British researcher John Yudkin, MD, examined another aspect of insulin, namely, its relationship with cortisol. He cited research that found that after two weeks of eating a high-sugar diet, volunteers had increased insulin and cortisol levels. Their fasting insulin levels rose 40 percent, but their cortisol levels shot up 300 to 400 percent! As we now know, cortisol works in concert with other chemicals to quicken fat storage and plump up cells, so controlling sugar consumption and getting a grip on insulin can help put a halt to excess fat.

Medication. There is another outside factor contributing to raised cortisol levels that you should know about. Some prescription drugs contain cortisol more potent than what your body produces. One example is the corticosteroid prednisone, whose cortisol is five times more powerful than your body's.

What the Fat Flush Plan Does for Stress as Fat Maker

By now you'll recognize features of the Fat Flush Plan designed to control cortisol and stress fat, including:

✓ Avoidance of caffeine, alcohol, and sugar, known cortisol boosters
✓ Protein at each meal to enhance fat burning
✓ Daily fat to reduce cravings and physiologic stress

As the preceding discussion makes plain, however, taking control of your weight involves more than taking control of your diet. The Fat Flush Plan incorporates various elements to manage stress, increase activity, and maintain cortisol at healthy levels.

Feel-Good Fat. As you know, the human brain contains more than 60 percent fat. It also happens to need more omega-3 fatty acids than any other organ or system in the body. According to the National Institutes of Health, omega-3s help to balance stress hormone levels and provide direct weight loss benefits. They can be supplied by ALA-rich foods found in the plan such as flax and walnut.

The omega-derived EPA and DHA fats from fatty fish like wild caught salmon, sardines, and anchovies are major players in regulating emotions and mood and warding off depression. In a number of clinical studies, these fats were shown to help to reduce aggression and hostility. They can help to fortify your system so you can mentally handle and cope with stress more efficiently to minimize the damage created by elevated levels of cortisol.

Exercise. The plan's moderate exercise regimen, based on the mini-trampoline, brisk walking, interval training, and, in phase 3, weight training to strengthen muscle mass, will help burn central fat and the fatty acids released during stress while increasing levels of the neurotransmitter hormone serotonin, which enhances mood and relaxation.

Exercise also teaches the body how to utilize cortisol better. Even though cortisol surges during exercise, the body uses this time to learn how to use cortisol more efficiently. Ultimately, exercise lowers cortisol levels, decreasing overall stress and the propensity for weight gain.

Sleep. A full seven to eight hours of sleep each night is important to reduce fatigue, provide growth hormone to help burn fat, and reduce cortisol levels. Strive for a 10 p.m. "lights-out" regimen to increase the likelihood of getting the quality sleep you need.

INSIDER TIP	My life has always been surrounded by the sound of music. I grew up singing all of the Broadway show tunes my mother would play day in and day out and later sung on stage for local musical productions and in the choir in both high school and college. Imagine my surprise to learn how healing singing is for your soul, as well as your stress levels. Mitchell L. Gaynor, MD, of the Cornell Center for Complementary and Integrative Medicine, has stated that you can lower your cortisol levels by as much as 25 percent when you listen to music for more than 15 minutes a day.

Keeping a journal helps to identify the emotions behind your overeating. It also helps to release negative feelings and to provide a handy distraction when temptations arise. Many Fat Flushers have told me that by keeping a journal they are able to follow the plan even better and they now understand what triggers their overeating. Understanding the reasons behind your behavior is an important step in gaining self-control.

I hope you will use many of the plan's features as the basis for rituals in your own life. When exercise, journaling, and regular sleep are daily habits, they become integrated into your permanent lifestyle plan. During these activities, your mind's healing powers can help repair some of the day's stress damage. What a plan!

3 Top 10 Hidden Weight Gain Factors #6 Through #10

I have no special talent. I am only passionately curious.

—ALBERT EINSTEIN

In Chapter 2, you learned about my original five hidden weight gain factors that were the underlying foundation for Fat Flush. As I worked with my online community and clients for the past 10 years since the publication of the first edition of *The Fat Flush Plan*, I became aware of even more subtle factors that were interfering with our most sincere weight loss efforts. The overwhelming evidence I have seen through the latest research and my own experience with clients has resulted in five more hidden weight gain factors. They are:

✓ Messy microbiome
✓ Poor quality bile
✓ Tuckered-out thyroid
✓ Hidden hitchhikers—parasites
✓ Missing magnesium

Functional medicine is on fire about the truly groundbreaking work being done around these issues, highlighting their repercussions for shrinking your waistline and expanding your health. Empowered with this new information, I am excited to offer you a newly fortified Fat Flush Plan for weight loss and well-being that I believe will guide you more confidently than ever before on the road to a happier, healthier you.

HIDDEN FACTOR #6: MESSY MICROBIOME

First, let's review. In the last chapter, you learned foundational, key concepts for developing optimal health and reaching a healthy weight. In short, you read that toxicity, fat-free eating, hormones, stress, and lack of sleep can hinder your body's functioning and lead to weight gain.

Now here's the doozy. Did you know you have an organ that you can't see? And this organ is so important that it actually plays a major role in every single one of the things I listed above.

Meet your microbiome.

Okay, so your microbiome is not actually an organ—or even human for that matter—but it has so many important functions in the body that some experts refer to it as one. The word *microbiome* refers to the trillions of bacteria that live on and within your body. You are currently housing at least 10,000 different species of bacteria, the majority of which live in your gut. In fact, you have so many of these microscopic friends that they outnumber your human cells 10 to 1.

Bacterial Best Friends: Probiotics

Bacteria have gotten a bad rap. You see soap and hand sanitizers lining supermarket shelves proudly advertising that their product kills 99.9 percent of all germs and bacteria. This implies the misguided assumption that *all* bacteria are breeders of illness that we should avoid at all cost. While some bacteria do cause illness, the majority that make up your microbiome are good bacteria, called probiotics, that support critical life-sustaining functions. Without your microbiome, you would not exist. Period.

Don't believe me? Your microbiome is integral to the immune response, the digestion and absorption of nutrients, and the manufacture of life-supporting substances such as enzymes, vitamins, hormones, and neurotransmitters. Your probiotic buddies do so much in the removal of toxins and waste from your system that some experts have called the microbiome the "second liver." Your microbiome also helps to control hormone and blood sugar levels, promotes quality sleep, influences hunger hormones, and regulates stress, especially through its influence on cortisol and adrenaline. Remember, excess cortisol, erratic blood sugar, lack of sleep, and haywire hunger hormones all cause weight gain, so your microbiome helps you both chill out and get out of your fat funk.

On top of that, these bacteria have epigenetic properties, meaning they moderate the expression of your genes. This means your microbiome has the ability to turn certain genes on and off, including the genes that affect metabolism and, in turn, your weight. Through its many functions, especially its epigenetic functions, the microbiome has a say in determining who you are, how you look, and how your body works.

However, modern microbiomes have found themselves in a state of despair. In a healthy gut, probiotic cells would number around 100 billion to 1,000 billion per millimeter of the digestive tract. This number ensures that good probiotics have a majority strong enough to maximize their ability to protect your health. Today, many Americans have probiotic counts as low as 5 per milliliter. Not 5 billion—just 5!

As a result of microbial assaults from your diet, the way that you were born, and medication (more about all these later), your microbiome cannot perform its job properly. Inflammation can get out of control. You cannot adequately digest and absorb nutrients. Critical vitamins, like B12 and K, and chemicals, like neurotransmitters such as serotonin, are not produced in sufficient quantities. Remember from Chapter 1 that low serotonin levels can lead to food cravings, weight gain, and depression. With these only being a few of the numerous consequences, a messy (dysbiotic) microbiome has been linked to Alzheimer's, diabetes, ADHD, depression, and obesity.

Belly-Busting Bacteria

Numerous studies have intimately linked a messy, unbalanced microbiome to weight gain and obesity. Its influential role in our metabolism gives our bacterial ecosystem substantial control over our weight. A damaged microbiome cannot properly perform its role in metabolizing blood sugar or regulating hormones (including hunger hormones) and may turn on genes that encourage obesity. As a matter of fact, scientists have started to attribute some of the weight loss associated with gastric bypass surgery to healthier gut bacteria that occur as a result of the procedure and an accompanying change in diet.

Researchers led by Jeffery Gordon at Washington University have proved the validity of the connection of gut bacteria to a bulging gut. The researchers took pairs of twins in which one was obese and one was at a normal weight and transferred the gut bacteria from both into mice. The mice that received the gut bacteria from the obese twin gained weight. The mice that received the gut bacteria from the thin twin stayed thin. Now here's the kicker: both groups of mice ate the same diet in the same amounts.

While these results are astonishing, there is one caveat: the mice who received the healthy microbiome had to eat a consistently healthy diet in order to sustain their leanness. When their diet went wacky, so did their weight.

Two critical features of your bacterial makeup have a significant impact on your weight: the diversity of your microbiome and your ratio of Firmicutes (fir-MIH-cue-tees) to Bacteroidetes (BAC-teer-OY-deh-tees).

Diversity. Study after study has shown that overweight people have a more homogenous microbiome than that of people with a lean body mass. Think of your microbiome as a system of checks and balance. Your microbiome requires a balance of probiotic and pathogenic bacteria to function properly, with good bacteria mitigating the effects of the bad. As diversity of the microbiome decreases, otherwise beneficial bacteria can lose their counterbalance, and their unchecked action in the body can turn them pathogenic. These overgrowths stress out the body, leading to inflammation and impaired microbiotic functions, and can create uncomfortable symptoms and conditions such as yeast infections. According to Gordon, a microbiome low in diversity can also lack crucial bacteria needed to maintain a normal metabolism and achieve a healthy weight.

The "Cutie" Ratio. The ratio of Firmicutes to Bacteroidetes, which I have nicknamed the "cutie" ratio because both of their names end in a kind of "cutie" sound, has a tremendous influence on your weight. It is very important that medical professionals use this ratio as an "obesity biomarker." These two bacteria are two of the most populous in your microbiome. They make up 90 percent of the bacteria in your colon.

Firmicutes have been called "fat-loving" bacteria because of their high level of efficiency at extracting calories from food, resulting in increased fat absorption. Higher levels of this calorie machine also turn on genes that raise the chance of obesity, diabetes, and heart disease. On the other hand, Bacteroidetes are especially good at breaking down plant starches and fibers into energy that the body can use in the form of shorter-chain fatty acids. A 2006 study from Washington University showed that people suffering from obesity have 20 percent more Firmicutes and 90 percent fewer Bacteroidetes on average. You can improve your cutie ratio by eating more dietary fiber.

Inflammation Squelchers

Your microbiome also influences your weight through its regulatory role in inflammation. About 70 to 80 percent of your overall immune system shares a home with your microbiome in your gut. This front line of pathogen defense has its own name: the gut-associated lymphatic tissue.

Part of this immune defense is your intestinal wall, which consists of a single layer of cells that create a judicious barrier between the substances, good and bad, in your intestine and the rest of your body. Think of it like a second skin. Second only to your skin, your intestinal wall is where your body encounters the most foreign material and organisms. Unlike your skin, your intestinal wall acts like a gatekeeper, controlling what substances can pass through its guard and gain entrance into the body. It also helps you to extract nutrients from your food and contains pathogen-fighting chemicals called immunoglobins that keep unhealthy substances out of your gut lining.

The bacteria in your gut work in tandem with your immune system, continually informing immune cells of the content of your intestines and directing now much your immune cells need to react to whatever you have ingested. That's right—your microbiome can tell your immune system what to react to, controlling inflammation. The bacteria also help maintain the integrity of your intestinal wall to help prevent unwanted substances from entering your body. The microbiome keeps your immune system sharp and able to quickly neutralize potential threats, as well as stops it from overreacting to benign foods and activating an autoimmune response. Your bacteria brothers and sisters, when healthy, can actually stop a chronic immune response.

Remember from our discussion of inflammation under Hidden Factor #4 in Chapter 2 that obesity is an inflammatory disease. When you have a messy microbiome, your bacteria cannot perform their crucial immune-regulating functions, and inflammation increases throughout your body. Your body stays under stress as your immune system stays on high alert. As a result, you gain weight.

Furthermore, many of the diseases associated with obesity actually have their roots in the changes in the microbiome that occur with large amounts of excess body fat. For example, take type 2 diabetes. Not only does it contribute to the inflammation at the onset of the disease, but a messy microbiome also cannot produce the by-products essential to maintain the health of the digestive system and effectively metabolize blood sugar. In other words, part of the reason the body cannot process glucose in people with insulin sensitivity and type 2 diabetes is a dysfunctional microbiome.

The microbiome is so critical to glucose regulation that Dr. M. Nieuwdorp from the University of Amsterdam successfully improved blood sugar in more than 250 patients with type 2 diabetes with fecal transplantations. Fecal transplantation effectively replaces the microbiome of one person with that of another by transplanting the fecal matter of the latter into the former. This treatment also worked for insulin sensitivity. No medication today can produce the same results.

Candida and Food Reactions: It's Overgrowth, Not Overweight. Among the most common reasons that food leaks through your intestinal wall and enters the bloodstream before it's fully digested is candidiasis, an overgrowth of the naturally occurring yeast *Candida albicans*. Candida normally lives alongside your microbiome, which controls its growth.

However, when your microbiome is thrown off balance and your immune system is weakened, candida can get out of control. It changes from a noninvasive spore form into a fungal form that grows threadlike mycelia. These structures bore through your intestinal lining, penetrate other cells, and extract nutrients. The candida migrates to other tissues, producing toxins such as acetaldehyde that stress the immune system. Candida also produces hormonelike substances that interfere with normal hormone production. For example, it may stimulate increased estrogen production and interfere with hormone signals to the immune system.

The holes in your intestine allow food macromolecules to enter the bloodstream—the trigger for food reactions. Studies in rats have found that candida also stimulates histamine production, another trigger in the classic allergic reaction. An estimated 80 percent of people with multiple allergies have candida overgrowth.

Many of the symptoms of candidiasis mimic those of food reactions: fatigue, headaches, bloating, nasal congestion, heartburn, and moodiness, among others.

The relationship between candidiasis and food sensitivities is made even stronger by consumption of sugars and refined carbohydrates. The foods you are most likely to crave as a result of food allergies are the ones most enjoyed by the candida—those sweets, chips, and pasta help create an environment that encourages yeast growth. This is compounded if you often consume food with a high yeast or mold content, such as dried fruit, bread, and beer.

A diet deficient in essential fatty acids, vitamins, and essential amino acids weakens your immune system and does not properly nourish your microbiome, creating the potential for candidiasis. In addition, candida overgrowth commonly develops in women taking birth control pills or in anyone taking antibiotics or cortisone-type medications, as the candida also disrupts the probiotic balance in your gut. The regular use of a quality probiotic can also help in battling candidiasis (Flora-Key is my daily go-to).

Making a Mess

Unfortunately, many people today have a messy microbiome. A healthy microbiome nurtures a rich diversity of bacterial species and has an overwhelming majority of good bacteria to bad bacteria. It works to reduce the effects of bad bacteria and promotes healthy immune, endocrine, digestive, and overall functioning. Typically, in a healthy microbiome, 85 percent of the bacteria are good, healthy bacteria that balance out the 15 percent that are pathogenic. When this sensitive internal ecosystem gets thrown out of whack, it loses diversity, the number of good bacteria decreases, and the number of pathogenic bacteria increases. The ratio of the two critical bacteria discussed earlier—Firmicutes and Bacteroidetes—gets off balance. You are left with your best probiotic partners struggling to get by.

Diet. When the microbiome is not nourished properly, it gets messy. It requires a diet high in quality fat, fiber, probiotics, and prebiotics (substances that encourage friendly bacterial growth) and low in sugar, processed fat, and refined carbohydrates to perform properly. Jeffery Gordon, the same Washington University researcher who performed the twin studies I talked about previously, also conducted a study that showed that a typical Western diet prevented good bacteria from having slimming effects.

Sugar, especially fructose, encourages the growth of bad, pathogenic bacteria, destabilizing the vital microbial balance. Like an artificial sweetener, this particular sugar found frequently in sodas, salad dressings, and fruit also decreases the production of leptin, so your body does not feel full as quickly and encourages you to keep eating. Ultimately, fructose can lead to the same metabolic disorders as real sugar, even though it does not raise insulin levels. This is because it creates a messy microbiome that cannot perform its part in regulating blood sugar and maintaining a healthy metabolism.

One of the worst bacterial offenders is gluten. Studies have shown that gluten activates a protein in the digestive track called zonulin. It has the job of regulating the opening of spaces between cells in the intestinal lining that allow molecules to flow in and out. The activation of zonulin increases the opening of these spaces, making the intestinal wall more permeable to a greater number of substances. This condition is called intestinal permeability, also known as leaky gut syndrome. Leaky gut syndrome hinders the intestinal wall's ability to act as a second skin and dictate what can and cannot enter your body. This leads to increased inflammation throughout the body, as more unwanted substances gain entrance into your system.

Birth Method. The sad truth is you will likely start off life with a messy microbiome if you were born via C-section. How you are born substantially influences your inflammation "set point," or the base level of inflammation you will have throughout your life, in part due to its influence on the development of the microbiome.

The fecal matter we encounter in our mother's birth canal provides the basis for our own bacteria that colonize our bodies throughout our life. If you are not born vaginally, you are never exposed to the healthy bacteria in your mother's body, and they do not colonize your body. Instead, you are colonized by the bacteria on the hands of your doctors, not the particularly balanced bacteria of your mother's gut. Formula feeding instead of breastfeeding has the exact same effect.

Babies born via C-section have 5 times the risk for allergies, an 80 percent increased risk of celiac disease, a 50 percent increased risk of becoming obese as an adult, and a 70 percent risk of developing type 1 diabetes.

Antibiotics. You can see the problem with antibiotics in its name. It is antibiotic, meaning it kills bacteria. While antibiotics have incredible, life-saving properties, they cannot distinguish good bacteria from the bad. They kill everything, maiming your microbiome.

An astounding 50 million pounds of antibiotics are used each year in the United States, and not only for people. Up to 18 million pounds are routinely placed in the food and water of even healthy livestock. This creates two distinct and popular methods of antibiotics overexposure: prescription medication and food products from animals that have been treated. You may not think of yourself as overexposed to antibiotics because you do not get sick very often and rarely get an antibiotic prescription. But consider how often you eat meat, especially from nonorganic sources. Now you see, there may be more antibiotics in your system than you realized.

The animals on factory farms receive low, subtherapeutic doses of "preventative" antibiotics for most of their natural lives in order to thwart the infection often caused by the conditions the animals live in. The antibiotics allow farmers to raise more animals in closer quarters without disease wiping out the herd. The antibiotics also make cows grow bigger, giving farmers a greater return on their investment. However, it's not only beef. Fish and poultry products also receive antibiotic treatment. Studies have shown that low levels of antibiotics increase the body fat of mice by 15 percent. To avoid antibiotics in your food, buy organic, pasture-raised meat.

When it comes to humans, antibiotics are often overprescribed. Experts estimate that doctors write 20 million unnecessary prescriptions a year for antibiotics when they will actually have little to no effect on treating the presenting ailments. Research shows that common maladies such as young children's ear infections are often better left to run their course. Yet even more research published in the *New England Journal of Medicine* found that this overprescribing extends to conditions like acute bronchitis, which, like the common cold, is often caused by a virus. Antibiotics have no power over a virus. Interestingly, the states with the highest antibiotic use, the southern states, tend to have the highest rates of obesity, and the states with lower antibiotic use tend to have lower levels of obesity. While a multitude of other factors are obviously at play, I think there is a clear connection between antibiotics, the microbiome, and obesity.

What the Fat Flush Plan Does for Your Messy Microbiome

The signature Fat Flush protocols are especially supportive of your microbiome. The plan carefully and systemically eliminates all simple sugars and processed grains, which feed yeast and fungus that can crowd out beneficial bacteria that keep you thin and healthy. The plan also eliminates all artificial sweeteners, which can enable certain fat-forming strains of bacteria to thrive. These in turn alter metabolism, slowing it down to a grinding halt. To add insult to metabolic injury (so to speak), consider that these unfriendly bacterial strains also have a tendency to trigger insulin resistance, encourage fat storage, and promote inflammation. Thankfully, the specific microbiome-friendly features of the new Fat Flush include the following:

✓ A prebiotic and probiotic special sweetener called Flora-Key that can be included in daily smoothies.
✓ A new sweetener known as yacon syrup, a prebiotic made from chicory, that will help fuel a healthy probiotic population. This new addition is introduced in phase 3, "The Lifestyle Eating Plan," along with the Flora-Key in all phases.
✓ Microbiome-nourishing foods like jicama, apples, pears, cauliflower, whey protein, broccoli, berries, cherries, onions, garlic, asparagus, Jerusalem artichokes, and leeks are included in each phase of the program. Special fermented foods like yogurt are introduced in maintenance (phase 3) along with umeboshi paste (pickled plum purée) for seasoning, sauces, dips, and corn on the cob.

Also noteworthy are the medium-chain fatty acids in coconut and MCT (medium-chain triglyceride) oil, which have powerful antifungal properties and leave the good bacteria intact. Coconut and MCT oil are now options for every phase of the program.

The Fat Flush eating plan provides a two-pronged approach: The first is cutting back on carb-rich foods in order to reduce yeast that can overgrow and outnumber your "skinny bacteria." The second is making use of the many therapeutic herbs and spices that are noteworthy for their yeast-destroying and microbiome-preserving benefits. In this regard, garlic is one such herb that comes to mind.

Garlic has been shown, especially in research from India, to be as effective as prescription meds in suppressing fungal overgrowth. Allicin, the ingredient in garlic that provides its distinctive flavor, also acts as a natural fungicide. You will find there is plenty of garlic in each and every phase of Fat Flush!

Fat Flush also cleans up a messy microbiome by providing a fiber-rich diet throughout the program. Soluble fiber, found in chia, flax, and hemp seeds as well as numerous fruits, vegetables, beans, and legumes, is fuel that friendly flora in your gut ferment into healing compounds that strengthen the entire microbiome.

HIDDEN FACTOR #7: POOR QUALITY BILE

Bile is brilliant! No conversation about weight is complete without discussing this yellowish-green liquid that the liver produces about a quart of every day. Bile is stored in the gallbladder, where it waits until it is transported to the intestines during digestion. Made from lecithin, cholesterol, and bilirubin, your bile has two jobs. First, it emulsifies and digests fat, breaking it down into small particles so that your intestines can absorb them. Second, it helps escort toxins that your liver has removed out of the body.

Your Buddy, Bile

No doubt, you've been hearing a lot about probiotics and the microbiome these days. But without all the good press is your body's brilliant bile—one of the liver's key detox methods introduced earlier. Simply put, without this important ally you will not receive the full benefits of the fat-flushing journey you are embarking on. Backed-up bile leads to hypothyroidism, weight gain, and nutritional deficiency.

Fat Digestion. I would be totally remiss to sing the praises of fat, and encourage you to eat it, if I do not first make sure your body is primed to reap its rewards. Fat is our best source of energy. Gram for gram, it yields more than twice as much energy as carbohydrates or protein. However, when you have thick, congested bile, your body cannot digest this dietary powerhouse. Without sufficient bile to break it down, your body has little use for fat, and so it stores it.

When bad bile keeps your body from digesting fats, not only does it make you gain weight, but it also leaves you without the nutritional benefits packed inside fat. Recall from Chapter 2 that fat supports brain function, creates healthy cell membranes, balances blood sugar levels, regulates hunger hormones, and serves as a building block for hormones such as estrogen and testosterone, as well as neurotransmitters such as serotonin. Furthermore, poor fat digestion impairs your ability to carry and store fat-soluble vitamins such as A, D, E, and K for healthy skin, reproduction, and blood clotting. Vitamin A, for example is a powerful infection-fighting vitamin and also functions as a powerful antiparasitic agent (more on this later). Without fat's help, you will be unable to conserve protein to rebuild vital tissues; maintain a normal body temperature; insulate and cushion your vital organs, nerves, and muscles against shock, heat, and cold; or seal in moisture for healthier skin, hair, and nails.

Detoxification. When the liver cleans the body, it dumps all the toxic waste into the bile, which then carries those toxins on their way to their ultimate excretion from the body. This renders high-quality, thin bile necessary to the detoxifying process. When bile flow is impeded, whether it be because you have a congested and fatty liver that cannot produce quality bile or your body is not receiving the proper nourishment to support the bile, your body cannot fully detoxify itself.

Remember from Chapter 2 the importance of promoting your liver's ability to cleanse the body. If the liver can't clear fats, then it most likely can't break down hormones or other metabolic waste products either, and you can end up with hot flashes, night sweats, acne, migraines, and even depression, plus the need to buy a larger sized wardrobe.

The lymphatic system assists the liver through its garbage disposal ability. When congested, waste can be recycled through the body and get stuck in the bloodstream, joint, and other tissues. A congested lymph impairs the body's ability to completely remove waste and is a major contributor to cellulite.

One important hormone that does not get broken down when bile is congested is estrogen. When the body reabsorbs estrogen, it can lead to estrogen dominance. As I explained in the previous chapter, too much estrogen in the system causes water retention, an increase in body fat, and hypothyroidism. In addition, excess estrogen causes cholesterol levels in the bile to rise, which results in thickened bile fluid.

Bile has such a substantial role in detoxification that there is already a 75 percent bile deficiency by the time allergies, arthritis, and inflammation in joints and muscles develop—conditions with a direct relationship to unnecessary toxins in the body. By the time cancer or chronic illness is diagnosed, a whopping 90 percent deficit has already occurred.

Keeping in mind all the new material that has already been covered in this book, you can see how bile deficiency depresses your overall health, prevents weight loss, and encourages weight gain. You know that erratic blood sugar levels, haywire hunger hormones, a tired, toxic liver, and poor detoxification prime the body to accumulate excess fat. Each of these factors are rooted to some degree in low quality bile as well as other causes. As a matter of fact, bile has such an important role in weight regulation that improving bile quality has been shown to increase metabolism by 50 percent. If you thin the bile, you thin the body. Period.

Think your bile might need a deep clean? Take a look at some of these signs and symptoms of low-quality bile:

✓ Queasiness after a fatty meal (impaired bile flow)
✓ Light-colored or floating stools (lack of bile output)
✓ Nausea (not enough bile)
✓ Dry skin and hair (lack of essential fatty acids)
✓ Constipation (inadequate bile for lubrication)
✓ Constant feeling of fullness
✓ Inability to lose weight
✓ Pain under the right rib cage (reflective pain from gallbladder)
✓ Hemorrhoids (congested liver)
✓ Varicose veins (pressure from constipation due to thickened bile)
✓ Pain between the shoulder blades (reflective pain from gallbladder)

✓ Bloating or gas
✓ Headache over the eyes (gallbladder meridian passes over this region)
✓ Bitter taste in mouth after meals (sign of bile regurgitation)
✓ History of prescription or recreational drug use (need for more liver and gallbladder support)
✓ Sensitivities to chemicals
✓ Easily intoxicated (need for more liver and gallbladder support)
✓ Fibromyalgia (sign of liver and gallbladder overload)
✓ Hypothyroidism (sign of deficient bile to stimulate active thyroid hormone in fat cells)

Where Is Your Gallbladder?

The technical answer is right underneath your liver; the gallbladder sits in this prime location to perform its duty of storing and regulating bile flow. It is in charge of releasing bile in response to your body's need to digest fat.

Despite its crucial role in bile regulation, what comes to mind when people think of the word *gallbladder* is gallstones, not fat digestion. The next thing people likely think of is gallbladder removal surgery, which doctors often use to fix gallbladder issues like gallstones and unresolved pain. Indeed, well over 20 million Americans have known gallbladder challenges, while millions more go undiagnosed. Gallbladder removal is the most common surgery in the United States, with 600,000 performed each year.

In light of everything you have just learned about the role of the gallbladder, it may seem strange that conventional medical professionals so readily resort to taking it out—yet, in some cases, the surgery is unavoidable. While this surgery can provide relief for some from their painful gallbladder-related symptoms, it also leaves a whole new battle of figuring out how to support a now unregulated bile. Without the gallbladder, your body loses the ability to regulate the release of bile. No matter how much you support your bile, it can never regain completely normal function; without a gallbladder, you continue to experience the consequences of bile deficiency.

Fortunately, you can get close. Taking an ox bile supplement (also known as bile salts) can greatly restore your body's ability to digest fats. While you may not be able to duplicate your body's remarkable wisdom of knowing just exactly when to release the exact right amount of bile, supplementation with a bile extract can go a long way in maximizing the process and assuring that your fat-soluble vitamins and essential fatty acids are being well-utilized. As the years progress, many find that they are woefully deficient in these important nutrients, but often do not connect the absence of the gallbladder with their symptoms. Without enough fat-soluble vitamin A, infection is more likely; without D, immunity is tamped down; without E, circulation is hampered; without K, calcium can be deposition in all the wrong places, like joint, arteries, and soft tissues.

Moreover, following the Fat Flush Plan serves not only as a successful weight loss program but also as lifestyle medicine, especially for gallbladder issues. Congested bile, insufficient fat consumption, stress, and food allergy lie at the foundation of many gallbladder issues. As a matter of fact, back in the 1960s and 70s Dr. James C. Breneman, chairman of the Food Allergy Committee of the American College of Allergists (now known as the American College of Allergy and Immunology), conducted a study in which the elimination of food allergies provided 100 percent relief to every single participant in the study experiencing gallbladder pain. Wow, gallbladder pain resolved with the elimination of common food allergies. Now that's a headline that would make big news in this day and age!

The major food offenders in his study were eggs (92.8 percent), pork (63.8 percent), onions (52.2 percent), chicken and turkey (34.8 percent), milk (24.6 percent), coffee (21.7 percent), and oranges (18.8 percent). The lifestyle plan I prescribe in this book will eliminate today's food allergens, support a healthy bile, and increase fat digestion, which will keep your gallbladder chugging along for the rest of your life.

HCl: Bile's Fat-Fighting Partner

HCl, which stands for hydrochloric acid, is the scientific name for stomach acid. For decades, scientists thought high stomach acid levels caused an array of gastric problems, as conditions like acid reflux became epidemic. But I am here to tell you to put down that Pepto. I can almost guarantee that you need more stomach acid, not less.

In a world where much of what we eat is contaminated (more on this when I talk about parasites in Hidden Factor #9), you need HCl more than ever. It functions as your front line of defense against potential parasites and pathogenic bacteria that may have hitched a ride with your breakfast. HCl also plays a significant part in absorption of nutrients—including fat.

Ideally, food should pass from your stomach into your small intestine, accompanied by a steady flow of bile. You need hydrochloric acid for this process to occur.

If you are not secreting enough hydrochloric acid, the opening to the small intestine, known as the pylorus, becomes spastic. A spastic pylorus keeps the bile from entering the small intestine, where it needs to go to carry out its fat-digesting duties. Denied entry to the intestines, bile backs up into the liver and gallbladder and leaves fat undigested. Your poor pancreas also suffers, resulting in not only poor regulation of blood sugar—that can lead to weight gain—but also problems with digestion and appetite.

In other words, bile and HCl are a package deal. Bile needs an HCl prompt to execute its role in the body. Not surprisingly, low hydrochloric acid levels are dramatically linked to a dysfunctional gallbladder. Low stomach acid levels are ridiculously common in the United States today. In fact, Dr. Johnathan Wright, a well-recognized expert on hydrochloric acid, has found that 90 percent of his patients suffer from too little hydrochloric acid.

Diet. Although I have always cautioned about those "crazy carbohydrates," especially in excess, do note that a low-carbohydrate diet, when not executed properly, can hinder stomach acid production. This is because people often compensate for fewer carbs with an excessive amount of protein. All the protein simply overwhelms HCl production as your stomach struggles to produce enough acid to break down the shear amount of this muscle-building nutrient. You will also not produce sufficient hydrochloric acid if you do not consume enough HCl-supporting nutrients in foods that contain sodium, iodine, and zinc. Think seafood and pumpkin seeds.

Not only does diet affect stomach acid production, but how you eat and drink has a big impact as well. Eating too much too quickly, eating irregularly, drinking large amounts of fluids with meals, not thoroughly chewing food, swallowing air when eating, and crowding in too much food at one time can all challenge your body's ability to produce HCl. Drinking water, especially cold water, within two hours of eating is particularly detrimental to stomach acid.

Stress. If a base weakens an acid, then, when it comes to stomach acid, stress is most definitely a base. Stress has an ability to stop HCl production in its tracks. This basic stress can come from the harsh eating habits I described above, life circumstances, or anything else that throws off or threatens the homeostasis of your body. Once again, controlling stress is tantamount to controlling your health.

What the Fat Flush Plan Does for Your Poor Quality Bile

Fat Flush is the only diet and detox program to focus on building up bile. It does so in several ways.

Bitter Is Better. First you will note that many of the vegetables and "legal" herbal teas function as dietary bitters. Bitters are a potent way to trigger the release of bile from the gallbladder. And if you no longer have your gallbladder, bitters will assist in fat digestion as well. Do note that many vegans can use digestive bitters instead of ox bile. These bitters include greens like arugula, radicchio, watercress, and escarole. Dandelion root tea is also considered a "bitter" and is legendary for assisting in bile thinning and decongestion—as are gentian and angelica.

In phase 2 you will be introduced to the number one bile-building vegetable—beets. Whether the beets are shredded raw or steamed, the betaine in beet will enhance bile flow and help digestive functions all around.

Bile-Thinning Beverages. On a daily basis, you will be consuming hot water and lemon. This morning beverage is designed to cleanse the bile while purifying the palate. Lemon is a liver-loving food par excellence.

Fat Flush also promotes the forgotten importance of lecithin—especially from non-GMO soy and sunflowers. Lecithin is an ingredient in bile that has detergentlike qualities. Daily lecithin in the Fat Flush Smoothies is your daily insurance for free-flowing bile.

Rituals. Castor oil packs, which have been recognized for decades for their ability to cleanse bile, are highly recommended in Chapter 9 on rituals. Once your bile is detoxed and decongested, the thickened sludgelike blockages will, it is hoped, dissolve. You will improve your body's ability to remove toxins via the bile route, which will in turn allow all your tissues and cells to release built-up wastes throughout your body.

HIDDEN FACTOR #8: TUCKERED-OUT THYROID

If the hypothalamus is the king of the endocrine system, then the thyroid is its highest-ranking general. The hypothalamus passes on commands to the pituitary gland, which in turn gives this tiny butterfly-shaped gland its marching orders. The interaction between these three parts of your body dictates much of your hormonal function. In fact, every single cell in your body has thyroid hormone receptor sites.

Because the thyroid has a decisive role in hormone regulation, its ability to function has consequences for every aspect of your health. This mighty gland regulates body temperature, as well as supports the immune system, the nervous system, and the intestines. It impacts the brain, muscles, heart, gallbladder, and liver. Thyroid hormones help strengthen hair, nails, and skin, and they support normal bone growth.

The thyroid's hormonal control makes it a significant part of metabolism. Rehabilitating your tuckered-out thyroid can be the key to finally inciting your metabolic burn.

Crossing Your Ts

In its body-regulating arsenal, the thyroid has a selection of mighty hormones that it produces and uses to relay commands and corral cellular function. For our purposes, we are concerned with two particularly important thyroid hormones: thyroxine (T4) and triiodothyronine (T3). They get their names from the number of iodine atoms they contain. T4 has four iodine atoms, and T3 has only three. These hormones control your body temperature, heart rate, and metabolism. When we talk about our "metabolic fire," these hormones serve as tinder for caloric burn.

The hypothalamus and the pituitary gland largely determine the amount of hormone your thyroid produces. When the hypothalamus senses that the amount of thyroid hormone in the body is too low, it sends a signal to the pituitary gland to produce thyroid-stimulating hormone (TSH). Following orders, the pituitary produces TSH, which triggers the thyroid to produce more thyroid hormone. When the hypothalamus senses that the body has enough thyroid hormone, it tells the pituitary to produce less TSH.

In response to the call of action from TSH, the thyroid produces and deploys T3 and T4 into the bloodstream. These metabolic soldiers reach every single cell in the body, giving each one directions on how much oxygen and nutrients to consume. In other words, T3 and T4 instruct cells whether to increase or decrease your metabolism.

Of the two thyroid hormones, T4 is the less active one. In fact, T3 packs three times the punch of T4. It is T3, not T4, that is actually responsible for revving up the body's metabolism. However, the thyroid produces substantially more T4 than T3, with T4 making up about 80 percent of the thyroid's hormonal output. Your body normally has a "reserve" of T4 ready to be converted into the more active hormone, T3. This conversion of T4 to T3 involves the removal of one iodine atom from T4 and occurs inside the cells of organs such as the kidneys, liver, and brain.

When T3 conversion fails to occur at adequate levels or the thyroid fails to produce enough thyroid hormone, hypothyroidism results. The conversion of T4 to T3 and the production of thyroid hormone can be blocked by many factors, including aging, illness, stress, high consumption of soy, and medications.

Hypothyroidism: A Thyroid Struggling to Keep Up

If the thyroid acts as an ignition that turns on and off your metabolism, then it follows that a tuckered-out thyroid leads to decreased metabolism and weight gain. Alongside a decreased metabolism, a sluggish thyroid may also lead your body to produce too much insulin, triggering low blood sugar along with intense cravings for carbs.

The condition of an underperforming thyroid is called hypothyroidism, and it has far more extensive consequences than excess body fat. Hypothyroidism's symptoms include:

✓ Swelling around the eyes
✓ Loss of appetite
✓ Extreme tiredness
✓ Cold hands and feet
✓ Muscle weakness and cramping
✓ Depression
✓ Hair loss
✓ Brain fog
✓ Poor eyebrow growth (especially the outer one-third of the brow)
✓ Inappropriate hair growth
✓ Dry, scaly skin
✓ Brittle nails
✓ Hot flashes
✓ Menstrual irregularities
✓ Insomnia
✓ Irritability
✓ Aching wrists, arms, and hands
✓ Fluid retention
✓ Decreased libido
✓ Increased cholesterol
✓ Constipation
✓ Difficulty swallowing pills, lump in throat
✓ Coarse voice
✓ Decreased blood pressure

✓ Premature graying of hair
✓ Inability to concentrate
✓ Dementia
✓ Infertility
✓ Muscle stiffness

According to the American Thyroid Association, nearly 30 million Americans have been diagnosed with a thyroid disorder—with the key word here being *diagnosed*. I believe that, in reality, many more people live their lives hindered by undiagnosed thyroid conditions. Thyroid disorders are notoriously hard to diagnose. People often do not take their symptoms seriously enough, attributing the constant fatigue and extra pudge to lifestyle factors such as chronic stress or aging. Furthermore, standard thyroid tests that look at T4 and TSH often miss telltale markers of a sluggish thyroid, so even those who get tested may still find themselves blind to the reason of their suffering.

Thyroid Overload

When you consider the prospect of living life overweight, depressed, and in a brain fog, the importance of taking care of your thyroid needs little explaining. If you want to lose weight, then the thyroid's role in metabolism makes it crucial to achieving your goals. However, the complex and extensive interaction your thyroid maintains with your entire body makes it sensitive to upsets on many different fronts. It takes vigilance and care on your part to make sure you do not accidentally overload your metabolic crusader.

Viruses. In his book that I reviewed and endorsed, *Medical Medium: Secrets Behind Chronic and Mystery Illness and How to Finally Heal* by Anthony William claims that viral overload may be the most powerful cause of thyroid dysfunction. He views viral overload as a precipitating cause of many modern-day maladies like fibromyalgia, rheumatoid arthritis, lupus, Lyme disease, and multiple sclerosis.

In regard to the thyroid, William points to one virus in particular as the main source of damage: the Epstein-Barr virus. EBV infiltrates your thyroid by literally twisting and spinning like a drill to burrow deep into the thyroid tissue, killing thyroid cells and scarring the organ as it goes. This results in hidden hypothyroidism in millions of women, from mild cases to the more extreme.

EBV is cunning, too, able to thwart your immune system's attempts to rid it from your system. Naturally, your immune system responds to an intruder with inflammation, but between EBV's neurotoxin, viral by-product, and poisonous corpses confusing things, and with EBV hidden in your thyroid, your immune system cannot tag the virus for complete destruction.

Next, the immune system may try to wall off the virus with calcium, creating nodules in your thyroid. However, EBV can outwit your body's plans. Most of its cells evade this attack and remain free. Even if your body does manage to catch a viral cell in a cocoon of calcification, EBV typically remains alive and turns its calcium prison into a comfortable home, where it feeds on your thyroid, draining it of energy. The virus cell might even eventually transform its prison into a living growth, called a cyst, that creates further strain on your thyroid. On top of it all, if you aren't eating enough calcium-rich foods as your body tries to attack EBV, it will extract calcium from your bones, which can lead to osteoporosis.

Stress and Adrenal Fatigue. Like every other part of your body, your thyroid is vulnerable to stress. In fact, stress can cause the spread of EBV. The virus feeds on the stress hormone adrenaline. It wants to activate the adrenal glands in order to obtain its main food source. Hence, the entire goal of EBV is to create stress in the body in order to promote its own growth.

The thyroid and the adrenal glands work closely together to help regulate your bodily functions. However, when under duress, this relationship can go sour. Stress, as you now know exceedingly well, increases cortisol levels. High amounts of cortisol can lead to underconversion of T4 to T3, meaning there is not enough of the more active T3 to ignite metabolic burn. Paradoxically, this triggers the body to increase cortisol production even more as a way to compensate for the decrease in metabolism. Do you see the cycle? Cortisol interferes with T4's conversion to T3, which decreases metabolism. The body then compensates by producing more cortisol, which in turn continues to hinder T4's conversion to T3. This cycle spins its way right into adrenal fatigue.

To meet the higher cortisol demand, the adrenal glands convert progesterone into cortisol. This can upset the estrogen-progesterone balance and lead to estrogen dominance. In response to the diminishing progesterone levels, the thyroid attempts to help out the adrenals by producing adrenal hormones. Now, in addition to adrenal fatigue, you also have a tuckered-out thyroid. This results in not only your hormones running in circles but also your body taking on a more circular shape.

Cortisol's impact on thyroid function extends beyond the underconversion of T3. In excess, cortisol can also exhaust the pituitary gland, hampering its ability to produce TSH. Without adequate TSH, the thyroid will not receive orders to create more thyroid hormone, and so it simply will not produce it, resulting in low levels of T3 and T4.

If the thyroid does manage to produce the proper amount of hormones, elevated cortisol levels and inflammation can still continue to interfere with its communication after those hormones have hit the bloodstream. Cortisol can cause thyroid-receptor site resistance as well. This means that even if the thyroid is producing all the right hormones, and those hormones are being properly converted, the cells in the body will not be able to receive those hormonal signals.

Poor Quality Bile. If you are not yet convinced of the significance of bile, then I am certain its role in thyroid function will remove all doubts. According to a study conducted at Tampere University Hospital in Finland, hypothyroidism is seven times more likely in people who experience reduced bile flow.

Why? A study conducted by researchers that included thyroid specialist Dr. Antonio Bianco showed that the release of bile triggered the release of an enzyme that converts T4 to T3. Recall that this is the very process that allows metabolism to take place in the body. Astoundingly, people in Bianco's study who improved their bile health saw a whopping 53 percent increase in their metabolism.

Elevated Estrogen. Hypothyroidism shares many of its symptoms with estrogen dominance. In fact, the late Dr. John Lee, my old friend who wrote seminal books on women's hormones, theorized that having too much estrogen and too little progesterone can cause thyroid dysfunction, even if thyroid hormone levels remain normal. In other words, regardless of whether you have a thyroid in prime fighting condition or not, having unbalanced estrogen and progesterone levels can still derail the thyroid's ability to function.

This is because high estrogen levels can elevate thyroid-binding globulin (TBG). TBG is a protein that transports thyroid hormone through the blood. If TBG levels are high, levels of unbound (free) thyroid hormone will be low, decreasing the availably of thyroid hormone. Excess estrogen can also thicken the bile, slowing the release of bile and its ability to produce the T4 converting enzymes.

Messy Microbiome. After learning about your microbiome's role in immunity, digestion, and hormones, it probably comes as no surprise that it also affects the thyroid as well. At least 20 percent of thyroid function relies on a healthy amount of quality beneficial bacteria. One strain in particular has been found to protect against the toxicity of gliadin, which is so problematic for thyroid patients. That strain is *B. lactis BI-04* and comes from the Bifidobacterium family.

Destructive Diet. Gluten has got to go. Gliadin, the protein found in gluten, highly resembles a crucial enzyme known as transglutaminase, which is concentrated in the thyroid. As the immune system attacks the gliadin, antibodies also attack the thyroid. The immune system can then go into overdrive, damaging the thyroid, sometimes for up to six months, and causing inflammation throughout the body, including in your brain.

It's not only gluten you have to worry about. A lack of protein can depress thyroid function, as thyroid hormones need protein to escort them to all bodily tissues. Raw cruciferous vegetables like broccoli, cabbage, brussels sprouts, kale, soybeans, and radishes contain substances called goitrogens that may block thyroid hormone production by interfering with the uptake of iodine. Recall that iodine is one of the main components of T3 and T4.

Speaking of iodine, three chemicals in particular compete with iodine for uptake in the thyroid: bromine, fluoride, and chlorine. Excessive amounts of these chemicals result in the thyroid absorbing less iodine, which in turn leads to decreased thyroid hormone production. Bromine, fluoride, and chlorine are contained in water, toothpastes, hot tubs, nonorganic foods, soft drinks, teas, commercial breads, some medications, and brominated vegetable oils.

What the Fat Flush Plan Does for Your Tuckered-Out Thyroid

The Fat Flush Plan amounts to a nap and rejuvenating spa day for your tuckered-out thyroid. You have already read about how the plan fixes things that damage your thyroid like poor quality bile, estrogen dominance, stress, and a messy microbiome, but the plan also has nutrients that will specifically nourish and support this hormonal sergeant in order to optimize its functioning.

Coconut Oil. Coconut oil really shores up thyroid functioning by 50 percent. Coconut is an excellent vegan source of saturated fat, and it is the one that does not require bile to break it down. It can actually bypass the gallbladder, and it has documented weight loss properties. As a rich source of lauric and caprylic acids, coconut functions as a marvelous antiviral, antifungal, and antiparasitic food. Furthermore, the medium-chain triglycerides in coconut oil can markedly improve the efficiency of your thyroid and boost metabolism over 50 percent. Add some coconut oil to dandelion root tea to boost energy and metabolism—and start your day off the Fat Flush way!

Increase Iodine. You read that bromine, fluoride, and chlorine can keep necessary iodine out of the thyroid. Without sufficient iodine to kick them out, these three chemicals can stockpile in your body and impede thyroid function. You can only avoid these substances by filtering your water and reading labels to see what foods they creep their way into.

In addition to avoiding the terrible thyroid trio, the plan will increase your iodine intake to support your thyroid. The best source of iodine? Sea vegetables. You will enjoy nori, a type of seaweed often used in sushi, that is a good source of vitamin C and meets 70 percent of your daily iodine needs with only one sheet. The plan also includes kelp, dulse, and seaweed gomasio, a seaweed blend you can use as a salty seasoning.

I do have one caveat about consuming sea vegetables. Do not consume sea vegetables that come from Japan, as the water is contaminated with toxic radiation due to the Fukushima nuclear disaster. I recommend getting your sea veggies from Maine or other parts of the northeastern United States. A company I particularly like is called Maine Seaweed.

HIDDEN FACTOR #9: HIDDEN HITCHHIKERS—PARASITES

Parasites can make you fat! I know this may sound like the strangest hidden factor of all, but it's true. Just like every other stressful, pathogenic, disruptive substance or organism I have discussed, parasites can sabotage any weight loss effort or attempt to create a healthier body.

Parasites place a major burden on the immune system and are especially toxic to the liver. By eliminating parasites first and foremost, your body can then reduce its toxic load, and your system can more efficiently clear pathogenic bacteria, heavy metals, fungus, and mold. Best of all, you just may lose weight once and for all.

In 2006, scientists found evidence supporting these bad bugs' connection to burly bellies. Researchers at Penn State uncovered a metabolic problem among the dragonfly population that looks eerily similar to the obesity epidemic in humans. These dragonflies harbored parasites similar to those that cause malaria and cryptosporidiosis. As a result, they experienced inflammation that impeded their metabolism of fat, resulting in increased fat accumulation around their muscles. Researchers believe that similar parasitic developments in humans may be partly responsible for the human epidemics of insulin resistance, type 2 diabetes, and obesity.

Sadly, parasites frequently go undetected, unsuspected, and therefore unrecognized. Many people in Westernized society operate under the common misconception that they live a life too clean and protected to ever acquire a parasite. However, the truth is that in random stool tests, 1 in 3 individuals have been found to carry some type of parasitic infection (I personally believe that that number is really closer to 2 out of 3). Over 130 various types of parasites have been identified in our country. Indeed, with more chemical-laiden food that is also more highly processed, traveling farther distances, and waiting on shelves for a longer time before it reaches our plates, parasites have more and more opportunities to hitch a havoc-wreaking ride into our bodies.

How Hidden Hitchhikers Hide

The truth is that no type of parasitic testing is always accurate, so it's impossible to use random stool testing as the "gold standard" for assessing true infection. In a study of diagnostic labs in the United States, researchers found that only one in ten correctly identified cases of amebic dysentery—a parasitic disease that can kill you.

On top of their ability to evade testing, parasites are the great masqueraders. Conditions that are linked to parasites can appear identical to a multitude of more common conditions. Take candida, for example. It is well recognized that candida can come from a sugary, yeast-rich diet, excess antibiotics, and too much alcohol. But who knows that the parasite giardia can also be a underlying trigger? If in fact you have giardia, you may be doing everything right to balance your microbiome, but you won't see the result you deserve because you have neglected to address the real culprit. If anything, that sounds like a true hidden weight gain factor to me.

Common Disguises. Besides being responsible for weight gain, over 130 different "hidden invaders" can account for over 385 diseases. Their symptoms go way beyond metabolism and the gastrointestinal tract. Parasites may be the underlying cause of some of the most prevalent insidious and mysterious disorders of our time like leaky gut syndrome—such a popular diagnosis today—as well as autoimmune problems, weight gain or weight loss, and viral conditions, to name just a few. And to name a few more:

✓ Chronic fatigue and candida can be a case of chronic giardia.
✓ Ulcerative colitis may be a case of undiagnosed amoeba.
✓ Migraine headaches and depression may be the result of toxoplasmosis. In fact, in one study, toxoplasmosis was found in nearly 50 percent of migraine sufferers. It is believed that toxoplasmosis may stimulate the trigeminal nerve controlling facial and head pain. Other symptoms included mysterious body aches, a fever that comes and goes, and fatigue.
✓ Roundworms have been connected to allergies and asthma. In particular, asthma has been related to roundworm going through the lungs, and even type 1 diabetes can have a parasite connection—tapeworm to be exact.
✓ I have seen ADD and ADHD clear up when pinworms were removed.
✓ Food and environmental allergies disappear when worms are eliminated.
✓ I have seen rashes and boils clear up when people do a comprehensive targeted colon cleanse.
✓ I have personally experienced how brain fog and hypoglycemia are "lifted" when thread worms are cleared from the system.
✓ We now know that some forms of arthritis can be connected to amoeba, while seizures can be triggered by a pork tapeworm infection.

The list goes on and on and can include constipation, diarrhea, gas and bloating, infectobesity, persistent flulike symptoms, anemia, secondary gluten intolerance, casein intolerance. lactose intolerance, Crohn's disease, sleep disturbances, and an enlarged liver or spleen.

Just remember one thing, above all else, as my reveared 106-year-old mentor, Dr. Hazel Parcells, taught me so many decades ago: parasites are the most immunosuppressive agent known to humans.

Unintended Vehicles

Many seemingly benign foods and activities we enjoy every day expose us to a whole host of microscopic and larger invaders. Following are the most prevalent twenty-first-century factors that may be the reason that so many of us are unwitting hosts of certain kinds of critters.

Travel. Travel may be the most obvious and well-known risk factor for parasites. Seeing new people, places, and cultures is a wonderful way to enrich your life and expand your mind, but with new places come new parasites.

With increasing globalization and ease of international travel, people bring parasites across national borders all the time. About a hundred cases of dengue fever occur every year in tourists coming back to the United States. At the same time, schistosomiasis, a parasitic worm, infects 200 million people worldwide and can cause anemia, chronic pain, diarrhea, fatigue, and poor nutrient absorption. One innocent swim in an inviting pool or lake that you find on vacation and that happens to be contaminated, and schisto-somiasis is yours.

Studies show that deadly parasites can even survive a transatlantic flight and attach themselves to the outside of an airplane. With more than 700 million passengers riding planes every year, it provides ample opportunity for parasites to cross the pond, the border, or the next city over.

Daycare. Daycares are notorious locales for the parasite giardia, which can cause chronic fatigue, persistent diarrhea, bloating, cramps, flatulence, and unintentional weight loss—due to diaper changing processes and inadequate sanitation. Giardia also takes up residence on counters, sinks, and chairs, as well as in lakes, rivers, and streams.

Restaurant Dining. In our consumer culture, we like to consume food, not cook it. In fact, in 2015, Americans spent more money dining out than they did on groceries. Unfortunately, the sparse oversight of local restaurants' hygiene standards amounts to little more than random inspections from the health department. This leaves restaurants at the frightening liberty to maintain dirty practices that could contaminate your meal, whether it be gourmet or fast food.

The emphasis on efficiency over cleanliness in the food service world only exacerbates this problem. Employees on bathroom breaks are pressured to get back work, sometimes at the expense of good hygiene. Or they feel the pressure to clean more dishes faster, not more thoroughly.

Raw and Undercooked Food. Most people are familiar with the ubiquitous restaurant warning that accompanies even the slightest chance of eating raw or undercooked meat. This warning comes with good reason.

You should never eat raw beef, as it can carry tapeworms that can dwell in your digestive system without causing obvious symptoms. Even rare beef is risky. It can contain a single-cell parasite that causes toxoplasmosis, also found in cat feces, which can cause birth defects, encephalitis, and migraine headaches. To ensure that the beef you eat is safe for consumption, turn up the cooking temperature to the magic number of 160 degrees Fahrenheit.

Unfortunately, it's not only beef. Eating a healthy diet of raw fruits and vegetables can increase your risk for contracting parasites. Parasites hop on vegetable leaves and fruit peels and are carried into any recipe in which these products are used in hopes of reaching their desired haven: your body. Berries, cherries, raspberries, strawberries, bamboo shoots, water chestnuts, watercress, spinach, parsley, lettuces, and celery are frequent homes to parasites if not properly washed.

Microwave Cooking. Never use a microwave as a primary method to cook food. Microwaves do not cook food evenly and mask undercooked parts of food with parts that are more thoroughly cooked. Anyone that has ever tried to cook in a microwave will know that just because the food is warm on the outside does not mean it's warm on the inside!

Although I do not recommend a microwave for cooking under any circumstances, as they all leak radiation, it is certainly better to use a microwave to reheat your food, as long as it has been fully cooked at an appropriate temperature before you reheat it.

Pork. Pork can carry both the trichina worm and pork tapeworm. Trichinosis is a well-known parasitic disease caused by the trichina worm that pigs acquire from contaminated garbage and infected rodents that causes flulike symptoms and intense muscle pain. Pork tapeworm can be found in ham, sausage, and pork and can cause serious brain damage. Pork should be cooked to an internal temperature of 170 degrees Fahrenheit in order to eradicate any of its parasitic partners.

Tap Water. In light of catastrophes like the lead contamination water crisis in Flint, Michigan, that prompted the state's governor to declare a state of emergency in January 2016, the United States is now well aware that the quality of tap water is shaky at best. According to researchers, more than a million Americans a year contract gastrointestinal illness from bad water, and about a thousand die. Because our climate is getting warmer, we are using more and more water, accompanied with a higher chance for contamination in a warmer world. This overly taxes municipal water suppliers, which often cannot keep up with the parasite crisis. In fact, the CDC recommends that those with compromised immunity and pregnant women always boil their water. Boiling water and/or adding an iodine preparation is key to avoiding waterborne parasites like giardia and cryptosporidium since chlorine does not kill either of these microscopic invaders. Note that bottled water is unregulated and therefore unreliable as a source of pure water. (See Chapter 15 for water filtration companies.)

Dogs and Cats. We love our pets as if they were our children, but like our children, they are also not always the cleanest. In fact over 200 diseases can be transmitted from animals to humans. All puppies are born infected with a dog roundworm called *Toxocara canis*. Half of all dogs may harbor parasites like hookworm, tapeworm, heartworm, and roundworm. Any park, road, lawn, or outdoor area frequented by dogs can be infested with these parasites through dog feces. Researchers have shown that up to 20 percent of soil in parks and playgrounds contains *Toxocara* from dogs.

What the Fat Flush Plan Does for Parasites

Cran-Water. The program helps to evict these unwelcome invaders. It primarily addresses them through the signature cran-water, which is consumed daily in all phases. Cran-water contains four unique acids that help with the digestion of wastes and, according to Dr. Parcells, are strongly antiparasitic. Cranberries, she contended, were consumed by Native Americans for that very purpose.

Vitamin Boosts. An antiparasite diet is rich in zinc and vitamin A—both of which are showcased in Fat Flush. Zinc fortifies your intestinal lining so that it can better thwart parasitic attacks. You can find it in beef, eggs, and seeds, like pumpkin seeds. Zinc-rich pumpkin seeds have been shown to help eliminate a variety of worms when eaten daily over the course of four to six weeks. Pumpkin seeds increase your body's ability to clear itself of parasites by up to 21 percent. Native Americans often chewed them as an effective deworming agent.

Crucially, vitamin A is a fat-soluble vitamin that increases a tissue's ability to resist penetration by parasite larvae. It exists in the greatest abundance in the oils of fatty fish. Because it is a fat-soluble substance, if you do not consume fat or your body cannot properly digest fat, you will have a hard time getting sufficient vitamin A—the anti-infection vitamin—in your diet. Other foods that provide beta-carotene, the precursor to vitamin A, include cooked carrots, sweet potatoes, yams, and greens.

Helpful Herbs. In addition, many spices and herbs are antiparasitic. This group of herbs includes garlic, thyme, and oregano. Garlic has been used since ancient times as a vermifuge (anthelmintic), an antiparasitic substance that rids the body of parasites by stunning or killing them. It contains a substance called allicin, a natural sulfur that reduces infection levels by 50 percent within five days of consuming it. All you need is two cloves of raw garlic per day in food preparation to ward off roundworms, pinworms, tapeworms, and hookworms.

Sorry, Sushi. You will note that in the Fat Flush Plan Away from Home sushi is a no-no. Sushi is not Fat Flush legal because of the very real danger of worms in undercooked fish. The use of microwaves is also highly discouraged—especially for beef, pork, and fish—because of an inadequate ability to thoroughly cook the food throughout.

HIDDEN FACTOR #10: MISSING MAGNESIUM

As far as the nutritional world is concerned, magnesium is to minerals as vitamin D is to vitamins: a superstar. Magnesium plays a starring role in Fat Flush as a critical mineral that helps turn food into fuel. Without enough of this vital catalyst, you lack a major nutritional component that triggers efficient fat burning.

In fact, magnesium is so important that vitamin D itself cannot function properly without it. Research findings show that low levels of magnesium (not just calcium) can lead to low levels of vitamin D. Because low magnesium levels create resistance to some of the effects of vitamin D, many individuals taking vitamin D may not be reaping the true benefits! Individuals over 50 are especially at risk, as most aren't reaching the USDA's daily average intake, let alone the Vitamin D Council's suggestion, of 5,000 IU/day for adults.

Magnesium is all about relaxation on a cellular level, so any condition related to overstimulation can be traced to magnesium deficiency. By overstimulation, I mean muscles contracting when they should not and neurons firing out of control—think anxiety, depression, muscle tension, heart palpitations, fatigue, asthma, and fibromyalgia, to name a few.

Metabolism. It's a shame that as many as three out of four of us don't get enough of marvelous magnesium. It is the "master mineral" and catalyzing star of over 300 key metabolic functions, including the utilization of energy (ATP), DNA, and vitamin D. That means magnesium promotes metabolism in 300 different ways, including the actual act of burning calories.

Magnesium really reigns supreme in the mineral kingdom. It acts as an electrolyte in the body and helps electrical processes like neural communication and the beat of your heart to occur. Your brain and your heart, the most electrical parts of your body, are the two places in your body with the highest levels of magnesium.

This mighty mineral also contributes to hormonal regulation. It prevents excess cortisol, increases insulin sensitivity, and aids in the production of thyroid hormone. Through only this one facet of its function, magnesium improves almost all of the hidden weight gain factors.

A lack of magnesium does not just spell trouble for weight loss. Magnesium has been linked to a litany of other conditions that also plague Fat Flushers. If high blood pressure, leg cramps, migraines, anxiety, irritability, depression, heart disease, unstable blood sugar, or insomnia is still challenging your well-being, then it's time to get on the magnesium bandwagon.

Heart Health. As the premier heart mineral, magnesium is absolutely key for cardiovascular health. In fact, one study states that magnesium should be available for immediate use in all emergency departments as a go-to method to stop a heart attack in its tracks. It is so important that many doctors and surgeons administer magnesium prior to some heart surgeries.

Magnesium's benefits for heart palpitations can reduce the occurrence of many life-threatening situations. However, up to 92 percent of hospitalized patients don't have their magnesium levels tested—this is a big concern considering that as many as 80 percent of patients in the ICU are considered magnesium deficient!

Studies dating back 100 years confirm magnesium's star power. Not only is this magnificent mineral essential for major metabolic functions; magnesium is also the *only* mineral linked to all of today's "fearsome foursome"—cancer, stroke, diabetes, and heart disease.

So Why Are So Many of Us *Still* Magnesium Deficient?

In this day and age, your body can require from 400–1,000 mg of magnesium a day, whereas in reality most of us only get one-half of that and lose it as rapidly as we take it in.

Today Americans depend upon magnesium to reduce depression, frequent nocturnal awakenings, and food cravings and, of course, to stabilize blood sugar. Fortunately, even more of us are eating healthier—think green smoothies, almonds, and sea veggies, which happen to be exceedingly rich sources of dietary magnesium.

By now you may also be supplementing with this miracle molecule, but chances are you're missing out because the type of magnesium supplement you're taking cannot get to the right places.

How Are We Losing It?

First, magnesium is a primo detox mineral. It is used up minute by minute to counteract stressors like food allergies and intolerances, prescription drugs, and exposure to heavy metals—especially aluminum. It also prevents kidney stone formation and even ADHD. You can see how easy it is to deplete yourself of magnesium simply by encountering the realities of everyday modern life.

Stress. Given our busier-than-ever lifestyles, the body's main use of magnesium is simply dealing with mental and physical stress. This adaptogenic mineral is being used up faster than we can possibly take it in. In times of high stress, our bodies ravenously consume magnesium to the point of deficiency to simply cope with the extra burden. As a matter of fact, low magnesium is considered a biomarker for chronic stress.

Subpar Supplements. Inefficient magnesium supplements with nonideal cofactors, combined with escalating environmental assaults, are leaving nearly 100 percent of us magnesium starved. Symptoms of magnesium deficiency range from facial twitches, to Alzheimer's, blood clots, chronic fatigue, and osteoporosis.

Dairy. Like estrogen and progesterone, and zinc and copper, magnesium exists in counterbalance to calcium. Contrary to popular belief, magnesium, not calcium, fortifies bones and prevents osteoporosis. You need magnesium to appropriately utilize calcium. Magnesium activates a hormone called thyrocalcitonin that stops bones from breaking down and aids in bone reformation. Calcium, on the other hand, can cause ectopic calcification when consumed in excess, inappropriately creating calcium deposits in soft tissue. This can lead to kidney stones; to hardening of the arterial walls, which can raise blood pressure and the risk of stroke and heart disease; and to stiffening of the bronchial tubes, which can lead to asthma.

Got milk? Mass media calls for people to consume massive amounts of dairy products on the basis that they provide a good source of bone-strengthening calcium. However, as you have now read, this mass consumption of calcium actually weakens bones without enough magnesium to counterbalance it. Furthermore, all this calcium in the body throws off the magnesium-calcium balance, tipping the scales dramatically toward calcium and exacerbating magnesium deficiency.

What the Fat Flush Plan Does for Missing Magnesium

To support our weight loss efforts, as well as stressed hearts and overworked brains, new research reveals most Americans may need to better optimize magnesium intake. Period. Luckily, I have just the plan that will do that. The Fat Flush diet, exercise, and ritual components all maximize magnesium intake and retention.

Green Smoothies. First, the diet plan includes daily greens as a key ingredient in the Fat Flush Smoothie. Greens such as romaine lettuce, escarole, kale, and spinach are some of the highest sources of magnesium. These magnesium-rich sources are not high in magnesium-competing calcium, which by the way is kept to a minimum, as calcium-rich dairy is an optional add-on to the program in phase 3.

Helpful Habits. Since the exercise plan is moderate and does not promote overdoing it, cortisol levels are kept in balance. This helps to retain key minerals like magnesium that are lost under any type of stress. Other sources of magnesium-depleting stress are also counteracted by daily meditation, journaling, therapeutic aromatherapy bathing, and special Epsom salt baths—especially high in magnesium sulfate for tired muscles.

4 Three-Day Ultra Fat Flush Tune-Up

*Let the highest and most important rule in eating for health
be to begin with food that contains the life force.*

—Dr. Hazel Parcells

This simple tune-up not only works quickly; it reignites your metabolism so you can keep right on losing weight as you proceed through all the phases! It is a quick start for those who want immediate results, and it can also be used to break a plateau between phases.

My metabolism-boosting Three-Day Ultra Fat Flush Tune-Up has all the right fats—including the slimming smart fats that you will be enjoying throughout the book. Many of my clients lose up to seven pounds in three days, and most shed at least three to four pounds with a flatter tummy and no more cravings or blood sugar highs and lows.

WHY IT WORKS

The Three-Day Ultra Fat Flush Tune-Up can be broken down into five factors.

Factor #1: Smart Flushing Fluids

You will be consuming three metabolism-boosting cocktails a day as well as three skinny smoothies.

Between meals, you can also drink lots of cran-water or plain, filtered water. Keeping well hydrated will elevate metabolism by at least 3 percent.

Factor #2: Hot Spices

The special booster cocktail contains just the right amount of fat-stoking cayenne pepper, mustard, turmeric, and ginger to raise heat production in the system, kicking fat burning into high gear.

Factor #3: No Grain Drain

For many individuals, grains can trigger fat-promoting and hunger-producing insulin. To replace grains, you will be filling up on delicious protein-based smoothies. Protein encourages the release of glucagon, which accesses stored body fat for energy. In addition, protein will stimulate metabolism by nearly 25 percent. But as you will see in phase 2 of the program, certain grains will be added back into the regimen for those who want the option of grain-based comfort foods.

Factor #4: Daily Detox

Ingesting Mother Nature's most purifying cleansing elements—especially chlorophyll-rich green leafy veggies and low-sugar fruits—can help your body eliminate toxins that inhibit fat burning. Since toxins from pollution and pesticides in food are stashed in the fat cells, the more we can cleanse, the more effectively our fat cells will shrink!

You can also snack on raw jicama, celery, and carrot sticks for even more veggie and fiber power. Jicama is a prebiotic that will feed your microbiome, ensuring you have plenty of "skinny bacteria" to keep you fit and trim.

Factor #5: Fire-Power Smart Fats

The tune-up is plenty low in calories; however, it provides all the slimming smart fats you need to satisfy satiety. And as they burn, they activate more metabolism-revving heat.

◆ ◆ ◆

I hope you will give this a try. Everything is so simple, and everything is right here so you can get started today!

Here is your daily tune-up menu to precede phase 1. These quick and easy liquid meals will help reset your digestive tract while spiking up fat burning on the double. Drink filtered, pure water (half your body weight in ounces) daily.

THE THREE-DAY PROTOCOL

DAILY MENU

Upon Arising	Fat Flush Metabolizer Cocktail (*see recipe on following page*)
Midmorning Snack	Fat Flush Smoothie (*see recipe on following page*)
	2 raw jicama, carrot, or celery sticks (*your choice*)
Lunch	Skinny Smoothie

Midafternoon Snack	Fat Flush Metabolizer Cocktail
	2 raw jicama, carrot, or celery sticks (*your choice*)
Dinner	Skinny Smoothie
Before Bedtime	Fat Flush Metabolizer Cocktail
	Drink at least 8 ounces of cran-water or pure water between all meals and snacks.

Fat Flush Metabolizer Cocktail

Makes 1 serving.

1 large ripe tomato, or 8 ounces low-sodium V8 or Knudsen's Very Veggie Juice (or bone broth)
¼ cup fresh-squeezed lime or lemon juice
½ cup filtered water (unless using juice)
Handful of fresh parsley
Handful of romaine lettuce or spinach
1 green onion, chopped
1 clove garlic, crushed
1/8 teaspoon cayenne pepper (or to taste)
1/8 teaspoon mustard
1/8 teaspoon turmeric
Pinch of ginger
2 teaspoons high-lignin flaxseed oil
1 tablespoon chia seeds
6 ice cubes

Combine all ingredients in a blender until desired consistency is reached.

Skinny Smoothie

Makes 1 serving.

8 ounces cran-water (1 ounce of unsweetened cranberry juice with 7 ounces of water)
Small handful of romaine lettuce, kale, or spinach or a scoop of green powder
½ cup frozen berries
1 scoop protein powder
1 tablespoon coconut oil
1 tablespoon ground flax seeds chia seeds, or hemp seeds
1 tablespoon non-GMO sunflower or soy lecithin granules
Ice cubes (optional)

Combine all ingredients in blender and blend until smooth.

5 The Fat Flush Plan: As Easy as 1–2–3

Your life does not get better by chance,
it gets better by change.

—JIM ROHN

The Fat Flush Plan has a rather basic and clear-cut mission: to increase metabolism, flush out bloat, speed up fat loss, and decrease inflammation throughout the body. At the core of the plan is the commitment to promote a balanced lifestyle and champion simple healthy habits that we all overlook or forget about as a result of everyday life. Every aspect of each phase of the plan is targeted like a guided missile to accomplish this goal: slimming smart fats [e.g., flaxseed oil, coconut oil, MCT oil, avocado, gamma-linolenic acid (GLA), and conjugated linoleic acid (CLA)], metabolism-raising protein (eight ounces or more plus whey or rice and pea vegan powders), high-fiber flax seeds, chia seeds, and hemp seeds, rainbow colored veggies, modest amounts of low-sugar fruits, calorie-burning condiments and spices (e.g., apple cider vinegar, coconut vinegar, mustard, cayenne pepper, ginger, cumin, turmeric, and cinnamon), liver- and lymph-cleansing beverages, exercise, journaling, and even sleep.

The Fat Flush Plan is all about whole food nutrition. It eliminates all weight loss–inhibiting foods and beverages such as white flour, white sugar, margarine, vegetable shortening, artificial sweeteners (e.g., aspartame), and caffeine in regular coffee, tea, chocolate, and many soft drinks.

In fact, the more meals you build around the Fat Flush foods on the plan, the more weight you will lose and the healthier you will be. That's right. Hunger will stop, food cravings will disappear, and even depression will noticeably lift, and triglyceride and cholesterol levels will balance out. Your circulation will increase, and you will look years younger as you feel reenergized, renewed, and refreshed.

The Fat Flush Plan is a springboard for a workable eating strategy. Each phase can be further individualized to target your personal needs by adding either more protein or more carbs sooner rather than later. For example, if you are a weight lifter or a large-framed, muscular individual, or if you have been suffering from severe stress due to an illness, you may need more than the 8 ounces of protein per day, perhaps even 12 ounces. Feel free to increase the meat, fish, poultry, or whey or pea and rice protein shake recommendations to fit your needs. Similarly, when you embark on the Two-Week Fat Flush but feel you absolutely must maintain your weekly high-intensity aerobic exercise and weight-strengthening program, then you may need to pop in a friendly carb or two right from the get-go.

The good news about the Fat Flush Plan is that you won't have to cut out your favorite foods forever, nor will you have to maintain a strict daily routine permanently. You just need to know the basic principles of fat flushing, which are discussed below, so that you can rely on the foods that will keep you lean with the help of the easy-to-follow menus and simple recipes.

For those who want instant results, I have created a Three-Day Ultra Fat Flush Tune-Up to kick-start your weight loss journey. This program combines some basic tenets of Fat Flush with a fast metabolizer cocktail to motivate you with daily weight and inch loss. This tune-up precedes phase 1, "The Two-Week Fat Flush." In phase 1, you will have not only 14 days of menus but more than 50 deliciously simple recipes to enjoy on the Two-Week Fat Flush. And you can always personalize any menu (breakfast, lunch, or dinner)—or recipe for that matter—to satisfy your own tastes based on the expanded lists of fat-flushing foods provided.

These cleansing diets will set the metabolic stage for phase 2, "The Metabolic Reset," as well as phase 3, "The Lifestyle Eating Plan." These two phases are discussed below.

Moreover, as so many of my clients have experienced, you can look forward to shedding unwanted pounds and feeling refreshed, cleansed, and nourished on all levels at every step of the plan. On the diet front, you will be putting a tight lid on, and counteracting, the effects of emotional eating, toxic foods, birth control pills, medications, and a stressful lifestyle. And this is important because your system likely has been overloaded and overburdened, creating havoc in your liver and lymph and decreasing your body's fat-burning ability. The Fat Flush Plan allows you to clean up and take control of your body and your life.

Here's what is in store for you to enjoy during every phase of the Fat Flush Plan:

✓ POWERFUL PROTEINS. Eight ounces or more a day of protein, such as lean beef, chicken, fish, and vegan-based brown rice and pea protein, tofu, and tempeh. They boost metabolism by up to 25 percent for about 12 hours to keep metabolic fires burning. Proteins are the tissue and muscle rebuilders par excellence. For every pound of muscle gained, you burn an extra 70 calories per hour. Subsequently, you will help stop hunger and keep blood sugar and insulin levels steady as well as support your system's detoxification process. And you'll actually be eating eggs with yolks on the diet because the sulfur-bearing amino acids in the yolks help the liver metabolize fats.

✓ **AMAZING OMEGAS AND SLIMMING SMART FATS.** Such as high-lignan flaxseed oil, flax seeds, chia, GLA-rich botanicals from evening primrose oil, borage, black currant seed oil, coconut oil, and avocado—all trigger fat-burning rather than fat storage. Flaxseed oil tops the satiety scale and can attract oil-soluble poisons that have been lodged in your fat stores and transport those poisons out of the system. The GLA oils can mobilize brown adipose tissue, which burns off excess calories and boosts energy.

✓ **COLORFUL, FRIENDLY CARBOHYDRATES.** Such as antioxidant-rich fruits and veggies. These are high in natural enzymes, vitamins, and minerals such as potassium and keep sodium out of your cells to banish water retention.

✓ **FLAVORFUL THERMOGENIC SPICES.** Such as anti-inflammatory ginger, cayenne, mustard, cumin, turmeric, and cinnamon, which raise your body temperature and kick your metabolism into high gear. In fact, studies show that some of these seasonings triple the body's ability to burn calories for fuel rather than store them as fat.

✓ **ELIMINATION OF METABOLISM BLOCKERS.** Such as wheat, milk, and yeast-based seasonings. By eliminating them you protect your fat-burning process and ward off those unsightly allergy-related symptoms, such as puffy eyes and dark circles under the eyes. Omitting them is vital to your weight loss success because they have a way of retaining fluid, slowing down metabolism, and making fat stick.

✓ **FIBER-RICH SEEDS.** To increase elimination, you'll enjoy flax seeds, chia seeds, and/or hemp seeds in daily smoothies filled with emulsifying enzymes from unsweetened cranberry juice diluted with water to help digest those fatty globules in the lymphatic system—your body's fat disposal dump, discussed in detail in Chapter 2. These high-fiber seeds increase fat excretion and bind toxins so that they are not reabsorbed into the body via bile.

BEFORE YOU BEGIN

The week before you begin the kickoff Three-Day Ultra Fat Flush Tune-Up is the best time to prepare your system for the entire Fat Flush Plan. Probably one of the most important preparations is to begin increasing your water intake between meals. Begin drinking at least two glasses between breakfast and lunch and two more between lunch and dinner. This will start increasing your hydration and create the new habit of power drinking to get more water into your system. After you feel confident that your hydration levels are increasing, begin to banish all trans fats from margarine, fried foods, and processed vegetable oils (see Chapter 6). Next, eliminate all the whites from your diet: white sugar, white rice, and white flour. Stock up instead on lots of fiber-rich veggies in all colors of the rainbow. Green, yellow, red, and orange veggies aid the cleansing process by providing natural fiber, which helps sweep out toxins, and pigment-based antioxidants aid the liver by keeping its detox pathways on the move. Adding a couple of pieces of fresh fruit also will help cleansing because fruits are a rich source of enzyme-activating potassium that starts to move accumulated fluids from your tissues.

By far the most important thing you can do to prepare your system for the plan is to gradually taper off all alcohol, coffee, tea, sodas (regular and diet), and energy drinks. This includes any regular or decaf coffee, aspartame, Splenda, and sugar alcohol–sweetened beverages. Even decaffeinated beverages have some caffeine, which can raise fat-storing cortisol. In addition, the acidity in decaffeinated coffee, for example, is higher than that in regular coffee because of the beans used to make decaf. Add to this the rancid oils and chemicals such as trichloroethylene or methylene chloride (drycleaning chemicals) used in the decaffeinating process, and you can see why decaf coffee is not the fat-flushing beverage of choice.

Thus, if you are a heavy coffee drinker (having more than two cups per day), here is what I suggest: Replace your coffee with dandelion root tea or dandelion root coffee, which gives you the taste and feel of the real deal. The beverages I enjoy and serve to my heavy-duty coffee-drinking friends not only are flavorful and satisfying but also are brewed like real coffee. Although there may be more types on the market, the one that lends itself best to the Fat Flush Plan is from the liver-loving dandelion.

I would cut down coffee consumption gradually by eliminating one cup every other day until you are down to just one cup a day, using the herbal coffees as a substitute for the other cups.

Taking these easy steps will help to prevent the withdrawal symptoms that about one in four Fat Flushers experience while on phase 1 during the first four days. Withdrawal from caffeine and sugar in particular can include such symptoms as headache, fatigue, irritability, and even increased hunger. These symptoms typically disappear by day five.

PHASE 1: THE TWO-WEEK FAT FLUSH

This initial phase based on an average of about 1,200 calories daily is designed to further accelerate weight loss and cleanse the system as a follow-up to the Three-Day Ultra Fat Flush Tune-Up. This two-week phase will transform your body by helping to target and shed fat loss from your body's favorite fat storage areas—your hips, belly, thighs, and buttocks. Some individuals report a loss of up to 12 inches during this first phase of the diet, whereas they may lose only 5 pounds. This means that they are losing fat and bloat, not muscle (as with so many other diet programs). Remember, muscle weighs more than fat, so dropping a couple of sizes can be more significant than losing 10 pounds on the scale.

Regardless of how much weight or how many inches you need to lose, phase 1 will continue to reset metabolism. Why? Because we all need the right nutrient support in order to continue and activate the fat-burning process—especially when it comes to encouraging bile production for breaking down dietary fats and carrying toxins out of the body. First and foremost, the Two-Week Fat Flush is a whole food–based cleansing program. The clean nourishment this approach provides helps to facilitate weight loss by giving your liver—the body's premier fat-burning organ—some well-deserved support to detoxify your body and digest fats with higher-quality, decongested, free-flowing bile. Many of my clients refer to this two-week phase fondly as "Fat Flush Boot Camp." And I agree. It is a program that is especially motivating if you have had difficulty losing weight before or if you have a lot of weight to lose.

While fat can be burned off by eating cleaner foods, taking thermogenic herbs, and working out, other weight loss regimens rarely rid your body of stored toxins. Unburned poisons often migrate from the shrinking fat reserves to the bloodstream, organs, and tissues, causing discomfort such as headache, irritability, and nausea. This is why most people find it difficult to stay on other weight loss programs and wind up not feeling well.

Phase 1, the Two-Week Fat Flush, counters this quite effectively by increasing the right kind of fats (in the form of flaxseed, coconut, MTC oil, and avocado), fiber, water, and exercise. While fiber, water, and exercise can flush out water-soluble toxins through the bowels, urine, and sweat, the oil, according to some researchers, can attract oil-soluble toxins that have been lodged in the fatty tissues of the body and carry them out of the system for elimination.

Now if you have a lot of weight to lose (over 25 pounds), you can stay on the initial phase of the program longer than two weeks. In fact, up to one month would be safe—and you can vary the program by extending phase 1 an additional two weeks. At this time, you can implement two smoothies per day as meal replacements for breakfast and lunch with a full meal in the evening. That's why there are so many smoothie options to choose from—fortified, as in the initial two weeks, with smoothie "add-ins" to supercharge the cleansing and healing benefits for collagen building, enhanced detox, electrolyte balance, blood sugar regulation, antiaging, and more carb control.

As an alternative, you may have more success moving to phase 2, where weight loss may even increase with the added fiber-rich foods and extended exercise prescription. Do note that in any case, phase 1 of this program is a bit too severe and rigorous for individuals who have kidney or liver disease, are pregnant or breastfeeding, have a history of eating disorders, or are under age 12.

PHASE 2: THE METABOLIC RESET

Phase 2, "The Metabolic Reset," is the next step for those individuals who have additional weight to lose and want to maintain a cleansing program but also enjoy more variety in food choices while still losing weight. This phase 2 program is designed for ongoing weight loss, with 1,200 to 1,500 calories each day, and is meant to be followed until you reach your desired weight or size.

Phase 2 is the perfect transition for those who are moving toward but are not quite ready for maintenance. This ongoing phase includes the foundational fat-flushing foods from phase 1 with up to two friendly and fiber-filled carbohydrate choices added into the menu plan one at a time each week. Easing them in this way will help you to determine whether the new food is helping or hindering your weight loss goals.

The slow but sure fiber increase introduced in this phase with the new choices of seedlike grains (quinoa and oatmeal) will help to further stabilize blood sugar and insulin. More fiber will also help to reduce fat storage cortisol and aid in decreasing excess estrogen by escorting it out via the bile.

Since more fiber can also mean more gas and bloating (sometimes even constipation), this phase takes fiber increase nice and easy to prevent these discomforting symptoms.

Interestingly, some individuals notice accelerated weight loss in this phase, while others have observed a slowdown in weight loss because of the additional carbs. Regardless, I recommend that you stay on phase 2 until you have achieved or nearly achieved your weight goal. For some, this may mean two weeks; for others, it may mean another four to six weeks; and for still others with a lot of weight to lose, it may mean months.

Journaling at this transition time is absolutely key. If you start adding on a pound or two, you will be able to track this immediately and cut out or reduce the amount of the offending food before it becomes a real challenge. Journaling also will help you in the phase 3 lifestyle plan to track which foods you can't tolerate. Symptoms such as a speedy pulse, bloating, gas, drowsiness, and the return of cravings are your body's private distress signals that should spur you on to take action—immediately!

Keep in mind that you can always go back to phase 1 if you need the structure of a more disciplined regimen.

PHASE 3: THE LIFESTYLE EATING PLAN

Phase 3, or lifestyle eating, is really the Fat Flush maintenance program for lifetime weight control. This phase offers over 1,800 calories daily, providing a basic lifelong eating program designed to increase your vitality and well-being for life. At this time, you will be using phase 2 as your foundational program, with its one or two friendly carb choices. You can now add up to two dairy products (or use coconut-based substitutes if you are dairy intolerant) as well as two more friendly carbs, making a grand total of four friendly carbs—weight and blood sugar permitting. Phase 3's friendly carbs include more choices from a variety of starchier, rainbow-colored veggies and nongluten seedlike grains (like wild rice, brown rice, buckwheat, and millet). As in phase 2, you will add these latest foods one at a time to make sure that you are tolerating the new additions without any food sensitivity symptoms.

Phase 3 is definitely more appropriate for both pregnant and breastfeeding women because of the higher calorie and calcium content from the additional starchy and nongluten grains and dairy products. My experience on the Fat Flush Plan has taught me that although leafy greens are also rich in calcium—for example, ½ cup of collard greens or turnip greens contains about 250 mg of calcium, compared with a cup of milk at 300 mg of calcium—and are widely available in all phases of the program, most dieters—without lactose or casein intolerances—prefer moderate amounts of pasture-raised, organic dairy calcium. And it makes menu planning a heck of a lot easier.

However, if you have noticed that cellulite has disappeared because you have avoided all dairy products (dairy, whether pasture raised or organic, still has hormones from the cow), then you can omit dairy entirely or use the coconut cream, yogurt, and milk alternatives.

To make sure that you don't gain back fat even if you gain back some weight during the phase 3 lifestyle program, the supplement CLA will be introduced. Remember that clinical trial I told you about in Chapter 2? To recap, in a research study of 80 overweight people who dieted had regained weight, it was discovered that those who took CLA put the pounds back on in a ratio of half fat to half muscle.

ALL THREE PHASES

To optimize the results of your food and exercise program on all phases of the plan, powerful nutrients that cleanse, support, and regenerate the liver as well as cleanse the bile are also recommended. These include dandelion root, milk thistle, Oregon grape root, methionine, inositol, choline, lipase, chromium, the nutrient L-carnitine (an amino acid shown to raise the body's fat-burning ability), bile salts, beet root, and taurine.

The Power of Ritual

Once you experience the cleansing aspect in the initial phases of the plan, you'll probably discover that you think more clearly and are more mentally alert. As one first-time Fat Flusher remarked, "We can't expect to have sharp minds and luminous spirits when our bodies are polluted." Many devotees find that when their bodies are cleansed, they are more willing—and better prepared—to deal with other facets of their being.

Because the Fat Flush Plan was designed originally as a seasonal detox, done four times a year at designated times, it taps into the power of ritual. Its practical, systemized approach creates a sense of not only order but also reassurance when it is so easy to become confused and overwhelmed by the sheer choices of eating plans.

Tuning in to Your Deeper Side

You'll discover journaling to be a vital companion to your Fat Flush experience. It helps you keep tabs on your food and eating habits. As a matter of fact, this in itself has been shown to be enough to prevent weight gain according to some experts. Your Fat Flush journal helps you track your food consumption, food responses (e.g., bloating, drowsiness, irritability, and headaches), and progress.

Once you graduate to phases 2 and 3, where you'll be adding more fiber, friendly carbohydrates, and some dairy or coconut-based foods, the journal will give you an opportunity to discover your body's distress signals, alerting you to negative food reactions.

However, I also believe that journaling nurtures your body and soul beyond the diet component. This is why you'll also be tracking emotions along the way, giving you a clear idea of the feelings behind your eating impulses so that you can handle them successfully. Journaling creates a safe, comfortable place where you can vent your feelings, chart your success, recognize patterns, and enter a private world of self-discovery. Because of this, journaling helps you eliminate one of the five hidden weight gain factors you've already read about in Chapter 2 that we all seem to share—stress! Besides, taking the time to write in your journal has been shown to actually reduce food consumption, which helps reduce your fat-gaining potential.

Tapping into the Power of Exercise

The exercise component of the Fat Flush Plan represents another progression beyond other exercise programs. The Fat Flush Exercise Plan (see Chapter 9), like the diet plan, centers on the lymphatic system, the body's built-in waste-processing plant. The lymphatic channels extract all types of viruses, bacteria, fats, and wastes from the cells and transport them out of the system, relying on muscle contractions for their flow via the thighs and arms. Lymph slowdown is much more common as we start to age, especially due to sedentary lifestyles, with too much sitting being the "new smoking." Since the lymph doesn't have a pump like the heart, it has to be "exercised" with either a bouncing action, deep breathing, or movement of the arms while walking briskly.

To help purify your lymph during all Fat Flush phases, you'll bounce on a mini-trampoline or rebounder for 10 minutes a day to gently ease waste materials and fat out of the lymph. By cleansing the lymph through gentle pressure on the thighs, lymphatic drainage is activated and fatty cellulite deposits begin to disappear. The greatest thing about this lymph-moving exercise is that virtually anyone can do it regardless of age or physical challenges. For instance, individuals who can't walk can still benefit from this exercise by sitting on the rebounder while someone else bounces on it.

On all three levels of the Fat Flush Plan, you'll enjoy moderate low-intensity exercise—starting with brisk walking done daily and later adding strength training twice a week to help tighten and tone the muscles. Strength training, in particular, will aid your weight loss efforts because it builds muscle (lean body mass), which is metabolically more active than fatty tissue. In phase 1 you'll do 30 minutes of brisk walking, dramatically swinging your arms back and forth to stimulate lymph flow and keep toxins moving. Then you'll graduate to 40 minutes in phase 2 and 60 minutes in phase 3.

Since so many of my clients have adrenal fatigue, I am not a proponent of more exercise during detox. Light to moderate is the key because overexercise can actually weaken taxed adrenals due to higher exercise-induced cortisol levels and increased inflammation. If cortisol levels are already elevated, then low-intensity movement is the exercise of choice to prevent accelerated tissue breakdown and metabolic slowdown. That's why walking is recommended along with your daily yoga and Pilates if you want.

Exercise keeps insulin levels low and can even improve your emotional health because it releases endorphins, those natural mood elevators in your brain that make you feel good. Without a doubt, you'll feel centered, focused, and more in control.

Learning the Beauty of Sleep

You'll also discover the value of getting the proper amount of quality sleep. Sleep reduces cortisol production—a key ingredient to stress fat—and helps restore the body physically. Throughout the program, you'll have a set bedtime (that magical time of 10 p.m.) and wake-up time, leaving you refreshed eight hours later!

All these fundamental elements weave together a splendid tapestry reflecting all the radiance and vitality of a balanced lifestyle. And let's face it, that's something we twenty-first-century men and women definitely need.

All the slimming details of the Fat Flush Plan are discussed in the following chapters. So let's get started!

6 Phase 1: The Two-Week Fat Flush

Courage is the first of the human qualities because it is the quality which guarantees all the others.

—WINSTON CHURCHILL

The Two-Week Fat Flush is a quick-start weight loss plan that tamps down inflammation while it cleanses the accumulated fats in your tissues, liver, and lymph and purges fluid buildup from your system. It also prevents new fats, in the form of triglycerides, from forming. This two-week program reestablishes a beneficial fat ratio for your body composition, which sets the stage for continuous fat burning and appetite control. The result is less hunger with steady weight loss, lowered insulin resistance, and improved glucose tolerance.

Without a doubt, weight loss is what pleases my Fat Flushers the most! In fact, one of my female participants, Jennifer K.—who had over 30 pounds to lose after her pregnancy—reported an impressive loss of 15 pounds in just 14 days. And then there was postmenopausal Linda L., who felt "10 years younger" after losing nearly 90 pounds following the basic Fat Flush protocol. Now you might be saying to yourself that in Jennifer's case it was merely "water weight" destined to come back the way it does after every other diet. But this is not so with Fat Flush. You see, both Jennifer and Linda remedied the underlying causes of their weight gain, primarily during phase 1 (as explained in Chapters 2 and 3). Then they continued to lose weight in phase 2 because they were still avoiding the gluten and dairy products and sugary foods that packed on the pounds in the first place. Linda's thyroid function greatly improved after she supplemented with nutrients to improve the quality and consistency of her bile, stoking her fat-burning fires. Many Fat Flushers have reported similar results whether after pregnancy or after menopause! They lose as many as 12 inches while dropping just 5 pounds. This seemingly small weight loss is actually a good sign, proving that fat cells are shrinking!

The key to your personal Fat Flush success is this: right from the beginning, set a goal for yourself, and track your progress in your Fat Flush journal daily. I truly believe that whatever your mind can conceive, you can achieve. So set different goals for each phase of the Fat Flush Plan. For instance, you can start with a goal related to whatever it is that is motivating you to change your eating habits. It may be to lose three inches around your hips, get rid of that cellulite in your thighs and buttocks, increase mental clarity, slim down your waistline or tummy, feel healthier and more energetic, get rid of bloating and water gain, cleanse your system, or any of the many other benefits that Fat Flush produces. Journaling will help you keep tabs along the way, mapping out an insightful, revealing chart that will help make you accountable while encouraging you.

Also please keep this in mind: If you are following the program mainly for weight loss, do yourself a favor and forget about hopping on the scale every day. Weigh yourself only once a week, or even consider bypassing the scale altogether. People don't lose weight at the same rate, and a variety of weight loss stumbling blocks (thyroid, bile, microbiome, a lack of magnesium) can be at play. You can get discouraged if you hit a plateau or are losing slowly while others have speedier results. And for those in perimenopause and beyond—weight loss does get more challenging as your overall system becomes more sluggish than when you were younger. Also, keep in mind that on the Fat Flush Plan you will decrease your body fat as you proportionally increase your lean muscle tissue. Since muscle weighs more than fat, you will be able to completely redistribute your weight and sculpt a slimmer silhouette without a dramatic loss on the scale. For these reasons, at least in the short term, weight is not the best measure of fat loss or increased fitness—and, in fact, can be misleading. There are simply too many important factors that the number on the scale doesn't account for, including the normal fluctuations that can occur in your body throughout the day, week, or month. Things like how recently you have used the bathroom or, if you are a female, whether you are menstruating can literally tip the scales.

GIVE YOUR LIVER A VACATION

The Two-Week Fat Flush is very supportive to your liver—that terribly overworked, often overlooked fat-burning organ you read about in Chapter 2. This phase of the Fat Flush Plan provides complete nutritional support for all the liver's varied functions—including quality bile production. Besides metabolizing fat (to slim you down) and lowering cholesterol, your liver is busy making and storing red blood cells, balancing hormones such as estrogen, bolstering your immunity, storing glycogen, and neutralizing all poisons. If poisons or excess fats clog your liver, it can't perform its fat-burning function via the bile, and symptoms such as constipation, fatigue, dry skin, and nausea can set in.

TWO-WEEK FAT FLUSH PROGRAM

Only certain foods are allowed on this accelerated part of the plan. Use them for your breakfast, lunch, and dinner as well as snacks! As you will see, the list is made up of whole foods (as GMO-free as possible). You will be banishing all fake fats that inhibit metabolism, dampen thyroid function, and promote inflammation. These include trans fats (in the form of margarine, processed vegetable oils, and shortening), canola oil, corn oil, sunflower seed oil, and soy oil as well as caffeine, diet and regular sodas, alcohol, aspartame, Splenda, sugar, coconut sugar, and most sugar alcohols like mannitol, sorbitol, and xylitol. The exception is erythritol, a sugar alcohol that is usually tolerated well by most people (but not by all—see the discussion below under "Fat Flush Sweeteners"). This alternative sweetener can be combined with monk fruit (a 0-calorie, low-glycemic-load sugar known for centuries in the Orient) in the Lakanto Monk Fruit Sweetener. The remaining foods to be eliminated are yeast-related vinegars including balsamic vinegar, soy sauce, and barbecue sauces. However, apple cider vinegar is part of the plan because it does not feed yeast. All of the above undesirable foods disrupt your liver by overloading the detoxification pathways, resulting in decreased fat burning. They also can stimulate fat-promoting insulin, which inhibits weight loss.

INSIDER TIP | The success of the Fat Flush Plan depends as much on what you don't eat as on what you do.

The herbs and spices provided in the menus are not there merely to enhance flavor. They are powerful anti-inflammatory diet aids that accelerate metabolism (e.g., cayenne pepper, dried mustard, ginger, and cumin), assist digestion (e.g., dill, garlic, anise, and fennel), improve insulin and glucose levels (e.g., cinnamon, cloves, bay leaves, and coriander), remove water weight (e.g., parsley, cilantro, fennel, anise, apple cider vinegar, and coconut vinegar), and protect against disease (cumin and turmeric).

I encourage you to avoid extremely hot spices such as heavy curries and chili peppers (cayenne is not a chili), because these types of seasonings can trigger water retention. In addition, many people get sleepy after consuming them. Similarly, black pepper is omitted because of its effect on the cellular pH, causing fatigue and drowsiness, and has become a primary food intolerance.

For this first two-week period, you also should avoid oils and fats of any kind other than the daily flaxseed or coconut or MCT oil; avocado; chia seeds, flax seeds, and hemp seeds; and essential fatty acid supplements from gamma-linolenic acid (GLA).

Use homemade or ready-made chicken and beef bone broths as well as vegetable broths (see Chapter 11 for specific brands) for sautéing, basting, cooking those eggs in the morning, and making soups. Bone broth is chock full of gelatin and collagen so important for strong, supple skin and a Fat Flush body that is cellulite-free.

Cut out *all* grains, bread, cereal, and starchy vegetables such as potatoes, corn, peas, carrots, parsnips, pumpkin, winter squash, and beans. The gluten-based grains from wheat, rye, barley, and spelt are common food sensitivity triggers creating water retention or "false fat." Other carbohydrates— the ones I call "friendly carbohydrates," such as peas, winter squash, beets, oatmeal, seedlike grains (quinoa, buckwheat, millet), and beans—will be added back gradually in phases 2 and 3. You also will notice that, for now at least, dairy products (with the exception of whey), such as milk, yogurt, kefir, and cheeses, are off limits. Dairy is one of the top five food allergens. The calcium in the Fat Flush Plan will be coming from the best nondairy sources— greens! The highest-calcium greens are kale, collards, escarole, watercress, broccoli, and mustard and turnip greens. I would recommend getting acquainted with at least two of these leafy vegetables and rotating them into your menus. They are great sources of both purifying chlorophyll and the most important mineral I know of that is a hidden factor in weight loss resistance—magnesium.

In the first two weeks, I not only dropped 15 pounds but I was able to wear one of my favorite outfits again. What really amazed me was how Fat Flush removed those cravings I used to wrestle with . . . I was a grazer and a craver! Everywhere I go, people tell me I look 10 years younger. Even my nails are stronger.

My profession is demanding, and I count on having the energy and stamina to stay on top. I own, produce, and do a radio show, which means a tremendous amount of work every day. Fat Flush revved up my energy levels and helped me keep in the game. If I can successfully work this remarkable program into my busy schedule—anyone can.

On my show, I've interviewed all the top diet gurus and tried their approaches—from Suzanne Somers to Dr. Atkins. I can honestly say that I've never had such dramatic results on any other program. It really jump-starts weight loss.

—FRANKIE BOYER, HOST OF THE BUSINESS OF BEING HEALTHY WITH FRANKIE BOYER

FATS AND OILS

Flaxseed, coconut, or MCT (medium-chain triglyceride) oil at 1 tablespoon twice daily, and ½ avocado daily plus avocado spray for cooking.

PURPOSE: Flaxseed oil is essential for its high–omega-3 fat-fighting and insulin-regulating potential. (If intolerant, then opt for omega-3–rich fish oil that is subtly flavored with lemon or orange.) Coconut oil, a rich source of medium-chain fatty acids, boosts metabolism by 50 percent and speeds up the thyroid. Avocado triggers adiponectin, the appetite hormone, for satiety and is also rich in glutathione to help with liver cleansing. MCT oil is a concentrated form of both coconut and palm oil that provides an even more potent source of energy for easy digestion, fat burning, and the brain.

FLUSH FLASH

A daily avocado provides an amazing amount of fiber—nearly 17 grams in 1 avocado. A great way to effortlessly and deliciously boost fiber intake.

FIBER-RICH SEEDS

DAILY INTAKE: 1 tablespoon twice daily of chia seeds, ground flax seeds, or hemp seeds.

PURPOSE: All three seed types provide soluble and insoluble fiber to help maintain regularity and provide satiety to meals and snacks. Their high–omega-3 content controls cortisol production, and in the case of flax seeds, the high lignan content (800 times more than in any other food) controls haywire hormones. Hemp seeds offer up skin-beautifying and -strengthening omega-6.

LEAN PROTEIN

DAILY INTAKE: 1 serving of whey or brown rice and pea protein powder, up to 2 eggs (optional), and a minimum of 8 ounces of cooked lean protein.

CHOOSE FROM: All varieties of fresh or frozen fish (with the exception of high-mercury swordfish and farm-raised tilapia) as well as canned fish (like Wild Planet Albacore and Skipjack Tuna, Vital Choice canned seafood, and Oregon Choice canned seafood), fresh or frozen seafood, lean beef, lamb, or skinless turkey or chicken; also tofu and tempeh, which may be consumed no more than twice per week. Use organic and grass-fed meat whenever possible. Choose hormone-free, unheated, undenatured, lactose-free, high-protein whey powders (like Fat Flush Vanilla and Chocolate Whey) with about 20 grams of protein per serving and negligible carbohydrates from nonmutated A2 milk. Choose non-GMO vegan protein powders (like Fat Flush Body Protein) with low carbohydrates and verification of low heavy metal content (especially arsenic and lead).

PURPOSE: Protein raises metabolism by 25 percent and activates the liver's detoxifying enzymes.

EGGS (OPTIONAL)

DAILY INTAKE: Up to 2 per day.

PURPOSE: For those without allergies or gallbladder issues, the omega-3–enriched eggs not only are delicious but also are brimming with antioxidants (e.g., lutein and zeaxanthin) for the eyes and brain, cholesterol-protective phosphatidylcholine, and sulfur to support your liver's cleansing process.

VEGETABLES

DAILY INTAKE: Unlimited (unless otherwise noted), raw or steamed. Put special emphasis on the bitter veggies (like arugula, watercress, escarole, and radishes) to help support liver and gallbladder health for greater cleansing power.

CHOOSE FROM: Arugula, endive, asparagus, green beans, broccoli, broccolini, broccoli rabe, brussels sprouts, cabbage, cauliflower, celery, Chinese cabbage, carrots (1), cucumbers, daikon, globe artichoke, Jerusalem artichoke, artichoke heart, fennel, eggplant, spinach, escarole, collard greens, rhubarb (1 cup), burdock, hearts of palm, kale, mustard greens, romaine lettuce, radicchio, endive, parsley, onions, watercress, chives, leeks, Swiss chard, bell peppers (yellow, orange, green, and red), jicama, mushrooms, olives (3), radishes, horseradish, okra, tomatoes, red or green loose-leaf lettuce, snow peas, zucchini, yellow squash, water chestnuts, bamboo shoots, garlic, spaghetti squash, and sprouts (alfalfa, broccoli, radish, and mung bean).

SEA VEGGIES: Agar-agar, hijiki, kombu, nori, wakame, or a sea veggie–based seasoning (like Eden Seaweed Gomasio, kelp granules, or dulse flakes from Maine).

PURPOSE: These fibrous and colorful phytonutrient-rich vegetables will help speed your liver's cleansing and provide valuable carotenoids. Broccoli sprouts are especially high in sulforaphane—a very powerful antioxidant that targets cellular health. Two ounces per day would be ideal. The sea veggies and seasonings provide iodine and trace minerals to help nourish the thyroid and counteract environmental pollutants.

FRUITS

DAILY INTAKE: Up to 2 whole portions daily.

CHOOSE FROM: 1 small apple, ½ grapefruit, 1 small orange, 2 medium plums, 6 large strawberries, 10 large cherries, 1 nectarine, 1 pomegranate, 1 peach, 1 pear, and 1 cup berries (blueberries, blackberries, or raspberries).

PURPOSE: Nature's cleansers are high in enzymes and minerals (e.g., potassium) and lowest in fructose—a sneaky fat promoter.

FAT FLUSH CRAN-WATER

DAILY INTAKE: 8 eight-ounce glasses per day

PURPOSE: The cranberry juice–water mixture eliminates water retention, cleanses accumulated wastes from the lymphatic system, and also helps to reduce the appearance of cellulite.

HOW TO: To prepare cranberry water, purchase Knudsen's, Trader Joe's, or Mountain Sun's Unsweetened Cranberry Juice. Then get two empty 32-ounce bottles. Fill each 32-ounce water bottle with 4 ounces of unsweetened cranberry juice and 28 ounces of water. Or purchase Knudsen's or Tree of Life Cranberry Concentrate and add 1½ tablespoons to each 32 ounces of water.

FLUSH FLASH

To make cranberry juice yourself, here's a simple recipe. Put a 12-ounce bag of cranberries into a large saucepan. Add about 4 cups of purified water, and boil until all the berries pop. Strain the juice, and if you like, you can add a touch of Stevia Plus to take the edge off the tartness (brave souls can take it straight). This recipe makes about 32 ounces of straight cranberry juice, enough for about 4 days.

FAT-FLUSHING HERBS AND SPICES

DAILY INTAKE: To taste.

CHOOSE FROM: Cayenne pepper, cumin, dried mustard, cinnamon, ginger, dill, garlic, anise, fennel, cloves, bay leaves, coriander, parsley, cilantro, apple cider vinegar, coconut vinegar, and cumin.

PURPOSE: Metabolism boosters.

LEGAL CHEAT

1 cup of organic coffee in the morning.

FAT FLUSH SWEETENERS

DAILY INTAKE: Organic SweetLeaf Stevia, Lakanto Monk Fruit Sweetener, or Uni Key Flora-Key.

WHAT MAKES THEM LEGAL: Both SweetLeaf Stevia and Lakanto are sugar-free and low-glycemic sweeteners. The plant-based stevia is 30 times sweeter than sugar, so a little goes a long way, and it is great for baking. According to the manufacturers, Lakanto can be used in a 1-to-1 ratio to replace sugar because it tastes, bakes, and looks like the white stuff. But I find that easily one-half that amount is a sweet-enough substitution. You might also want to consider reducing the amount of Lakanto due to the presence of erythritol, which causes some folks to experience loose stools and digestive upsets. That's why I also recommend the prebiotic and probiotic sweetener Flora-Key as another alternative. This immune-boosting probiotic formula contains various strains of acidophilus, bifidus, and a special prebiotic, rather sweet-tasting substance known as inulin to stimulate the growth of the beneficial bacteria. This product helps to ward off toxins and aids in the synthesis of key vitamins and minerals while helping to support the good bacteria in the gut. It can be used in your morning smoothie, and is an optional ingredient in several of the recipes for the Fat Flush Plan. Flora-Key should only be used in nonheat recipes, as heating will destroy the beneficial bacteria, whereas both stevia and Lakanto can be used in recipes that require heat.

BESIDES THE DAILY DIET

BEFORE BREAKFAST: Drink an 8-ounce cup of hot water with the juice of ½ lemon to assist your kidneys and liver and thin the bile.

BREAKFAST AND DINNER: Take supplements rich in fat-burning, skin-beautifying, and anti-inflammatory GLA in a total daily amount of 360 mg per day.

CHOOSE FROM: Straight GLA supplements from black currant seed oil contained in the Fat Flush Kit, or purchase GLA supplements made from black currant seed oil at your favorite health food store. Each capsule in the kit contains 90 mg of GLA, and you take 2 capsules 2 times daily.

DAILY: You can also take the additional supplements from the Fat Flush Kit or from your current regimen to optimize your results, like the Fat Flush Dieters' Multi (with or without iron) and the Fat Flush Weight Loss Formula. The Fat Flush Dieters' Multi provides a balanced multivitamin and mineral supplementation during detox. The Fat Flush Weight Loss Formula contains liver- and bile-supporting herbs such as milk thistle and blood sugar–stabilizing berberine containing Oregon grape root, as well as carbohydrate controllers like chromium and fat burners such as L-carnitine, methionine, choline, inositol, lipase, and lecithin. If you do not have a gallbladder or have had a history of symptoms related to poor fat digestion, hypothyroidism, or estrogen metabolism, then you might wish to consider the Fat Flush Bile Builder. To review, you can supplement with the following if you choose your own supplements:

✓ A balanced multivitamin and mineral supplement for general nutrition insurance

✓ A weight loss formula containing liver-supporting herbs such as dandelion root and milk thistle

✓ Carbohydrate controllers such as chromium

✓ Fat burners and liver- and gallbladder-supporting elements such as L-carnitine, methionine, choline, inositol, lipase, and lecithin

✓ Bile-supporting nutrients such as ox bile salts and beet root.

Full Disclosure: I have been a spokesperson and formulator for Uni Key Health Systems for nearly 25 years. Uni Key Health Systems (see Chapter 15) has been distributing the official Fat Flush Kit for my clients and readers for over 15 years.

In regard to the Fat Flush Kit, I couldn't find fat-flushing supplements in the health food stores with all the right dosages or the right ingredients, so I developed this kit. While many of my clients find it easier to use the kit, you can also choose to put together your own combination of supplements. Other appropriate supplements to complement both the Fat Flush Kit supplements and comparable formulas are listed in Chapter 15.

> *Ten years ago, I lost weight following the Fat Flush Plan. I even helped moderate Ann Louise's online forum for a while and went on a couple of her Fat Flush cruises! However, over the years, due to the stress of caring for my ailing parents (and the emotional eating that went along with that), the scale started moving in the wrong direction.*
>
> *At the same time, I developed hypothyroidism. As a nurse, I figured that was an easy fix . . . just take the thyroid medication prescribed by my doctor. Yet, even though I took the medication religiously, follow-up blood tests showed that my thyroid function was continuing to decline. And, the weight wasn't budging, no matter how little I ate. After I began having attacks of gallbladder pain, I knew that I had the risk factors for needing my gallbladder removed. Wanting to avoid surgery, I e-mailed Ann Louise looking for advice.*
>
> *My start date with the updated protocols of the Fat Flush Plan was on my 62nd birthday. Within two days, my intense carb cravings were gone and the scale was already showing movement! There were no hunger pangs; no feelings of deprivation; no calorie counting; no points to add up. During the first three months, I lost 31 pounds. After six months, I had lost another 22 pounds. And, now, at the age of 63, I am 93 pounds lighter than when I started this journey!*
>
> *—LINDA LEEKLEY*

TWO-WEEK FAT FLUSH MENU PLAN

Here is a helpful 14-day menu program to get you going on Fat Flush. Each metabolism-boosting menu incorporates the nutritional philosophy conveyed in the preceding chapters. Breakfast, lunch, and dinner feature the best fat-flushing, fat-burning, and diuretic foods, beverages, and seasonings. The more you build around these foods, the easier it will be to pare off the pounds.

Keep in mind that these menus are not set in stone. I know that many of you are working guys and gals, just like me. Although it's best to follow the menu plans as precisely as possible, you can always find something that will work if you're at a restaurant. Simply mirror the Fat Flush concept. This could be as easy as ordering something like salmon, turkey, a hamburger (without the bun), fresh seafood (e.g., crab, shrimp, scallops), steak, roast beef slices, or that old reliable standby, chicken—and then adding a side of veggies. Or order a Caesar salad without the croutons and dressing, asking the chef to toss in some onions and parsley. Then have it topped with some broiled shrimp, salmon, turkey, or chicken. Don't forget to "lemonize." Delicious. I encourage you to lemonize your salad by simply squeezing a lemon (or lime) over it instead of a restaurant dressing if you haven't brought your own.

Also be sure to give your personal touch to the menus. You can alter them to suit your individual taste. Just remember to refer to Chapter 13 and then exchange one food for another from the same food grouping.

Substitutions

Let's say you're not keen on kale. Not a problem. In fact, it's a great opportunity to expand your horizons and try some of the other great chlorophyll-rich greens listed. In fact, many (like kale) will be your main source of calcium on Fat Flush. Thus, if plain old lettuce has been your standard thing, be daring and live it up. Try arugula with its peppery mustard flavor and radish-leaf appearance; bok choy, that mild-flavored Asian green; radicchio, the Italian red-leafed veggie with a faint bitter taste and crisp leaves; watercress, with its slight bitter, pepperlike taste; mustard greens, the dark-leaf greens with a pungent mustard taste; or one of the many other deliciously slimming and slightly bitter greens such as Belgian endive, romaine lettuce, red or green loose-leaf lettuce, spinach, or escarole. Blend different ones together—your taste buds just might be pleasantly surprised, and your liver will really thank you.

INSIDER TIP	Recipes for the dishes in the menu plan that are marked with asterisks can be found in Chapter 13.

Here's the Thing

✓ It's up to you to keep in mind daily protocols for each phase. For example, don't forget to include at least two tablespoons daily of chia seeds, flax seeds, or hemp seeds in soups, salads, and sides to total 2 tablespoons per day to "fiber up" your metabolism. This is true for all the food requirements.

✓ Breakfast, lunch, and dinner are interchangeable.

✓ Make sure to consume your daily quota of 64 ounces of Fat Flush Cran-Water. To satisfy additional thirst, enjoy plain water or dandelion root, ginger, fennel, or peppermint tea—along with your 1 cup of organic coffee. All of the above are best enjoyed plain, but you can get creative and use a tablespoon of coconut oil to "bulletproof your coffee" if you would like. Some of my most creative Fat Flushers pop a teaspoon of cocoa or high-flavanol (at least 70 percent cocoa) cacao powder twice a week in a beverage of their choice. (High-copper foods like cocoa and cacao are limited due to copper's connection with estrogen dominance that leads to weight gain and bloating.) You can also enjoy cacao nibs up to twice per week if you prefer.

✓ Vegans and vegetarians can substitute ½ cup beans per day for nonvegan entrees. Choose from legumes such as ½ cup red or green lentils, chickpeas, aduki beans, pinto beans, black beans, or split yellow or green peas. Ideally, these should be soaked from 12 to about 24 hours to neutralize both enzyme inhibitors and mineral-leaching phytates. See Chapter 13 for recipes. Include 4 ounces of non-GMO organic tofu or tempeh twice a week to further support protein levels.

Phase 1 Sample Menu

WEEK 1

DAY 1

Breakfast	Cinnaberry Smoothie*
Midmorning snack	Mashed avocado in celery stalks with a squeeze of lemon
Lunch	Broiled sole brushed with 1 tablespoon coconut oil, parsley, and garlic; warm asparagus; mixed-greens salad with hearts of palm, 1 tablespoon chia seeds, and cucumber
4 p.m. snack	Apple slices rolled in flax seeds
Dinner	4 ounces broiled veal chop with Fat Flush Seasoning*; Savory Spaghetti Squash*; grated daikon, carrot, and fennel salad with a dash of lime

DAY 2

Breakfast	Whey Pancakes* drizzled with 1 table-spoon coconut oil and topped with 1 cup mixed berries
Midmorning snack	Snow peas sprinkled with 1 tablespoon hemp seeds
Lunch	Beef stir fry with lean beef and greens, bok choy, mushrooms, carrot, water chestnuts, and bean sprouts stir-sautéed in broth with ½ teaspoon ginger and a dash of cayenne; romaine salad with shredded jicama, avocado, 1 tablespoon ground flax seeds, and sliced radishes with lemon juice

| 4 p.m. snack | 1 nectarine |
| Dinner | Slow Cooker Cuban Ropa Vieja* (make enough for next day); medley of Cauliflower Rice*, yellow squash, 1 tablespoon hemp seeds; escarole with 1 tablespoon flaxseed oil |

DAY 3

Breakfast	Eggs scrambled with red and green peppers, onions, avocado, and 2 tablespoons hemp seeds
Midmorning snack	10 large cherries
Lunch	Leftover Slow Cooker Cuban Ropa Vieja*; steamed Swiss chard and okra with 1 tablespoon flaxseed oil; shredded red and green cabbage with 1 tablespoon flaxseed oil
4 p.m. snack	1 pear
Dinner	Baked halibut brushed with 1 tablespoon coconut oil, dill, garlic, and lemon; Egg Drop Cilantro Soup*; braised greens in bone broth

DAY 4

Breakfast	Strawberry Peach Smoothie*
Midmorning snack	Hard-boiled egg with a dash of dried mustard
Lunch	Broiled shrimp with garlic and ginger; steamed broccoli; tomato, parsley, avocado, and cucumber salad with apple cider vinegar
4 p.m. snack	Fat Flush Bone Broth* with toasted nori and 1 tablespoon hemp seeds
Dinner	Marinated flank steak; roasted red, orange, and yellow peppers brushed with broth; collard greens stir-sautéed in vegetable broth with 1 tablespoon flaxseed oil

DAY 5

| Breakfast | Asparagus-mushroom omelet with artichoke hearts and a dash of onion powder |
| Midmorning snack | 1 Granny Smith apple |

Lunch	Scallops sautéed in broth with scallions, minced garlic, and fresh parsley topped with 1 tablespoon flax seeds; warm green beans; tricolor salad of arugula, endive, and radicchio with 1 tablespoon flaxseed oil
4 p.m. snack	Avocado mashed with cucumber and lime juice
Dinner	Portobello Burger*; pan-tossed zucchini, kale, and onions; mixed baby greens salad with grated daikon and 1 tablespoon flaxseed oil and 1 tablespoon flax seeds

DAY 6

Breakfast	Green Goddess Smoothie*
Midmorning snack	Mashed tofu with 3 flax crackers
Lunch	Yummy Crab Cake*; tossed salad with grated carrot, olives, avocado, cucumbers, 1 tablespoon chia seeds, and apple cider vinegar
4 p.m. snack	1 peach
Dinner	Eggplant Delight*; steamed blend of yellow squash, water chestnuts, and okra; greens sautéed in broth with garlic

DAY 7

Breakfast	Savory Spaghetti Squash Pancakes* topped with 1 cup mixed berries
Midmorning snack	2 plums
Lunch	Tuna fish salad with avocado and Fat Flush Mayo*; green beans and water chestnuts on a bed of pan-seared greens sautéed in bone broth; Orange-Scented Roasted Brussels Sprouts*
4 p.m. snack	5-Star Artichoke Dip*
Dinner	Broiled lamb chops marinated in lemon juice, dried mustard, and garlic; steamed asparagus; Jicama Salad* with 2 tablespoons hemp seeds and 1 tablespoon flaxseed oil

WEEK 2

DAY 1

Breakfast	Plum Passion Smoothie*
Midmorning snack	Hard-boiled egg with avocado
Lunch	Grilled turkey burger with fennel; steamed medley of broccoli, carrot, cauliflower, parsley, and lemon
4 p.m. snack	1 nectarine
Dinner	Broiled chicken with lime and garlic; sautéed spinach and mushrooms in bone broth; leafy green salad with 1 tablespoon flaxseed oil and topped with 1 tablespoon chia seeds

DAY 2

Breakfast	Eggs over easy on steamed spinach drizzled with 1 tablespoon flaxseed oil
Midmorning snack	1 cup berries with 1 tablespoon hemp seeds
Lunch	Avocado stuffed with chicken salad; 1 tablespoon Fat Flush Mayo*; green beans
4 p.m. snack	1 pear cut up in chunks and rolled in 1 tablespoon flax seeds
Dinner:	Baked chicken with lime and garlic; steamed kale and pearl onions drizzled with 1 tablespoon flaxseed oil

DAY 3

Breakfast	Choco-Cherry Smoothie*
Midmorning snack	1 nectarine
Lunch	Grilled salmon brushed with broth; chopped parsley, tomatoes, scallions, 1 tablespoon ground flax seeds, and 1 tablespoon Fat Flush Vinaigrette*
4 p.m. snack	Avocado mashed with 3 flax crackers
Dinner	Chicken Kabob* with peppers, onions, and cherry tomatoes; sautéed collard greens; 1 carrot in vegetable broth with garlic and apple cider vinegar

D A Y 4

Breakfast	Veggie scramble with tofu, kale, green peppers, scallions, parsley, and 1 tablespoon hemp seeds
Midmorning snack	½ large grapefruit
Lunch	Grilled tempeh brushed with 1 tablespoon coconut oil with a dash of coriander; salad of Bibb lettuce, black olives, avocado, and watercress with mung bean sprouts, shredded carrot, and cucumber slices with 1 tablespoon chia seeds and 1 tablespoon flaxseed oil and apple cider vinegar
4 p.m. snack	6 large strawberries
Dinner	Slow Cooker Beef Stew* (make enough for next day's lunch); steamed yellow squash with 1 tablespoon flaxseed oil and ½ teaspoon cinnamon

D A Y 5

Breakfast	Raspberry Harmony Smoothie*
Midmorning snack	Fat Flush Bone Broth* with toasted nori strips
Lunch	Leftover Slow Cooker Beef Stew; steamed broccolini, zucchini, and okra with 1 tablespoon flaxseed oil
4 p.m. snack	Avocado mashed on Fabulous Chia Crax*
Dinner	Succulent Sea Scallops*; Roasted Veggie Medley*; steamed escarole with 1 tablespoon hemp seeds

D A Y 6

Breakfast	Cherry-Vanilla Smoothie*
Midmorning snack	Celery, jicama, avocado, and carrot sticks
Lunch	Portobello Burger* with 5-Star Artichoke Dip* topped with 1 tablespoon hemp seeds
4 p.m. snack	1 apple
Dinner	Basic Stir-Fry* (with ground lamb and cinnamon); Egg Drop Cilantro Soup*; braised greens in broth with 1 tablespoon flaxseed oil

D A Y 7

Breakfast	Scrambled eggs with cilantro, avocado, tomatoes, 2 tablespoons hemp seeds, and a dash of cumin
Midmorning snack	1 peach
Lunch	Cider Turkey with Mushrooms*; steamed green beans with ½ cup diced jicama drizzled with 1 tablespoon flaxseed oil
4 p.m. snack	Fabulous Chia Crax* with 1 cup berries
Dinner	Grilled chicken with Dijon mustard and parsley; sautéed kale in bone broth; baked yellow squash with a touch of cloves and 1 tablespoon flaxseed oil

7 Phase 2: The Metabolic Reset

Surround yourself with only people who are going to lift you higher.

—Oprah Winfrey

Congratulations! You just completed the most challenging phase of the entire Fat Flush Plan. Now it's time to step up to the next phase of Fat Flush and continue releasing stubborn fat, as you recalibrate and revitalize your system from head to toe. You'll continue to lose weight and maintain your cleansing momentum—but with more everyday food choices. To accomplish this, you will be making several changes.

As in phase 1 you will continue the hot water–lemon juice mixture, cran-water, a cup of coffee, and acceptable herbal and spiced teas. All these will continue to enable your liver to fulfill its filtering tasks and build healthy bile. Your liver and bile will metabolize your body's waste products without having to do the work of the kidneys. More water in all of these beverages is the tickets to accelerating your liver's metabolic removal of stored fats, resulting in healthy weight loss.

The next change, I just know you're going to love! You'll be adding one or two "friendly carbohydrates" back into your diet. This means that you can have quinoa and steel-cut oatmeal—the two most highly requested complex carbs on my program. Quinoa is the perfect wheat substitute, and its nutty, light flavor lends itself well to many dishes. Considered to be the highest-protein grain—although it is technically a grainlike seed—its quality protein content is superior to that of other grains. It also contains more collagen-building and virus-preventing lysine than wheat, and it ranks highest in iron with a whopping 8 mg in ½ cup. On top of it all, its fiber content, weighing in at 5 grams of fiber in ½ cup, is not too shabby either.

Oatmeal is another welcome, new friendly carb addition—unless, of course, you are highly gluten intolerant or have celiac disease. Oat products are typically manufactured in facilities that also process wheat and can become contaminated. For this reason, you must read labels on packaging very carefully to be assured there is no wheat processing in the same facilities. That being said and understood, do take note that this all-time comfort food has been a staple on diabetic diets for years—and with good reason. Its high fiber content with a mix of 45 percent insoluble to 55 percent soluble fiber stabilizes blood sugar, brings down cholesterol, and offers up a special kind of immune booster known as beta-glucan to supercharge immunity.

Steel-cut oats and rolled oats, not the processed or "instant" fast-cooking-time variety, can be soaked overnight in a thermos or on low heat in the oven. Raw oats are often the main ingredient in a variety of granolas these days, and when moistened with hot water or even a protein powder mixed with water (I like whey protein for this one), they make a perfectly acceptable snack!

Now all you have to do is decide when and how you are going to expand your new friendly carb choices. After working with literally thousands of Fat Flushers, I can say from practical experience that your best bet is to add back just one friendly carb (such as a ½ cup of oatmeal in the morning) one day at a time and then track your body's responses in your Fat Flush journal. That way you will be able to pinpoint whether or not the addition of this familiar cereal is creating any negative response, such as gas, bloating, sleepiness after eating, or headaches.

Then add another friendly carb in the second week, noting your responses. These carbohydrates are the ones most unlikely to precipitate insulin response or weight gain. And they are also considered to be moderate on the glycemic index, which rates foods based on their effect on blood sugar.

For that second week, you may gradually reintroduce one of the following friendly carbs into your Fat Flush diet. I suggest beginning with just ¼ cup, journaling your reactions. If you experience any of the negative responses mentioned earlier, or if your clothes are a bit tight, then cut out that particular food immediately. You can choose a sweet potato, green peas, cooked carrots, butternut squash, acorn squash, or beets.

The new friendly carb choices are noteworthy in several respects. They have been chosen because they are least likely to trigger sensitivity symptoms. If you can cultivate an appreciation of beets, your liver and gallbladder benefit. Beets, besides providing a source of nitric oxide so helpful in warding off circulatory issues, are also a primary source of betaine, a substance that decongests and thins out bile. Beets also trigger the release of bile from the gallbladder for those of us fortunate enough to still have that much-underrated organ!

Along with your new friendly carb additions, I have added in some favorite fruits to your daily fruit selection, like banana and pineapple. Why? The fiber these mineral-rich gems provide helps to maintain regularity and ferry toxic wastes out of the system.

Since the Fat Flush Cran-Water is somewhat diuretic, additional potassium (over 400 mg in a banana, for example) will help to keep your muscles from cramping and your heart beating nice and steady. Besides, there is nothing like a banana to complement a bowl of morning oatmeal on a cold wintry day!

When it comes to pineapple, think manganese. Manganese is a key trace mineral that was one of Dr. Atkins's favorites for stabilizing glucose levels. It also functions as part of the SOD (superoxidase dismutase) molecule, a key antioxidant to ward off oxidative stress. Skin, cartilage, and healthy bone formation all depend upon manganese, making pineapple a welcome addition to renewing your body from the inside out.

> *Fat Flush has shown me that the detox process doesn't need to be coupled with deprivation, and I can help my system lighten its load while also keeping well-fueled with fresh and delicious food.*
>
> —ELISA B.

THE METABOLIC RESET FLUSH DAILY PROTOCOL

FATS AND OILS

DAILY INTAKE: Flaxseed, coconut, or MCT (medium-chain triglyceride) oil at 1 tablespoon twice daily, and ½ avocado daily plus avocado spray for cooking.

PURPOSE: Flaxseed oil is essential for its high–omega-3 fat-fighting and insulin-regulating potential. (If intolerant, then opt for omega-3–rich fish oil that is subtly flavored with lemon or orange.) Coconut oil, a rich source of medium-chain fatty acids, boosts metabolism by 50 percent and speeds the thyroid. Avocado triggers adiponectin, the appetite hormone, for satiety. Also rich in glutathione to help with liver cleansing, MCT oil is a concentrated form of both coconut and palm oil and provides an even more concentrated source of energy for easy digestion, fat burning, and the brain.

FLUSH FLASH

Daily avocado provides an amazing amount of fiber—nearly 17 grams in 1 avocado. A great way to deliciously and effortlessly boost fiber intake.

FIBER-RICH SEEDS

DAILY INTAKE: 1 tablespoon twice daily of chia seeds, ground flax seeds, or hemp seeds.

PURPOSE: All three seed types provide soluble and insoluble fiber to help maintain regularity and provide satiety to meals and snacks. Their high omega-3 content controls cortisol production, and in the case of flax seeds, the high lignan content (800 times more than in any other food) controls haywire hormones. Hemp seeds offer up skin-beautifying and -strengthening omega-6.

LEAN PROTEIN

DAILY INTAKE: 1 whey or rice and pea protein serving, up to 2 eggs (optional), and a minimum of 8 ounces of cooked lean protein.

CHOOSE FROM: All varieties of fresh or frozen fish (with the exception of high-mercury swordfish and farm-raised tilapia) as well as canned fish (like Wild Planet Albacore and Skipjack Tuna, Vital Choice canned seafood, and Oregon Choice canned seafood), fresh or frozen seafood, lean beef, lamb, or skinless turkey or chicken; also tofu and tempeh, which may be consumed no more than twice per week. Use organic and grass-fed meat whenever possible. Choose hormone-free, unheated, undenatured, lactose-free, high-protein whey powders (like Fat Flush Vanilla and Chocolate Whey) with about 20 grams of protein per serving and negligible carbohydrates from nonmutated A2 milk. Choose non-GMO vegan protein powders (like Fat Flush Body Protein) with low carbohydrates and verification of low heavy metal content (especially arsenic and lead).

PURPOSE: Protein raises metabolism by 25 percent and activates the liver's detoxifying enzymes.

EGGS (OPTIONAL)

DAILY INTAKE: Up to 2 per day.

PURPOSE: For those without allergies or gallbladder issues, the omega-3–enriched eggs not only are delicious but also are brimming with antioxidants (e.g., lutein and zeaxanthin) for the eyes and brain, cholesterol-protective phosphatidylcholine, and sulfur to support your liver's cleansing process.

VEGETABLES

DAILY INTAKE: Unlimited (unless otherwise noted), raw or steamed. Put special emphasis on the bitter veggies (like arugula, watercress, escarole, and radishes) to help support liver and gallbladder health for greater cleansing power.

CHOOSE FROM: Arugula, asparagus, green beans, broccoli, broccolini, broccoli rabe, brussels sprouts, cabbage, cauliflower, celery, Chinese cabbage, carrots (1), cucumbers, daikon, globe artichoke, Jerusalem artichoke, artichoke heart, fennel, eggplant, spinach, escarole, collard greens, kale, mustard greens, romaine lettuce, rhubarb (1 cup), burdock, hearts of palm, radicchio, endive, parsley, onions, watercress, chives, leeks, Swiss chard, bell peppers (yellow, orange, green, and red), jicama, mushrooms, olives (3), radishes, horseradish, okra, tomatoes, red or green loose-leaf lettuce, snow peas, zucchini, yellow squash, water chestnuts, bamboo shoots, garlic, spaghetti squash, and sprouts (alfalfa, broccoli, radish, and mung bean).

SEA VEGGIES: Agar-agar, hijiki, kombu, nori, wakame, or a sea veggie–based seasoning (like Eden Seaweed Gomasio, kelp granules, or dulse flakes from Maine).

PURPOSE: These fibrous and colorful phytonutrient-rich vegetables will help speed your liver's cleansing and provide valuable carotenoids. Broccoli sprouts are especially high in sulforaphane—a very potent antioxidant that targets cellular health. Two ounces per day would be ideal. The sea veggies and seasonings provide iodine and trace minerals to help nourish the thyroid and counteract environmental pollutants.

FRIENDLY CARBOHYDRATES

DAILY INTAKE: Start with small increments (even half a serving), and work your way up gradually to the following portions, especially with the starchy vegetables:

WEEK 1, PHASE 2: 1 serving per day.

WEEK 2, PHASE 2: 2 servings per day.

CHOOSE FROM: 1 small sweet potato, ½ cup green peas, ½ cup cooked carrots, ½ cup butternut or acorn squash, ½ cup beets, ½ cup oatmeal, and ½ cup quinoa.

FRUITS

DAILY INTAKE: Up to 2 whole portions daily.

CHOOSE FROM: 1 small apple, ½ grapefruit, 1 small orange, 2 medium plums, 6 large strawberries, 10 large cherries, 1 nectarine, 1 peach, 1 pear, 1 cup berries (blueberries, blackberries, or raspberries), 1 pomegranate, ½ or 1 small banana, and ½ cup pineapple.

PURPOSE: Nature's cleansers are high in enzymes and minerals (e.g., potassium) and low on the glycemic load.

FAT FLUSH CRAN-WATER

DAILY INTAKE: 8 eight-ounce glasses per day

PURPOSE: The cranberry juice–water mixture eliminates water retention, cleanses accumulated wastes from the lymphatic system, and also helps to reduce the appearance of cellulite.

FAT-FLUSHING HERBS AND SPICES

DAILY INTAKE: To taste.

CHOOSE FROM: Cayenne pepper, dried mustard, cinnamon, ginger, dill, garlic, anise, fennel, cloves, bay leaves, coriander, parsley, cilantro, turmeric, apple cider vinegar, coconut vinegar, and cumin.

PURPOSE: Metabolism boosters.

LEGAL CHEAT

1 cup of organic coffee at breakfast.

FAT FLUSH SWEETENERS

DAILY INTAKE: Organic SweetLeaf Stevia, Lakanto Monk Fruit Sweetener, or Uni Key's Flora-Key.

WHAT MAKES THEM LEGAL: Both SweetLeaf Stevia and Lakanto are sugar-free and low-glycemic sweeteners. The plant-based stevia is 30 times sweeter than sugar, so a little goes a long way, and it is great for baking. According to the manufacturer, Lakanto can be used in a 1-to-1 ratio to replace sugar because it tastes, bakes, and looks like the white stuff. But I find that easily one-half that amount is a sweet-enough substitution. You might also want to consider reducing the amount of Lakanto due to the presence of erythritol, which causes some folks to experience loose stools and digestive upsets. That's why I also recommend the prebiotic and probiotic sweetener Flora-Key as another alternative. This immune-boosting probiotic formula contains various strains of acidophilus, bifidus, and a special prebiotic, rather sweet-tasting substance known as inulin to stimulate the growth of the beneficial bacteria. This product helps to ward off toxins and aids in the synthesis of key vitamins and minerals while helping to support the good bacteria in the gut. It can be used in morning smoothies and is an optional ingredient in several of the recipes for the Fat Flush Plan. Flora-Key should only be used in nonheat recipes, as heating will destroy the beneficial bacteria, whereas both stevia and Lakanto can be used in recipes that require heat.

BESIDES THE DAILY DIET

BEFORE BREAKFAST: Drink an 8-ounce cup of hot water with the juice of ½ lemon to assist your kidneys and liver and thin the bile.

BREAKFAST AND DINNER: Take supplements rich in fat-burning, skin-beautifying, and anti-inflammatory gamma-linolenic acid (GLA) in a total daily amount of 360 mg per day.

CHOOSE FROM: Straight GLA supplements from black currant seed oil contained in the Fat Flush Kit, or purchase GLA supplements from black currant seed oil at your favorite health food store. Each capsule in the kit contains 90 mg of GLA, and you take 2 capsules 2 times daily.

DAILY: You can also take the additional supplements from the Fat Flush Kit or from your current regimen to optimize your results, like the Fat Flush Dieters' Multi (with or without iron) and the Fat Flush Weight Loss Formula. The Fat Flush Dieters' Multi provides a balanced multivitamin and mineral supplementation during detox. The Fat Flush Weight Loss Formula contains liver-and bile-supporting herbs like milk thistle and blood sugar–stabilizing berberine containing Oregon grape root, as well as carbohydrate controllers like chromium and fat burners such as L-carnitine, methionine, choline, inositol, lipase, and lecithin. If you do not have a gallbladder or have had a history of symptoms related to poor fat digestion, hypothyroidism, or estrogen metabolism, then you might wish to consider the Fat Flush Bile Builder. To review, you can supplement with the following if you choose your own supplements:

✓ A balanced multivitamin and mineral supplement for general nutrition insurance
✓ A weight loss formula containing liver-supporting herbs such as dandelion root and milk thistle
✓ Carbohydrate controllers such as chromium
✓ Fat burners and liver- and gallbladder-supporting elements such as L-carnitine, methionine, choline, inositol, lipase, and lecithin
✓ Bile-supporting nutrients such as ox bile salts, taurine, and beet root

Full Disclosure: I have been a spokesperson and formulator for Uni Key Health Systems for nearly 25 years (see Chapter 15). They have been distributing the official Fat Flush Kit for my clients and readers for over 15 years.

In regard to the Fast Flush Kit, I couldn't find fat-flushing supplements in the health food stores with all the right dosages or the right ingredients, so I developed this kit. While many of my clients find it easier to use the kit, you can also choose to put together your own combination of supplements. Other appropriate supplements to complement both the Fat Flush Kit and comparable supplements are also listed in Chapter 15.

● ● ●

Use phase 1 as your foundational program, building on it with the phase 2 food list (see Chapter 11, "The Fat Flush Master Shopping List"). Below are some simple examples of how to "upgrade" breakfast and lunch for the ongoing Fat Flush. You also may want to use the dinner menu ideas from phase 1. *And remember that all recipes identified by an asterisk are found in Chapter 13.*

Here's the Thing

✓ It's up to you to keep in mind daily protocols for each phase.
✓ Breakfast, lunch, and dinner are interchangeable.
✓ Make sure to consume your daily quota of 64 ounces of Fat Flush Cran-Water. To satisfy additional thirst, enjoy plain water or dandelion root, ginger, fennel, or peppermint tea—along with your 1 cup of organic coffee. All of the above are best enjoyed plain, but you can get creative and use a tablespoon of coconut oil to "bulletproof your coffee" if you would like. Some of my most creative Fat Flushers pop a teaspoon of cocoa or high-flavanol (at least 70 percent cocoa) cacao powder twice a week in a beverage of their choice. (High-copper foods like cocoa and cacao are limited due to copper's connection with estrogen dominance that leads to weight gain and bloating.) You can also enjoy cacao nibs up to twice per week if you prefer.

✓ Vegans and vegetarians can substitute ½ cup beans per day for nonvegan entrees. Choose from legumes such as ½ cup red or green lentils, chickpeas, aduki beans, pinto beans, black beans, or split yellow or green peas. Ideally, these should be soaked from 12 to about 24 hours to neutralize both enzyme inhibitors and mineral-leaching phytates. See the recipes in Chapter 13. Include 4 ounces of non-GMO organic tofu or tempeh at least twice a week to further support protein levels.

SAMPLE MENU

DAY 1

Before breakfast	Fat Flush Lemon Water
Breakfast	Blueberry Smoothie*
Midmorning snack	Mashed avocado with 3 Fabulous Chia Crax*
Lunch	Portobello Burger* with Fat Flush Mayo* and Fat Flush Pickles*; Jicama Salad*
4 p.m. snack	1 nectarine
Dinner	Roasted turkey with Fresh Cranberry Chutney*; spaghetti squash, peas, and green beans topped with 1 tablespoon hemp seeds

DAY 2

Before breakfast	Fat Flush Lemon Water*
Breakfast	Whey Pancakes* drizzled with 1 tablespoon coconut oil and topped with 1 cup mixed berries
Midmorning snack	Jicama sticks with a dash of lime and cayenne
Lunch	Stir-fry with ground beef, mushrooms, black olives, water chestnuts, zucchini, and bean sprouts stir-sautéed in bone broth with ¼ teaspoon ginger; romaine salad with 1 tablespoon flaxseed oil, avocado, and 1 tablespoon chia seeds
4 p.m. snack	1 pear
Dinner	Grilled chicken breast with Fat Flush Seasoning*; Quinoa Tabbouleh* with 1 tablespoon hemp seeds; steamed snow peas with dill

DAY 3

Before breakfast	Fat Flush Lemon Water*
Breakfast	Scrambled tofu with turmeric, onions, parsley, and spinach
Midmorning snack	10 large cherries
Lunch	Tuna fish salad with avocado and 1 tablespoon Fat Flush Mayo*, lemon, cumin, and a dash of mustard; steamed broccoli
4 p.m. snack	Toasted nori strips with carrots
Dinner	Grilled mahi-mahi; ½ cup baked butternut squash with 1 tablespoon hemp seeds and a pinch of seaweed gomasio; steamed broccoli with lemon

DAY 4

Before breakfast	Fat Flush Lemon Water*
Breakfast	Poached eggs on Cauliflower Rice* with 1 tablespoon hemp seeds
Midmorning snack	1 orange
Lunch	Grilled shrimp on a bed of mixed greens, shredded beets, cucumbers, olives, and scallions with 1 tablespoon flaxseed oil and 1 tablespoon ground flax seeds
4 p.m. snack	10 large cherries
Dinner	Lettuce wrap bison burger; 1 small sweet potato; wilted red cabbage salad with cilantro, avocado, and 1 tablespoon each of freshly squeezed lime juice and flaxseed oil

DAY 5

Before breakfast	Fat Flush Lemon Water*
Breakfast	Asparagus-mushroom omelet with a dash of cayenne pepper
Midmorning snack	½ banana
Lunch	Shrimp salad with 1 tablespoon Fat Flush Mayo* on a colorful salad of arugula, endive, radicchio, and shredded beets with 1 tablespoon ground flax seeds and drizzled with apple cider vinegar

| 4 p.m. snack | Mashed avocado on Fabulous Chia Crax* |
| Dinner | Veal medallions cooked with Fat Flush Bone Broth*; pan-tossed zucchini, kale, and yellow squash; mixed baby greens salad with grated daikon, 1 tablespoon hemp seeds, and 1 tablespoon flaxseed oil |

DAY 6

Before breakfast	Fat Flush Lemon Water*
Breakfast	Piña Colada Smoothie*
Midmorning snack	Mashed tofu stuffed in snow peas
Lunch	Mushroom Tempeh Chili*; tossed salad with grated carrots, shredded beets, cucumbers, avocado, 1 tablespoon chia seeds, and 1 tablespoon flaxseed oil
4 p.m. snack	½ grapefruit
Dinner	Turkey cutlets with Dijon mustard; steamed spaghetti squash; greens sautéed in broth with garlic

DAY 7

Before breakfast	Fat Flush Lemon Water*
Breakfast	Spaghetti Squash Peach Pudding*
Midmorning snack	2 plums
Lunch	Grilled chicken breast; warm green beans, cucumbers, and tomatoes on a bed of greens with 2 tablespoons hemp seeds and 1 tablespoon flaxseed oil
4 p.m. snack	Mashed avocado with 3 flax crackers
Dinner	Stir-fry with chicken, peas, bok choy, bean sprouts, celery, steamed artichoke, and 1 tablespoon coconut oil

8 Phase 3: The Lifestyle Eating Plan

Digestion exists for health, and health exists for life.
—G. K. Chesterton

Way to go—you have graduated to the Lifestyle Eating Plan. And this means that you have overcome many of your former eating habits, have stabilized your weight, and can better cope with real-life challenges. Perhaps your journaling experience has even revealed some emotional eating patterns that you are now better equipped to handle. Isn't it interesting that the health-sabotaging, stress-promoting foods—the breads, pastas, mashed potatoes, and sweets—are the very ones we tend to gravitate toward when we need comfort foods?

The basic Fat Flush principles you embraced during the initial phases of the plan are still at work here with many welcome additions. This also will be an important time to continue tracking your food choices in your journal. This will help nip in the bud cravings or weight gain from any new food and will facilitate its elimination pronto.

While there are some more liberal choices in the fats and oil and fruit categories in phase 3, the most significant add-ons include dairy products (if you can tolerate them) and even more "friendly carbs" to choose from. Gluten-free options such as brown rice, buckwheat, millet, amaranth, beans, baked potato, and GMO-free corn on the cob are added to those you started to include during phase 2. Of course, this doesn't give you license to make a meal of just high-carb rice and beans or a baked potato (as you probably know by now). Measured amounts of these new friendly carbs can accompany your proteins and fats in special combinations.

For the first week of phase 3, I suggest adding only one dairy product and eating it every day that week. Note your responses in your journal. If you experience symptoms that may be due to dairy intolerance such as bloat, weight gain, gas, or phlegm, or if you have to clear your throat a lot, then

117

omit that dairy product immediately. If not, keep your cheese, and eat it too until you are enjoying two dairy servings per day.

During the second week of phase 3, substitute a new friendly carb for one of the carbs you are presently eating. Again, observe your responses.

Weight permitting, many of you may ultimately include up to four servings per day from each of the friendly carb selections, while others will need to scale back accordingly.

And this leads me to another important aspect of phase 3 lifestyle eating: food combinations. The Lifestyle Eating Plan incorporates the fat-flushing food combination rules I first learned about from my mentor Dr. Hazel Parcells, long before food-combining principles became popular. Dr. Parcells's landmark research at Sierra State University revealed that when foods were eaten in very precise combinations, people did not gain weight regardless of calorie count. In addition, gas, bloating, diarrhea, and constipation were greatly relieved. I have further developed and elaborated on her guidelines based on my own experience with thousands of clients.

THE FAT-FLUSHING FOOD COMBINATIONS

✓ One protein at a meal. This means no double-protein combos. Have each individual protein food, such as beef, fish, poultry, seafood, or tofu, by itself. No mixtures such as shrimp and scallops or steak and lobster together at one meal. Digestion is impaired, and toxicity results.

✓ Eggs are the exception to the protein rule. They are considered neutral and can be added to the above-mentioned proteins. They go particularly well with dairy products (as in a quiche) and add to the protein value of bean dishes.

✓ Beans are considered a starch *and* protein and combine well with dairy products and veggies but not with meat, fish, or chicken.

✓ Proteins such as fish, fowl, and beef do not combine well with gluten-rich grain starches (e.g., wheat, rye, oats, and barley). An example of this is a burger on a bun. Proteins do combine well with other friendly carbs, such as a baked potato, a sweet potato, corn, or peas—provided a green leafy salad is included in the meal.

✓ In general, vegetables and fruits should not be eaten together (unless they are broken down through the blending process in juices or in a smoothie).

✓ Milk and meat (e.g., a glass of milk and a steak) shouldn't be consumed together. Dairy fats, however, such as butter, cream, and sour cream are regarded as fats and do combine with other protein foods (e.g., beef stroganoff).

✓ Flaxseed oil, because of its unique metabolic makeup, combines well with dairy (e.g., cottage cheese or ricotta cheese and yogurt), friendly carbs, and vegetables.

✓ Water should not be taken with meals before food is swallowed. While water is necessary for many metabolic processes, including digestion, saliva activity is weakened when large amounts of water are used to wash down food. Extremely hot or cold water depresses gastric juices and acts as a shock to the system.

You will also be pleased to note that more fermented foods are part of the Lifetime Eating Protocol, which do wonders to support the microbiome. You'll be enjoying a delightful seasoning known as umeboshi plum paste (from fermented plums) for taste and fuel for flourishing skinny gut bacteria. In addition, occasional tamari (gluten-free soy sauce) and miso can also be enjoyed.

> *Before I started the Fat Flush Plan I was not only overweight—I was fatigued, my metabolism was sluggish and I also suffered with frequent hot flashes, mood swings and digestive problems. Fat Flush has not only helped me lose weight (25 pounds so far!), but thankfully, my hormones have regulated and my digestive problems have disappeared. At 57 I have more energy than ever! Fat Flush has become a lifestyle guide for me, and I'm forever grateful to Ann Louise!*
>
> —TERESA P.

THE LIFESTYLE EATING PROTOCOL

FATS AND OILS

DAILY INTAKE: Up to 3 tablespoons of oil daily; ½ avocado daily plus avocado spray for cooking.

CHOOSE FROM: Flaxseed oil, coconut oil, olive oil, MCT (medium-chain triglyceride) oil, sesame oil, avocado oil, or macadamia nut oil.

PURPOSE: Flaxseed oil is essential for its high–omega-3 fat-fighting and insulin-regulating potential. (If intolerant, then opt for omega-3–rich fish oil that is subtly flavored with lemon or orange.) Coconut oil, a rich source of medium-chain fatty acids, boosts metabolism by 50 percent and speeds the thyroid. Avocado triggers adiponectin, the appetite hormone, for satiety and is also rich in filling omega-9 and glutathione, which helps with liver cleansing. MCT oil is a concentrated form of coconut oil and palm oil that provides an even more potent source of energy for easy digestion, fat burning, and the brain. Sesame seed oil can help heart health by regulating insulin and preventing atherosclerotic lesions with the antioxidant and anti-inflammatory compound known as sesamol. Sesame seeds contain anticancer compounds including phytic acid, magnesium, and phytosterols. Macadamia nut oil is high in monounsaturated fatty acids, including oleic acid (omega-9), as well as collagen-boosting omega-7—all of which are very moisturizing, regenerating, and softening to the skin. All these fatty acids also have anti-inflammatory properties, which dial down hunger hormones.

BONUS FOODS: To replace a tablespoon of oil, you can choose from a handful of nuts (almonds, walnuts, or macadamias), a couple of tablespoons of seeds (e.g., pumpkin, sunflower, or tahini or sesame), a tablespoon of nut butter, 2 tablespoons of shredded coconut, 1 tablespoon of ghee (clarified butter), or 3 ounces of full-fat coconut milk. A pat of butter, a smear of cream cheese, and a dollop of sour cream (or coconut cream) are all tasty add-ons, and when enjoyed in the specified amounts, they are "free" add-ons. Unsweetened organic almond milk, organic almond flour, organic coconut flour, and organic shredded coconut are fine once a day.

FIBER-RICH SEEDS

DAILY INTAKE: 1 tablespoon twice daily of chia seeds, ground flax seeds, or hemp seeds.

PURPOSE: All three seed types provide soluble and insoluble fiber to help maintain regularity and provide satiety to meals and snacks. Their high omega-3 content controls cortisol production, and in the case of flax seeds, the high lignan content (800 times more than in any other food) controls haywire hormones. Hemp seeds offer up skin-beautifying and -strengthening omega-6.

LEAN PROTEIN

DAILY INTAKE: 1 whey or rice and pea protein powder serving, up to 2 eggs (optional), and a minimum of 8 ounces of cooked lean protein. Can add nitrate-free turkey bacon once or twice a week for added flavor. Since it contains a minimal amount of protein grams (6 grams in one strip), turkey bacon does not have to be included in daily totals.

CHOOSE FROM: All varieties of fresh or frozen fish (with the exception of high-mercury swordfish and farm-raised tilapia) as well as canned fish (like Wild Planet Albacore and Skipjack Tuna, Vital Choice canned seafood, and Oregon Choice canned seafood), fresh or frozen seafood, lean beef, lamb, or skinless turkey or chicken; also tofu and tempeh, which may be consumed no more than twice per week. Use organic and grass-fed meat whenever possible. Choose hormone-free, unheated, undenatured, lactose-free, high-protein whey powders (like Fat Flush Vanilla and Chocolate Whey) with about 20 grams of protein per serving and negligible carbohydrates from nonmutated A2 milk. Choose non-GMO vegan protein powders (like Fat Flush Body Protein) with low carbohydrates and verification of low heavy metal content (especially arsenic and lead).

PURPOSE: Protein raises metabolism by 25 percent and activates the liver's detoxifying enzymes.

EGGS (OPTIONAL)

DAILY INTAKE: Up to 2 per day.

PURPOSE: The omega-3–enriched eggs not only are delicious but also are brimming with antioxidants (e.g., lutein and zeaxanthin) for the eyes and brain, cholesterol-protective phosphatidylcholine, and sulfur to support your liver's cleansing process.

VEGETABLES

DAILY INTAKE: Unlimited (unless otherwise noted), raw or steamed. Put special emphasis on the bitter veggies (like arugula, watercress, escarole, and radishes) to help support liver and gallbladder health for greater cleansing power.

CHOOSE FROM: Arugula, asparagus, green beans, broccoli, broccolini, broccoli rabe, brussels sprouts, cabbage, cauliflower, celery, Chinese cabbage, carrots (1), cucumbers, daikon, globe artichoke, Jerusalem artichoke, artichoke heart, fennel, eggplant, spinach, escarole, collard greens, kale, mustard greens, romaine lettuce, radicchio, endive, rhubarb (1 cup), burdock, hearts of palm, parsley, onions, watercress, chives, leeks, Swiss chard, bell peppers (yellow, orange, green, and red), jicama, mushrooms, olives (3), radishes, horseradish, okra, tomatoes, red or green loose-leaf lettuce, snow peas, zucchini, yellow squash, water chestnuts, bamboo shoots, garlic, spaghetti squash, and sprouts (alfalfa, broccoli, radish, and mung bean).

SEA VEGGIES: Agar-agar, hijiki, kombu, nori, wakame, or a sea veggie–based seasoning (like Eden Seaweed Gomasio, kelp granules, or dulse flakes from Maine).

PURPOSE: These fibrous and colorful phytonutrient-rich vegetables will help speed your liver's cleansing and provide valuable carotenoids. Broccoli sprouts are especially high in sulforaphane—a very potent antioxidant that targets cellular health. Two ounces per day would be ideal. The sea veggies and seasonings provide iodine and trace minerals to help nourish the thyroid and counteract environmental pollutants.

FRUITS

DAILY INTAKE: Up to 2 portions daily.

CHOOSE FROM: 1 small apple, ½ grapefruit, 1 small orange, 2 medium plums, 1 cup berries (e.g., strawberries, blueberries, blackberries, or raspberries), 10 large cherries, 12 large grapes, 1 nectarine, 1 peach, 1 small kiwi, 1 pear, 1 pomegranate, ½ banana, ½ cup mango, ½ cup papaya, and ½ cup melon (e.g., cantaloupe, honeydew, or watermelon), ½ cup pineapple.

SPECIAL OCCASION: Dried fruits (1 large fig, 2 dates, 2 tablespoons raisins or currants, 2 dried plums or prunes, 3 dried apricot halves), 2 tablespoons unsweetened fruit preserves, and ½ cup unsweetened juice.

PURPOSE: Nature's cleansers are high in enzymes and minerals (e.g., potassium) and low in fructose.

DAIRY (OPTIONAL)

DAILY INTAKE: Up to 2 servings per day.

CHOOSE FROM: 1 ounce hard cheese, ½ cup full-fat cottage or ricotta cheese, 4 tablespoons Romano cheese, 4 tablespoons Parmesan cheese, ½ cup buttermilk, or 1 cup plain full-fat or Greek yogurt.

PURPOSE: Dairy foods provide calcium, protein, and saturated fats for energy.

| INSIDER TIP | If dairy sensitive, choose coconut alternatives when possible. |

FRIENDLY CARBOHYDRATES

DAILY INTAKE: Work up to 4 servings per day or as many servings as you can tolerate.

Week 1, Phase 3: Substitute a new friendly carb for one of those from phase 2, adding no new servings, to gauge the body's response.

Week 2, Phase 3: Add 1 serving, making 3 servings total per day, noting the body's response.

Week 3, Phase 3: Add 1 serving, making 4 servings total per day, noting the body's response.

CHOOSE FROM: A handful of tigernuts (small root vegetables); 4 large chestnuts; 1 Ezekiel 4:9 Sprouted Tortilla; 1 non-GMO corn tortilla; ½ cup peas; ½ cup cooked carrots; 1 small sweet potato; ½ cup acorn or butternut squash; ½ cup beets; ½ cup cooked turnips, rutabaga, parsnips, or pumpkin; 1 small corn on the cob; 1 small baked potato or ½ cup red potatoes; ½ cup chickpeas, pinto beans, adzuki, black beans, or kidney beans; ½ cup brown rice, oatmeal, quinoa, buckwheat groats, millet, or amaranth; 3 cups popcorn.

| INSIDER TIP | Tigernut flour is a gluten-free, nut-free, and dairy-free flour substitute. It is an exceptionally rich source of resistant starch, which is a prebiotic fiber that is not digested, but instead functions as food for probiotics in your gut. |

| INSIDER TIP | If bloating, gas, or weight gain is noted, omit the new carb serving and revert to the diet of the previous week. After the symptoms have subsided, add back 1/4 cup (or other incremental amount) of a different carbohydrate and monitor your response until you reach your tolerance level. Also, note that tigernuts are chock-full of potassium, magnesium, and fiber and are delightful in gluten-free cookies. |

FAT FLUSH CRAN-WATER

DAILY INTAKE: 8 eight-ounce glasses per day

PURPOSE: The cranberry juice–water mixture eliminates water retention, cleanses accumulated wastes from the lymphatic system, and also helps to reduce the appearance of cellulite.

BEVERAGES

Drink spiced teas (ginger, fennel, and peppermint), dandelion root tea, or red tea (rooibos tea).

FAT-FLUSHING HERBS AND SPICES

DAILY INTAKE: To taste.

CHOOSE FROM: Cayenne pepper, dried mustard, cinnamon, ginger, dill, garlic, anise, fennel, cloves, bay leaves, coriander, parsley, cilantro, turmeric, apple cider vinegar, coconut vinegar, cumin, basil, oregano, rosemary, and thyme. You also may add other flavorful spices (like curry in small amounts) and any other herb as you wish, but keep these as your main focus.

PURPOSE: Metabolism boosting.

LEGAL CHEAT

1 cup of organic coffee at breakfast.

SALT

DAILY INTAKE: 350–400 mg per meal from Selina's Celtic Sea Salt. Due to environmental, political, and ecological concerns, I prefer Selina brand salt products rather than Himalayan salt. If on a low-sodium diet, then check out the Selina Makai Sea Salt, which is lower in sodium and higher in potassium than any other type of sea salt on the market.

SPECIAL OCCASION: ½ tablespoon of low sodium tamari and capers, rinsed and drained.

FAT FLUSH SWEETENERS

DAILY INTAKE: Organic SweetLeaf Stevia, Lakanto Monk Fruit Sweetener, Uni Key Flora-Key, and yakon syrup.

WHAT MAKES THEM LEGAL: Both SweetLeaf Stevia and Lakanto are sugar-free and low-glycemic sweeteners. The plant-based stevia is 30 times sweeter than sugar, so a little goes a long way and is great for baking. According to the manufacturer, Lakanto can be used in a 1-to-1 ratio to replace sugar because it tastes, bakes, and looks like the white stuff. But I find that easily one-half that amount is a sweet enough substitution. You might also want to consider reducing the amount of Lakanto due to the presence of erythritol, which causes some folks to experience loose stools and digestive upsets. That's why I also recommend the prebiotic and probiotic sweetener Flora-Key as another alternative. This immune-boosting probiotic formula contains various strains of acidophilus, bifidus, and a special prebiotic, rather sweet-tasting substance known as inulin to stimulate the growth of the beneficial bacteria. This product helps to ward off toxins and aids in the synthesis of key vitamins and minerals while helping to support the good bacteria in the gut. It can be used in morning smoothies and is an optional ingredient in several of the recipes for the Fat Flush Plan. Flora-Key should only be used in nonheat recipes, as heating will destroy the beneficial bacteria, whereas both stevia and Lakanto can be used in recipes that require heat. Yakon syrup is made from chicory root and can be used as a honey substitute in recipes in equal measure. It is considered a prebiotic and will feed the skinny gut bacteria.

SPECIAL OCCASION: 1 tablespoon raw honey, maple syrup, date sugar, or blackstrap molasses. (This replaces one fruit each.)

ALCOHOL

WEEKLY INTAKE: Should you choose to indulge, you may have 1 drink per week and on special occasions, of course.

CHOOSE FROM: Organic wine or grain-free hard liquor.

INSIDER TIP	When alcohol is used for cooking, most of it is burned off while the flavor remains. Alcohol burn off takes about one half hour when food is simmering is soups and stews. It burns off in three minutes when used to sauté. Try to avoid "cooking wine," which contains added salt. The term "cooking wine" refers to an earlier time when wine set aside for use in food was purposely salted to prevent the cook from drinking it.

BESIDES THE DAILY DIET

BEFORE BREAKFAST: Drink an 8-ounce cup of hot water with the juice of ½ lemon to assist your kidneys and liver and thin the bile.

BREAKFAST AND DINNER: Take supplements rich in fat-burning, skin-beautifying, and anti-inflammatory gamma-linolenic acid (GLA) in a total daily amount of 360 mg per day.

WITH ALL MEALS: Take a 1,000-mg conjugated linoleic acid (CLA) capsule 3 times per day to maintain your fat loss progress. As you recall from Chapter 2, CLA not only reduces the body's ability to deposit fat but also promotes the use of stored fat for energy.

CHOOSE FROM: Straight GLA supplements from black currant seed oil contained in the Fat Flush Kit, or purchase GLA supplements from black currant seed oil at your favorite health food store. Each capsule in the kit contains 90 mg of GLA, and you take 2 capsules 2 times daily.

DAILY: You can also take the additional supplements from the Fat Flush Kit or similar formulas from your current regimen to optimize your results, like the Fat Flush Dieters' Multi (with or without iron) and the Fat Flush Weight Loss Formula. The Fat Flush Dieters' Multi provides balanced multivitamin and mineral supplementation during detox. The Fat Flush Weight Loss Formula contains liver- and bile-supporting herbs like milk thistle and blood sugar–stabilizing berberine containing Oregon grape root, as well as carbohydrate controllers like chromium and fat burners such as L-carnitine, methionine, choline, inositol, lipase, and lecithin. If you do not have a gallbladder or have a history of symptoms related to poor fat digestion, hypothyroidism, or estrogen metabolism, then you might wish to consider the Fat Flush Bile Builder. To review, you can supplement with the following if you choose your own supplements:

✓ A balanced multivitamin and mineral supplement for general nutrition insurance
✓ A weight loss formula containing liver-supporting herbs such as dandelion root and milk thistle
✓ Carbohydrate controllers such as chromium
✓ Fat burners and liver- and gallbladder-supporting elements such as L-carnitine, methionine, choline, inositol, lipase, and lecithin
✓ Gallbladder- and bile-supporting nutrients such as ox bile salts, taurine, and beet root

Full Disclosure: I have been a spokesperson and formulator for Uni Key Health Systems for nearly 25 years. Uni Key Health Systems (see Chapter 15) has been distributing the official Fat Flush Kit for my clients and readers for over 15 years.

In regard to the Fat Flush Kit, I couldn't find fat-flushing supplements in the health food stores with all the right dosages or the right ingredients, so I developed this kit. While many of my clients find it easier to use the kit, you can also choose to put together your own combination of supplements. Other appropriate supplements to complement both the Fat Flush Kit supplements and comparable formulas are also listed in Chapter 15.

• • •

Use phase 1 as your foundational program, building on it with the phase 2 food list (see Chapter 11, "The Fat Flush Master Shopping List"). Here are some simple examples of how to "upgrade" breakfast and lunch from phase 2. You also may want to use the dinner menu ideas from phase 1.

THE LIFESTYLE EATING PLAN

Below is a sample one-week menu program to show you how to include the new foods you have learned about that will support your body. Although I suggest that you introduce one new food per week, for the sake of more varied and creative menu planning, this sample menu incorporates just one dairy selection. Although in this menu you add just two friendly carbs, you can ultimately add up to four friendly carbs per day, weight permitting. The majority of individuals I have worked with seem to tolerate these amounts of dairy and friendly carbs without gaining weight or going backward. The portions are given in full, but you can always cut them in half and work up to the full amount. Keep using those Fat Flush Bone Broths from phases 1 and 2 for veggie dishes (especially good with kale, collards, and bok choy) or even as a snack between meals! Bone broths are great for omelets and other egg dishes when the menu doesn't specify cooking oil such as olive or sesame oil. Lastly, *recipes for the dishes marked with asterisks can be found in Chapter 13.*

Here's the Thing

✓ It's up to you to keep in mind daily protocols for each phase. The menus are just a basic template for you to consider.

✓ Breakfast, lunch, and dinner are interchangeable.

✓ Make sure to consume your daily quota of 64 ounces of Fat Flush Cran-Water. To satisfy additional thirst, enjoy plain water and dandelion root, ginger, fennel, or peppermint tea—along with your 1 cup of organic coffee. All of the above are best enjoyed plain, but you can get creative and use a tablespoon of coconut or MCT oil to "bulletproof your coffee" if you would like. Some of my most creative Fat Flushers pop a teaspoon of cocoa or high-flavanol (at least 70 percent cocoa) cacao powder twice a week in a beverage of their choice. (High-copper foods like cocoa and cacao are limited due to copper's connection with estrogen dominance that leads to weight gain and bloating). You can also enjoy cacao nibs up to twice per week if you prefer.

✓ Vegans and vegetarians can substitute ½ cup beans per day for nonvegan entrees. Choose from legumes such as ½ cup red or green lentils, chickpeas, aduki beans, pinto beans, black beans, or split yellow or green peas. Ideally, these should be soaked from 12 to about 24 hours to neutralize both enzyme inhibitors and mineral-leaching phytates. See the recipes in Chapter 13. Include 4 ounces of non-GMO organic tofu or tempeh no more than twice a week to further support protein levels.

Sample Menu

DAY 1

Before breakfast	Fat Flush Lemon Water*
Breakfast	Spiced Mocha-Choca Smoothie*
Midmorning snack	Handful of almonds with ½ cup cottage cheese
Lunch	Salmon salad with celery, scallions, and parsley with Macadamia Mayo*; baked potato drizzled with 1 tablespoon flaxseed

	oil and 1 tablespoon ground flax seeds; leafy green salad with avocado and apple cider vinegar
4 p.m. snack	½ banana
Dinner	Slow Cooker Beef Stew* (make enough for next day's lunch); steamed yellow squash, beets, ½ teaspoon cinnamon, and 1 tablespoon hemp seeds

DAY 2

Before breakfast	8 ounces Fat Flush Lemon Water*
Breakfast	Sweet Potato Hash* with poached eggs topped with 1 tablespoon hemp seeds
Midmorning snack	Celery stalks stuffed with 1 tablespoon almond butter and sliced avocado
Lunch	Leftover Slow Cooker Beef Stew*; steamed broccoli, zucchini, and okra with 1 tablespoon flaxseed oil
Midafternoon snack	1 cup mixed berries; 1 ounce string cheese
Dinner	Baked halibut with lemon, parsley, and ginger; ½ cup brown rice drizzled with 1 tablespoon sesame oil and 1 tablespoon ground flax seeds; spinach sautéed in bone broth with garlic

DAY 3

Before breakfast	Fat Flush Lemon Water*
Breakfast	½ cup melon cubes and handful of chopped walnuts blended in ½ cup ricotta cheese
Midmorning snack	Celery, jicama, and carrot sticks
Lunch	Sardines (or mackerel or tuna fish) with chopped tomato, avocado, parsley, 1 tablespoon chia seeds, and scallions; 1 small corn on the cob rubbed with ½ teaspoon umeboshi paste
Midafternoon snack	2 plums
Dinner	Slow Cooker Cuban Ropa Vieja* (make enough for next day's lunch); medley of warmed hearts of palm, yellow squash, and

1 tablespoon hemp seeds; escarole with ½
cup quinoa

DAY 4

Before breakfast	8 ounces Fat Flush Lemon Water*
Breakfast	Strawberry Banana Rhubarb Smoothie*
Midmorning snack	1 apple; 1 ounce Swiss cheese
Lunch	Leftover Slow Cooker Cuban Ropa Vieja*; steamed Swiss chard and okra; shredded red and green cabbage with 1 tablespoon olive oil
Midafternoon snack	1 warmed or toasted Ezekiel 4:9 Tortilla with butter
Dinner	Bombay Curry Tofu* over ½ cup brown rice with toasted pumpkin seeds; mixed greens salad with 1 tablespoon flaxseed oil, avocado, and 1 tablespoon hemp seeds

DAY 5

Before breakfast	Fat Flush Lemon Water*
Breakfast	Poached eggs and avocado topped with 1 tablespoon salsa on 1 warm corn tortilla drizzled with 1 tablespoon flaxseed oil
Midmorning snack	1 cup Greek yogurt with ¼ teaspoon vanilla extract, 1 tablespoon toasted sunflower seeds, and 1 tablespoon chia seeds; 1 small kiwi
Lunch	Broiled sea bass with lemon and garlic; sliced cucumbers and tomatoes with dill and 1 tablespoon olive oil with ½ cup millet; 1 cup miso soup
Midafternoon snack	Fat Flush Hummus* with celery sticks
Dinner	Friendly Italian Wedding Soup*; vegetable mélange of asparagus tips, 1 tablespoon ground flax seeds, ½ cup baby carrots, and green beans drizzled with 1 tablespoon flaxseed oil

DAY 6

Before breakfast	Fat Flush Lemon Water*
Breakfast	Cherry-Vanilla Smoothie*

Midmorning snack	½ cup cantaloupe cubes with 1 tablespoon almond butter
Lunch	Chicken salad with 1 tablespoon Macadamia Mayo* with tarragon, steamed artichoke, 1 tablespoon hemp seeds, and ½ cup peas; baby greens with lemon juice
Midafternoon snack	1 toasted Ezekiel 4:9 Tortilla with ½ cup cottage cheese and sliced avocado
Dinner	Grilled lamb chops with cinnamon and coriander; ½ cup steamed peas and romaine lettuce, hearts of palm, and tomato salad with apple cider vinegar and toasted sesame seeds

DAY 7

Before breakfast	8 ounces Fat Flush Lemon Water*
Breakfast	½ grapefruit; scrambled eggs with mushrooms and onions and 1 slice melted cheddar cheese, topped with 1 tablespoon chia seeds
Midmorning snack	1 Granny Smith apple
Lunch	Tofu and vegetable stir-fry: tofu, water chestnuts, bok choy, avocado, and bamboo shoots sautéed in 1 tablespoon sesame oil; ½ cup brown rice with 1 tablespoon hemp seeds
Midafternoon snack	Fruity Fruit Sorbet*
Dinner	Basic Stir-Fry* sautéed in 1 tablespoon coconut oil; spaghetti squash with toasted sunflower seeds; baby greens with lemon juice

The fiber with cran-water has regulated me. It made me aware of the damage I was doing to my body by thinking that a bowel movement every few days was okay and allowing the toxins to be reabsorbed into my body. Also, I used to eat ice all day long—even with meals. I had no idea that was shocking my body to hang on to toxins.

—Shelia C.

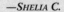

9 The Power of Ritual

*So many times I am asked for the secret of my longevity.
I can assure you, there are no secrets. There is only the
understanding of nature and the everyday practice
of nature's laws.*

—DR. HAZEL PARCELLS, ON HER 106TH BIRTHDAY

Now that you understand the foundation of the Fat Flush Plan, let me introduce you to another equally important aspect of the program. Four distinct rituals—moderate exercise, sleep, journaling, and therapeutic bathing—are included to help maximize your individual weight loss journey. Practicing them faithfully will empower you to do your best and reach your goals—and feel and look better than ever!

Please practice the pleasure principle. Fat Flush rituals will help you accomplish this: the basic nurturing of your body through the body-mind connection, a primary focus. This means giving yourself permission to enjoy the full gamut of self-care, from health-promoting food and physical fitness to stress relief, proper sleep, aromatherapy, and advanced wellness practices.

Your physiology and your psychology are a part of a complex interplay that largely determines your overall health. You know that stress is stress, regardless of whether it has a physical or psychological origin, and excessive stress can make you sick. No matter what you do to improve your physical health, if you ignore things like anxiety and depression, you will likely not achieve whole body health nor be able to fully enjoy the benefits of a healthy body.

The good news is that you can use the mind-body connection to your advantage. Taking care of your physical health will improve your psychological health, and tending to spiritual, emotional, and mental health will improve your physical health right down to your DNA. Every time you do something kind for your body—eating right, exercising, journaling, getting enough sleep—you send a subconscious signal to yourself that you *are* a worthwhile person who deserves to be taken care of.

Reclaiming the right to care for yourself is fundamental to a successful, rewarding life. It also is the stepping-stone toward enjoying positive, meaningful interactions with others and with yourself. Nurturing your Fat Flush experience with these prime rituals will help you to stay focused, reduce stress, and develop better lifestyle management habits so that you don't have to be on a perpetual diet for the rest of your life. And isn't that a welcomed relief?

EXERCISE

When it comes to exercising on the Fat Flush Plan, less is definitely more—and with good reason. It's true that exercise might very well be a form of potent medicine to level out blood sugar and encourage your cells to become less insulin resistant. Regular, moderate exercise heightens endurance, increases muscle tone and flexibility, encourages disease resistance, and acts as a natural antidepressant. Bumping up your workout to a more strenuous level, however, doesn't increase these benefits. In fact, mounting evidence suggests that strenuous exercise can endanger your health and can even be deadly—particularly if your cortisol levels are already sky high. High-intensity aerobic exercise halts metabolism and can speed up tissue breakdown.

Getting more than two hours of strenuous, nonstop activity on a daily basis can elevate cortisol levels, encouraging weight gain and heightened stress levels—the exact opposite of the Fat Flush Plan's goals! For women, extended exercise of this type can impede estrogen production and result in a loss of bone strength, particularly in thin or slight-framed women. And even if exercise is reduced and estrogen levels become more regulated, a woman is still left with a 20 percent bone loss. Repeating this cycle along with a diet rich in mineral "robbers" (such as sugar, coffee, and soda) creates a stage for premature bone thinning before menopause even starts. This is one of the reasons why moderation is the key to smart exercise and diet during your twenties and thirties—before you cross the threshold of the forties and fifties, where the bone-protecting benefits of estrogen and progesterone wane.

There are, however, other reasons why women should think twice about overexercising. Maintaining a strenuous workout regimen also increases the loss of body fat. I know, that sounds like a good thing, but loss of body fat can cause hormones to plummet. If a hormonal deficiency occurs, bone loss can be expected. Also, the increase in fat loss drains estrogen stores, producing irregular menses or a cessation of menses altogether. You frequently will see this unfortunate scenario in professional athletes, such as body builders, runners, and ballet dancers, who are able to turn their periods on or off with a three- to five-pound weight gain or loss.

As a matter of fact, it would be wise for any woman addicted to exercise in her teens and twenties, and who missed around one-third or more of her regular menses, to have her bone density checked. It's not unusual for women in their late twenties and early thirties to confuse this hormonal imbalance resulting from overexercise with the onset of perimenopause.

Another factor in support of moderate workouts is that overexercising, like canola oil and other polyunsaturated fats, augments oxidative stress in your body. This creates free radicals—those mad molecules that damage tissue in your body. High-intensity training generates a superabundance of these malevolent free radicals, found to be the cause of over 50 diseases. In time, they debilitate your immune system and make you more vulnerable to premature aging, heart attacks, cataracts, infections, and a number of cancers.

I will never forget the startling research I came across from Kenneth Cooper, MD—the "father" of the fitness movement and previous proponent of strenuous exercise—that appears to strongly support findings that show the dangers of overexercising. President and founder of the Cooper Aerobics Center in Dallas, Texas, he discovered that the damage done by free radicals generated during periods of overexercise could contribute to premature aging. His extensive findings were so revealing that he took a U-turn from his earlier belief in hard workouts, declaring that only 30 minutes of low-intensity exercise three to four times per week actually is healthier. Cooper's research shows that low- to moderate-intensity exercise is just as beneficial as high-intensity exercise—but without the rigorous wear and tear on the system.

Cooper's groundbreaking work in his book, *The Antioxidant Revolution*, describes his concern over the early onset of cancer and untimely deaths of world-class and other highly trained athletes. Jim Fixx, the highly regarded marathon runner, is one such example. Fixx suddenly dropped dead after a 4-mile run in Vermont. According to his autopsy, his arteries were almost blocked. This probably sounds surprising for a man who ran 37,000 miles in nearly 20 years and 60 miles per week up until his death. The cause of his death could be traced to an overproduction of exercise-induced free radicals, which can instigate coronary artery disease along with other deadly conditions.

Another major reason that the Fat Flush fitness prescription only recommends light to moderate exercise is that many women already have compromised adrenals. Compromised adrenals create high cortisol levels, and more exercise will add injury to insult. Even though exercise can reduce cortisol levels over time, it does increase them in the short term. The more strenuous the exercise, the greater the cortisol production. Keeping the exercise light allows for the body to experience its positive, stress-busting benefits without the detrimental and counterproductive effects of overexertion.

Most of all, you won't be doing strenuous exercises on the Fat Flush Plan because your body will be undergoing cleansing as it sheds those extra pounds. It is important to conserve antioxidants rather than expel them through strenuous exercise because they are your best tool for helping cleanse your liver. Thus, they are, in reality, your fat-burning friends. And since your caloric intake is lower on the first two phases of the program, you won't have the energy you need to tackle harder workouts. Instead, you will start with low to moderate activity designed to help you accelerate weight loss, and then you will graduate to a longer—yet moderate and balanced—routine that includes weight resistance.

Fat Flush Exercise Plan

You are entirely welcome to maintain your current yoga and Pilates practice. In addition to these, you'll find the plan's exercises simple, enjoyable, effective, and healthy—the direct opposite of overexercising. And you can do them right at home, easily fitting them into your schedule. You'll start off with bouncing and brisk walking in phases 1 and 2 and then add weight training in phase 3. Here are some of the ways the Fat Flush Exercise Plan benefits your weight loss goals:

✓ IT KEEPS CELLULAR WASTES MOVING, CAUSING BETTER ELIMINATION. In particular, the exercises targeting your lymph system—like rebounding or jumping on a mini-trampoline—help stop toxins from overrunning your body. Rebounding may also aid in diabetes prevention according to new studies measuring fasting blood sugar, A1C levels, and blood pressure. Exercise allows you to enjoy a sense of well-being and makes you less prone to weight gain. Consequently, your liver can operate optimally doing what it does best: burn fat. Exercise also helps blood, nutrients, and fresh oxygen reach each body cell to keep your body humming along. It also aids digestion, absorption, metabolism, and food assimilation and improves enzyme stores.

✓ IT BURNS THROUGH CALORIES. A 30-minute brisk walk burns 300 calories, adding up to 2,100 calories a week. This is a sufficient amount to oxidize almost a pound of fat—or 35 pounds annually. And since exercise increases muscle mass, it further helps burn calories because muscle tissue uses more of them for energy.

✓ IT REVS UP YOUR METABOLISM, MAKING YOU FEEL REVITALIZED. Recent research indicates that aerobic routines keep your metabolism elevated for 4 to 12 hours after you quit exercising, burning nearly as many calories as your workout did. And when you exercise, your body releases natural mood elevators called endorphins. They make you feel good and in control, which reduces your potential for overeating because of depressed emotions.

✓ IT HELPS CURB CRAVINGS. According to a California State University study, going for a 10-minute brisk walk prior to every meal can quench those snack impulses. Exercising also suppresses those cravings tied to uncomfortable emotions and stress. It encourages serotonin, dopamine, and norepinephrine production; these neurotransmitters help tranquilize the body up to four hours after working out. Anxiety is relieved, and you keep your appetite in control. In addition, exercise reduces blood sugar levels, increasing the effectiveness of insulin for muscle and fat cells. Steady blood sugar levels balance hormones, reduce the desire to snack on those problem carbohydrates, and prevent insulin-related fat storage.

✓ IT BUMPS UP YOUR ENERGY LEVEL. It enhances your circulation and stimulates hormone production, such as testosterone, a hormone that invigorates everyone—men and women. When your body is energized, you stay active. And when you're active, you are less likely to be hanging out in the kitchen.

✓ IT REDUCES STRESS. As I have alluded to, exercise bathes your brain with a burst of endorphins, your body's own version of the painkiller morphine, creating a serene feeling that runners affectionately call a "runner's high." While the act of exercising raises cortisol levels, exercise, when done in an appropriate amount, actually decreases cortisol levels in the long run. During exercise, your body learns to metabolize cortisol more efficiently—a skill it carries into the rest of every area of life, even when not exercising. Exercise also indirectly lowers cortisol levels by improving your ability to sleep and by building a healthier body with less vulnerability to stress.

FLUSH FLASH

Before beginning this or any other exercise program, please consult your physician.

> *I'm a 43-year-old woman, who has always been looking toward better health. But through life's many transitions, I have found myself depressed, unfocused, bloated, and eventually gaining 10 pounds on my once toned body frame. Lately, I've been exhausted, tired, and lacking any motivation to do regular activities or even pursue anything new. Fat Flush came at a critical time when I needed to shift from what was becoming an unhealthy cycle. Exercise has always been in my regimen, but that alone wasn't working, so I started your program. I notice a huge, huge difference! I've lost weight, gained energy, and am much more alert.*
>
> —SUZANNE P.

Phase 1 Exercise Program

Goal: Working the Lymphatics

✓ WARM-UPS AND STRETCHING. Whenever you're going to exercise, even if it is just going for a walk, be sure to always begin your session by warming up your muscles for 5 to 10 minutes by marching in place and swinging your arms back and forth. Then spend 5 to 10 minutes gently stretching your muscles, ligaments, and tendons to improve flexibility and prevent potential injury, muscle strains, and stiffness. Stretch your arms, your legs, your inner thighs, etc., by holding each stretch pose for 15 seconds and building up to a minute as you gain more flexibility.

✓ BOUNCING OFF FAT. As you learned in Chapter 2, purifying the lymphatic system is vital for ridding your body of cellulitelike deposits during phase 1 of the Fat Flush. Since it doesn't have a pump like the heart, the lymphatic system has to be exercised, relying on muscle contractions for its flow via the thighs and arms. The best way to do this, and to help dissolve those fatty deposits, is by cleansing your lymphatic system either with a bouncing action or by moving your arms while walking briskly.

To give your lymphatic drainage system a complete cellular cleansing during all phases of Fat Flush, I'd like you to consider purchasing a mini-trampoline (or small rebounder). These units typically stand 8 inches from the floor and are anywhere from 36 to 40 inches in diameter. You'll bounce on it every day for five minutes to gently ease waste materials out of the lymphatic system. The greatest thing about this lymph-cleansing exercise is that virtually anyone can do it, regardless of age or certain physical challenges. Individuals who can't walk can still benefit from this exercise by sitting on the rebounder while someone else bounces on it.

Use of a mini-trampoline (or rebounder) has proved to be an efficient form of exercise with virtually no harmful side effects. Your cardiovascular fitness will excel, and you will be toning your body at the same time. Bouncing fires up cellular metabolism, energizing every cell with fresh oxygen and nutrients. The low impact (such as the light pressure on the thighs) stimulates drainage, easing waste material out of the lymphatic system. In approximately two weeks, you should notice that your legs, buttocks, and ankles are becoming toned and those orange peel–like cellulite deposits are smoothing out.

You can help improve your lymph flow by (1) breathing deeply through your nose, letting oxygen into the lower part of your lungs, (2) not sitting for extended periods, which restricts lymphatic flow in your thoracic cavity, and (3) not overdoing your exercise routine, which augments oxidative stress.

I think you'll find bouncing to be a lot of fun. The great thing about it is that you can do it anywhere you live—an apartment or home—and you can even take your mini-trampoline outside.

Bouncing Tips

✓ CLOTHING. No special clothing is required. Select comfortable apparel that won't interfere with your bouncing routine or get caught in the unit.

✓ FEET. Bounce barefoot for freer movements and control. Avoid wearing socks, nylons, or slippery shoes or slippers. If you must wear shoes, choose ones with rubber, nonskid soles.

✓ TECHNIQUE. Strive for at least 100 jumping jacks (approximately five minutes) for the first half of the rebounding workout. With legs together and arms down at your sides, leap up. As you come back down to the trampoline, spread your legs and throw your arms above your head. Keeping that position, jump up again—but this time when you come down, go back to your beginning position of legs together and hands to your sides.

✓ PLACEMENT. Keep your mini-trampoline handy so you'll be encouraged to use it. Bounce in a well-lit area. Exercising in front of a mirror is a good way to perfect your technique.

Walking for Health. The next part of your phase 1 exercise regimen is a 20-minute brisk walk, which I would like you to get into the habit of doing every day or at least five times per week. Walk briskly with your arms swinging along your sides in sync with your pace to keep the lymphatic system moving. Distance is not important—your time, however, is.

An aerobic exercise, brisk walking keeps your heart and lungs strong, promoting cardiovascular health, energy, endurance, and the production of endorphins. As a matter of fact, the United States and Japan released studies demonstrating that individuals who walked habitually had two times the reduction in mortality rate and complications related to coronary artery disease of their more sedentary counterparts.

A Note About Running. During this gentle Fat Flush phase, I do not want you using your energy reserves for any kind of overly strenuous movement. For this reason, I am asking you not to run. Too strenuous an exercise, like running or heavy weight lifting, distracts your body's resources from its primary job of cleansing. Use phase 1 as a relaxing reward for a body that usually works so hard. I promise, your increased energy and enhanced performance during your workouts will justify giving your body this short, restorative reprieve. Don't worry; you will start to reincorporate cardio of a higher intensity in phase 2.

Monitoring Intensity. As I have said, phase 1 is a critical period for your body's rejuvenation. So to maximize its benefit, it is a good idea to monitor the intensity of your workout. You can do this a number of ways.

An easy method is to pace yourself, walking approximately 1 to 1.5 miles in 20 minutes. Walking any quicker stimulates additional oxidative stress. Breathe deeply and regularly through your nose during your workout to help reduce potential damage from free radicals.

If you are walking on a treadmill, keep your pace generally between three and four miles per hour. Everyone has a different body and fitness level, so definitions of "brisk" can vary from person to person. On a scale of 1 to 10— 1 meaning sitting and 10 meaning maximum exertion—you should be between 3 and 4.

You may even want to try a more technical approach, which I will strongly encourage in phase 3. You can track your pulse rate while exercising to ensure that the intensity of your workout falls within certain zones of your maximum heart rate, called max HR.

You can do this quite easily by first figuring your max HR, which requires nothing more than subtracting your age from 220. For instance, if you are 32 years old, your max HR would be 188 beats per minute.

For phase 1 of your Fat Flush exercise program, I recommend keeping your heart rate at 50 percent of your max HR or slightly above. Thus, if your max HR is 188 beats per minute, then 50 percent of this number would equal a heart rate of 94. (If you don't want to do the math, look up your age in Table 9.1. Column 2 shows your max HR; columns 3, 4, and 5 show the pulse

Table 9.1 Assessing Your Heart Rate

ASSESSING YOUR HEART RATE				
AGE, YEARS	MAXIMUM HEART RATE, BEATS PER MINUTE	TARGET HEART RATE, BEATS PER MINUTE		
		50 PERCENT	60 PERCENT	70 PERCENT
15–19	201	100	121	140
20–24	196	98	118	137
25–29	191	96	115	133
30–34	186	93	112	130
35–39	181	91	109	126
40–44	176	88	106	123
45–49	171	86	103	120
50–54	166	83	100	116
55–59	161	81	97	113
60–64	156	78	94	109
65–69	151	76	91	106
70–74	146	73	88	102
75–80	141	71	85	99

rates for the 50, 60, and 70 percent zones. Use the number in column 3, the 50 percent zone, for phase 1 of the exercise plan.)

How can you determine your heart rate (beats per minute)? Just check your pulse rate while exercising. You can do this by using a heart rate monitor strapped around your chest, a smart watch with a built-in monitor, or an app on your phone, or you can feel your pulse rate via your radial artery on the underside of your wrist. With this last method, you place your index and middle fingers on the thumb side of your wrist, count the beats for 30 seconds, and multiply that number by 2. (A quicker but less accurate method is to take your pulse for 6 seconds and then add a zero after that number. For example, 14 beats with a zero added at the end is 140.)

Keeping within the 50 and 60 percent zones is especially good for people who are walking or for individuals who are breaking into an exercise program for the first time, even though it isn't intense enough to reap broader cardiovascular benefits. Also, exercising within these zones has demonstrated an ability to reduce body fat, cholesterol, and blood pressure levels and lessen the potential for strains, injuries, and degenerative disease. At this intensity level, 85 percent of the calories you burn are fat, 10 percent are carbohydrate, and 5 percent are protein.

Rule of Thumb. Whatever your target heart rate is, you should exercise only at a level that lets you breathe and move comfortably—and that is safe for your body.

When you actually take your walk is entirely up to you. However, mornings before breakfast seem to be the best fat-burning choice for most of us. Before breakfast, the level of glycogen (carbohydrate storage of fuel in the liver) runs low, causing your body to choose fat instead for its energy. As it is busy using up these stored fatty acids, your body becomes a fat-eating machine.

PHASE 1 FAT FLUSH EXERCISE WRAP-UP

Warm-up and stretching	At least 5 minutes every session
Bouncing	10 minutes daily
Brisk walking	20–30 minutes, 5–7 times a week
Cool-down	At least 5 minutes every session

I was on the program for a few days when I noticed the cellulite lumps on my upper arms had noticeably diminished! Now I can see those triceps I've been exercising so hard for.

—ANN V. LEIGH

The Fat Flush Plan has worked a true miracle on me. I'm 28 and quite overweight. I sit behind a computer under fluorescent lights all day. I lost 16 pounds, my skin cleaned up, my eyes are brighter, and my hair looks better than it's looked in a while.

—GEORGIA ANNA RODRIGUEZ

Phase 2 Exercise Program

Goal: Building Endurance

During this phase of your Fat Flush Plan, you will continue your phase 1 exercise routine, but you will add another 10 minutes to your brisk walking time. You will also start to add high-intensity interval training (HIIT) into your workout to effectively increase cardiovascular strength with less impact on your body.

If you are keeping tabs on your heart rate, you may want to try upping your exercise intensity slightly, to 60 percent of your max HR. Using the preceding example, if your max HR is 188 beats per minute, your pulse rate while exercising would be 60 percent of that, or 112 beats per minute. If you are using a treadmill, keep the pace between 3.4 and 4.0 miles per hour. On the exertion scale, you should be at a 4 or 5.

Working within this zone helps your body to access stored fat for energy. As a result, you will burn more calories while at the same time helping your cardiovascular system become more fit. Approximately 85 percent of the calories you burn will be fat, along with 10 percent carbohydrates and 5 percent protein.

Runners rejoice! In phase 2, I want you to practice HIIT one to two times per week for 5 to 10 minutes. HIIT consists of alternating intervals of all-out exertion and little to no exertion. Studies have shown that a short period of HIIT is equally as effective as 30 to 45 minutes (if not more) of moderate exercise in increasing cardiovascular and respiratory fitness, as well as providing many of the other benefits of exercise. That's right—in a fraction of the time, HIIT increases endurance and improves insulin sensitivity. Incredible.

You will use intervals of 30 seconds, meaning 30 seconds of maximum exertion followed by 30 seconds of low exertion or rest. This can be done with a variety of different activities. For our purpose, I recommend running or cycling. I still want you to warm up, stretch, and cool down with every HIIT session. You can even incorporate HIIT intervals into your brisk walking, adding them before or after a walk.

Though they may be short, HIIT intervals are hard. Do not feel the need to overexert yourself. You are still in the cleansing process and should treat your body gently. If five intervals once a week is what feels right, start there. You have the rest of your life to work up to more intervals, more frequently.

PHASE 2 FAT FLUSH EXERCISE WRAP-UP

Warm-up and stretching	At least 5 minutes every session
Bouncing	10 minutes daily
Brisk walking	30–40 minutes, 5–7 times a week
HIIT	5–10 minutes, 1–2 times a week
Cool-down	At least 5 minutes every session

I have followed the Fat Flush Plan with great success! I don't know how much weight I've lost—I don't weigh myself—but I now have great muscle definition, more energy, and skin that is getting more radiant every day. Thank you!

—KATIE M.

Phase 3 Exercise Program

Goal: Strengthening Muscle Mass

Now that you have graduated to the lifestyle phase of the Fat Flush Plan, you are ready to build on your phase 1 and 2 foundation. The endurance you have developed over the last several weeks, along with the added fuel from the foods you are reintroducing, lays the groundwork for expanding your exercise regimen.

Your brisk walk also will extend 10 minutes, to a total of 40 minutes five times a week. And if you haven't already been doing it, now is the time to watch your target heart rate for the entire walk.

Try to move up to 70 percent of your max HR (the figure in the last column of Table 9.1). Training at 70 percent or slightly higher (to 80 percent) puts you in the aerobic zone, where half your burned calories are from fat, almost half are from carbohydrates, and less than 1 percent are from protein.

If you are a runner, cycler, or any other kind of higher-intensity athlete, you can begin to ease back into your training regime, replacing your walks with your activity of choice.

HIIT intervals increase to 10 to 15 minutes, two to three times per week. Consider practicing your intervals with new activities. If you usually complete your HIIT workouts running on a treadmill or sprinting outside, maybe hop on a bicycle or try indoor spinning. Bored of cycling? Try rowing. You can apply the HIIT concept to almost any form of exercise.

Varying your activities will help both enhance your fitness by challenging your body in new ways and keep you from getting bored with your same old exercise routine. When trying any new activity, be sure to get proper instruction on how to do it correctly. Improper execution of any kind of exercise can lead to injury.

You'll also be topping off your lifestyle regimen with a new exercise to tone and sculpt your body: weight training.

Weight Training.   I am not talking about bulking up here. Even using two- to five-pound dumbbells can help you build lean muscle mass. And remember, muscle accelerates metabolism and burns calories longer, even while you sleep.

Maintaining lean muscle mass is especially important for women, because we tend to lose ¼ to ⅓ pound of muscle every year past age 35. And if you're a woman who is thinking that you'll soon have Mr. America–type arms, don't. High testosterone levels are responsible for those muscular physiques. Since women don't have to contend with high levels of this hormone, weight training actually will help to improve the tone and strength of your muscles as well as strengthen your musculoskeletal system.

You should weight-train at least twice a week or up to every other day. Start out by following a regimen created by a professional. You don't have to sign up for a personal trainer; you could find programs online, download an app, buy a video or book, or even go to the library to access the information.

Weight-training routines tend to isolate certain muscle groups. Typically, your workout would focus on different groups at least once a week. You may want to consider varying your routine over time to work your muscles differently.

If you start with lower weights (2 to 5 pounds), you will have to do more repetitions than if you were already lifting 10-pound weights (your goal). As you increase your muscle mass—and fat-burning potential—your actual weight may not budge a whole lot, because muscle weighs more than fat. This is okay, because you are reducing body fat, which is your objective. Studies reveal that weight-training women generally add 3 to 5 pounds of muscle and lose the same amount of fat pounds. Quite often women drop one or two dress sizes, thanks to their more toned bodies.

Weight-Training Tips

✓ CLOTHING. Choose apparel that doesn't impede movement. Dress for the room temperature.

✓ SHOES. Wear comfortable shoes with good traction.

✓ WATER. Drink plenty of water before, during, and after your workout to avoid dehydration. Feel free to drink more than your allotted 48 ounces of plain water on phase 3 for this purpose. In warm weather or dry climates, drink sufficient water before you begin exercising to replace what will be lost in perspiration. Generally, figure on drinking a quart of water per 100 pounds of body weight.

✓ ROUTINE

- Follow a program designed by a certified expert.
- Work different muscles on different days, taking a day off in between. Try working your chest, shoulders, and biceps one time, then your triceps and back two days later. Then, two days after that, target your lower body.
- Keep your back straight while lifting.
- Lift weights of a reasonable amount slowly with proper form. Quality is better than quantity, and strong is better than injured.
- Breathe out when you lift, and breathe naturally to keep muscles oxidized. Avoid holding your breath as you lift, since it hinders the flow of blood in and out of the brain.
- Take three or four seconds to lift the weights and even longer to lower them.
- Start with lighter weights, increasing poundage by either 1-pound, 2-pound, or 5-pound increments each workout to a total of 10-pound weights.

Double Your Fat-Burning Power. Lifting weights uses glycogen for energy. Thus, after you're done using your weights, it would be a good time to do some aerobic exercise to burn even more fat—such as taking a brisk walk. The aerobic activity causes your body (now low in glycogen from lifting weights) to use fatty acids for fuel, similar to how it reacts to exercise before breakfast.

You may want to consider moving your combination weight training and brisk walk to later in the afternoon to accelerate calorie loss another notch. Apparently, our muscles and joints tend to be more limber between 3 and 5 p.m., which is the same time our airways are more open and we breathe more easily. This combination causes us to feel good and actually burn through a higher amount of calories per minute—with less effort.

PHASE 3 FAT FLUSH EXERCISE WRAP-UP

Warm-up and stretching	At least 5 minutes every session
Bouncing	10 minutes daily
Brisk walking	40–60 minutes, 5 times a week
HIIT	10–15 minutes, 2–3 times a week
Weight training	10–15 minutes, at least twice a week or every other day
Cool-down	At least 5 minutes every session

Dr. Ann Louise is a wealth of knowledge on all things nutrition and health. As a woman's health and fitness expert, I like to keep abreast of all the current research to stay well informed so I can better serve my clientele. If I have an unanswered question on nutrition or health, I can always look to Ann Louise and trust she will have the answer, because she is always on the leading edge. I own a copy of every book she has ever written and highly recommend them. Dr. Ann Louise has been a mentor to me and a huge inspiration in the direction I have taken my health and fitness career and for that I will be forever grateful. I was honored to collaborate with Ann Louise on the fitness portion of her book Fat Flush for Life. *Ann Louise Gittleman is the top expert in her field, and she is always my first go-to when I want to catch up on the latest scientific breakthrough.*

—LINDA MITCHELL, CEO OF CHICKFIT AND
AUTHOR OF THE SISTERHOOD OF S.W.E.A.T.

SLEEP

You may not think of sleep as a key component of weight loss, but it definitely is. Our bodies run on a biological clock. Every cell is tuned in to this biorhythmic clock, relying on it for metabolic processes, such as your hormone levels, blood sugar levels, metabolic rates, sodium and potassium levels, and even your body temperature and your immune functions—all of which greatly influence the hidden weight gain factors.

Getting to bed and rising at specific times are vital to the success of these body functions. If your lifestyle isn't in sync with your biological clock, your health, well-being, and (believe it or not) weight loss goals suffer. Without sleep, your internal sensors go awry, which actually can cause you to overeat. According to statistics, poor sleepers consume approximately 15 percent more food than their sleep-nourished counterparts. Without proper sleep, they often feel tired and grab high-carbohydrate "comfort" foods, which are also high in sugar, to boost energy. Their bodies also begin to store fat, taking the fatigue as a signal that a crisis is approaching.

When you get a restful, deep sleep, energy levels are restored and hormones are reset. However, poor sleep does more than cause a drop in your energy level—it also creates problems with your hormones. In fact, University of Chicago researchers say that lack of sleep could even make you flabby. Some scientists believe that poor sleep impedes surges of growth hormone, which is needed to promote lean muscle tissue and reduce body fat, resulting in a deficiency.

Compounding the problem, insufficient sleep puts your body under stress, forcing your cortisol level to rise. As you learned in Chapter 2, cortisol works in concert with other hormones to quicken fat storage, targeting the central fat cells. It releases glucose and fatty acids so that muscles have energy—and consequently stimulates your appetite to encourage you to replenish fuel. When your twenty-first-century lifestyle causes you to become sleep-deprived (thanks to having a crazy work schedule, juggling two jobs, getting a degree, and managing a family), your cortisol level stays elevated. As a result, you may find yourself wanting to grab a late-night snack, such as some sugary food. Unfortunately, that only aggravates the situation by promoting even more cortisol production.

For most of us Americans, this spells trouble because we have embraced a new 24-hour mentality. We are busy around the clock nowadays—spending more time shopping at all-night convenience stores, grocery markets, or national-chain superstores. And, of course, there is the Internet. Online shopping is an addiction in a class all its own. I have friends who stay up deep into a night lit by little more than a computer screen, combing designer discount sites for the perfect deal. We use this never-ending wireless ecosystem to stay connected with others through social media, play online games, do our banking, take courses, make travel arrangements, search an infinite number of topics, chitchat with friends, and read articles into the wee hours of the morning. With the now global takeover of handheld devices that have access to the Internet, we have little reason to look up from our screen anymore, much less do something radical like close our eyes and get an adequate amount of sleep.

According to a poll conducted by Gallup in 2013, 40 percent of Americans get less than 6 hours of sleep per night. That's almost half the people in the country putting undue stress on their bodies and functioning at a suboptimal level. Moreover, Gallup has consistently found this number since 1990. The average amount of sleep that all Americans get falls short as well, coming in at around 6.8 hours since 1990. Keeping in mind these statistics, the persistence and severity of the obesity epidemic in the United States might make a little more sense.

It is a vicious cycle that strikes a familiar chord, especially in women, who tend to suffer the most. Their sleeping habits are often affected by hormonal changes, menses, responsibilities of parenting, and stress from family and work. Joyce A. Walsleben, PhD, director of the Sleep Disorders Center at the New York University School of Medicine, says that "women are probably the most sleep-deprived creatures on earth. . . . The average woman aged thirty to sixty sleeps only six hours and forty-one minutes during the workweek. . . . Most people need at least eight hours of sleep to function at their best."

The founder of the *Huffington Post*, Arianna Huffington, used to be one of these sleep-deprived creatures. A workhorse like so many modern women, Huffington survived on a frighteningly meager three to four hours of sleep a night in an attempt to juggle booming success at her media empire with a personal life full of parenting two daughters. In 2007, she collapsed of exhaustion and broke her cheekbone.

For Huffington, passing out from exhaustion was the jolt she needed to get back into a healthy sleep routine. She completely changed her life to prioritize quality rest. Inspired by the benefits she experienced, she wrote a book called *The Sleep Revolution*. In a *New York Times* article, Huffington says her goal is nothing short of rekindling our romance with sleep. She views sleep as a performance enhancer, and I completely agree. In 2011, Huffington, who is also the author of 15 books, sold the *Huffington Post* to AOL for $315 million. This is certainly rich proof that getting enough sleep does not make you lazy—and, in fact, is a wise and responsible practice to help bring about your own success.

These are Arianna Huffington's "12 Tips for Better Sleep":

1. Keep your bedroom dark, quiet, and cool—between 60 and 67 degrees.
2. No electronic devices starting 30 minutes before bedtime.
3. Don't charge your phone next to your bed. Even better: gently escort all devices completely out of your bedroom.
4. No caffeine after 2 p.m.
5. Remember, your bed is for sleep and sex only—no work!
6. Sorry, Mr. Snuffles: No pets on the bed.
7. Take a hot bath with Epsom salts before bed to help calm your mind and body. [I especially love this tip of Arianna's. You will see why soon!]
8. Pajamas, nightdresses, and even special T-shirts send a sleep-friendly message to your body. If you wore it to the gym, don't wear it to bed.

9. Do some light stretching, deep breathing, yoga, or meditation to help your body and your mind transition to sleep.
10. When reading in bed, make it a real book or an e-reader that does not emit blue light. And make sure it is not work-related: novels, poetry, philosophy, anything but work.
11. Ease yourself into sleep mode by drinking some chamomile or lavender tea.
12. Before bed, write a list of what you are grateful for. It's a great way to make sure your blessings get the closing scene of the night.

Fat Flush Sleep Program

It is really quite simple. You will follow your internal biological clock, in sync with your daily rhythm of cortisol. This means going to bed by that magical hour of 10 p.m., when your cortisol levels diminish to their lowest levels, three hours after sunset. And you'll rise when your cortisol levels peak in the early morning, a refreshing eight hours later.

Understandably, you may have times when your hectic day makes it difficult to unwind. Here are some bedtime tips you may find helpful to protect your beauty rest:

Fat Flush Sleep Tips

AVOID:
Eating two hours before bedtime.
Taking a nap after 4 p.m. or for more than an hour.
Exercising too close to bedtime.
Lying in bed awake. Instead, try reading, putting on some calming music, or even meditating until you can fall asleep.
Maintaining extreme temperatures in your bedroom.

TRY:
Sleeping in a cooler room, ideally between 60 and 67 degrees Fahrenheit. A warm room impedes sleep and causes more awakenings. Use a fan or air-conditioner to keep you cool and comfortable.
Keeping your bedtime peaceful and restricting your bedroom for sleep-related activities only.
Making sure that you have a comfortable bed to sleep on.
Getting to bed and waking up the same time every day.
Waking up with the sun, if possible, to reset your internal biological clock daily. Getting an hour of morning sunlight (or using extremely bright lights in the morning) could help with falling asleep at night.
Taking a warm bath. Researchers suggest that taking a 15-minute bath in 105 degree Fahrenheit water approximately 90 minutes before going to bed is helpful. The rise in body temperature, followed by the decline in the core temperature, signals the body that it's bedtime.

JOURNALING

As I have previously encouraged you to do, the best way to keep tabs on yourself throughout your Fat Flush journey is to keep a journal. Hands down, journaling has proved to be a helpful factor in attaining weight loss goals. This certainly was the case for participants in a research study conducted by the National Weight Control Registry. These individuals, who had to lose more than 30 pounds and maintain the loss for one year at minimum in order to take part in the study, found that keeping a diet journal proved elemental to their success.

Their achievement might very well be linked to the fact that journaling creates the perfect place to discover what motivates your food desires, what triggers those cravings, and what's really going on beneath those surface feelings. By taking the time to write these things down, you'll reduce anxiety and stay in touch with yourself. Stress researcher Ann McGee-Cooper, EdD, suggests that by writing through emotions, you actually may be less likely to fall prey to stress. And since stress can lead to weight gain, journaling through those feelings could keep you from abandoning your weight and fitness objectives. Additional recent studies support this fact, indicating that 15 minutes of journaling each day can cut stress levels and even bolster the immune system by 76 percent.

So if a coworker gets you worked up, grab your Fat Flush journal, not those doughnuts. By the time you write through it, you'll feel the stress ease away and that desire for junk food fade.

Besides tracking meals, supplements, exercise, and sleep and helping you through stressful times, journaling provides numerous other opportunities for insight. You can jot down personal concerns, note changes in your health and emotions, trace the origins of specific food reactions as you reintroduce quality carbohydrates and dairy into your diet, and even find something you did each day to deserve a personal pat on the back—food related or not. Most important, journaling will help you learn more about and connect with the most important person in your life: you.

Journaling will help you improve not only your ability to function physically but also your ability to function emotionally. Health is not completely health if you don't take care of the whole self—mind, body, and spirit.

Journaling Basics

The primary tenet of journaling centers on that tried-and-true adage "Honesty is the best policy." So don't be timid. Jot down whatever words and thoughts come to mind, recording everything and anything. For instance, if you're hungry, write it down. It's not a crime. In fact, it is a rather typical response as you get started on phase 1.

And this holds true for other responses as well, such as your sinuses draining, your digestive system getting a bit upset, or your skin breaking out. Don't fret over these things. Just write them all down, because these side effects are actually good signs—and not at all unusual. They mean that your body is cleansing itself and Fat Flush is working!

Journaling will be of special help as you begin to add back foods (in phases 2 and 3). It's not uncommon for some people to notice food reactions, such as gas, bloating, sleepiness, headaches, or cramps, which can occur anywhere from 10 minutes to 12 hours after you've eaten. By honestly tracking these types of responses, you'll be able to clearly identify which foods are hidden sources of weight gain and take control of your weight loss goals.

When you journal is really up to you. Some Fat Flushers like to write things down as they occur, so they carry their journals with them throughout the day. You can also find a few moments at the end of the day if you can properly recall what you ate. In the end, you determine what will work best for your lifestyle.

Regardless of when you journal, the most important thing you can do is be kind to yourself. Don't be critical. Go back every few days, and read what you wrote and how you were feeling. This will help you learn who you are and identify positive trends you may otherwise be missing. It also will help you learn to become your own best friend.

How to Create Your Fat Flush Journal

There are several ways to get started. You can use a notebook, pick up an inexpensive journal book with blank pages at your local bookstore, or create your own journal pages on a computer to print out and insert in a nicely colored project folder.

There are several categories that I think would be especially helpful to have in your daily Fat Flush journal. However, please feel free to pick and choose whichever areas mean the most to you. I've provided a sample page from one of my Fat Flushers near the end of the chapter to give you an idea of how your journal could look. Be sure to leave yourself enough room in each category, particularly the ones where you may be inclined to write more. And always date every page for accurate referencing. There are some blank journal pages provided in the Appendix for you to photocopy and use if you wish.

Here are some areas and categories that have worked for Fat Flushers in the past:

✓ PHASES. At the top of each journal page, title it according to the Fat Flush phase you're in: "Accelerated Weight Loss" (for those in phase 1), "Metabolic Reset" (for those in phase 2), or "Lifestyle Eating" (for those in phase 3).

✓ GOALS. Determine a goal for each phase of your Fat Flush journey. Maybe you want to drop three to six inches off your hips, fit into that favorite outfit hanging in the back of your closet, decrease your anxiety, or get rid of that ugly cellulite on your thighs and buttocks. Decide what is most important to you at each phase.

Set your Fat Flush goal, visualize it, and then follow the program with your goal in front of you. Based on my experience of working with thousands of individuals, those who set goals enjoy a number of benefits. They appear to be more contented with their performances and actually perform better. Goal-oriented people also appear more self-confident, tend to worry less, and display better concentration.

Reality Check. Be good to yourself by setting realistic goals. A 40-year-old can't expect to look 25 again. Set goals that are attainable for your age, stage of life, and body frame. Tables 9.2 and 9.3 present two helpful charts to determine the average weight for women and men.

✓ REWARDS. Your awesome efforts deserve recognition, so you may want to think of a way to reward yourself for reaching the goal of each phase. Choose something you would really look forward to, such as treating yourself to a spa manicure and pedicure, buying some new clothes, or doing something else that is special. You might even want to schedule time in that busy day planner of yours to soak in a relaxing bubble bath with lighted candles and soothing music.

✓ MEALS, BEVERAGES, AND SNACKS. Jot down everything you eat, from cran-water and hot water with lemon juice to every snack and meal. Tracking your food gives you good cause to adopt the "mindful eating" approach. Instead of eating on the run or eating while doing something else—such as watching TV or reading a book—focus on your meal. Set the table, making it and your meal visually appealing. Take the time to chew the food, savoring every bite. By staying "in the now" when you eat, you'll be less likely to overeat because you'll recognize when you are full instead of mindlessly munching on more helpings. If you stay aware of your eating, you also will be able to discern why you are eating in the first place. Is it emotional or physical? Identifying the reason and writing it down empowers you to finally address the reason behind your hunger. Best of all, you will truly get pleasure from the flavor of your food as you take time to notice the flavorful sensations. What's the point of eating good food if you don't enjoy it?

✓ SUPPLEMENTS. Keep track of what you're taking and how much. Did you remember to take your multivitamin? Gamma-linolenic acid (GLA)? Bile builder? Fat burner?

✓ WEEKLY MEASUREMENTS. Once a week, measure your chest, waist, hips and thighs. Some Fat Flushers like to measure their arms, above the elbows. Remember, losing inches is the key to a slimmer you, not pounds on a scale. Inch loss reveals true fat loss, a real assessment of your progress. The scale will tend to move up and down occasionally for other reasons—such as having your period, for example.

✓ FOOD FOR THOUGHT. Jot down whatever is going on with you that is food related. For instance, did you spend the afternoon with food on the brain? Have you noticed your cravings fading away? Did you notice your-

Table 9.2 For Women

Aged 25 to 59 years Weight in pounds, per frame type (with indoor clothing weighing 3 pounds and wearing 1-inch-heeled shoes)			
HEIGHT	SMALL FRAME	MEDIUM FRAME	LARGE FRAME
4' 10"	102–111	109–121	118–131
4' 11"	103–113	111–123	120–134
5' 0"	104–115	113–126	122–137
5' 1"	106–118	115–129	125–140
5' 2"	108–121	118–132	128–143
5' 3"	111–124	121–135	131–147
5' 4"	114–127	124–138	134–151
5' 5"	117–130	127–141	137–155
5' 6"	120–133	130–144	140–159
5' 7"	123–136	133–147	143–163
5' 8"	126–139	136–150	146–167
5' 9"	129–142	139–153	149–170
5' 10"	132–145	142–156	152–173
5' 11"	135–148	145–159	155–176
6' 0"	138–151	148–162	158–179

Table 9.3 For Men

Aged 25 to 59 years Weight in pounds, per frame type (with indoor clothing weighing 3 pounds and wearing 1-inch-heeled shoes)			
HEIGHT	SMALL FRAME	MEDIUM FRAME	LARGE FRAME
5' 2"	128–134	131–141	138–150
5' 3"	130–136	133–143	140–153
5' 4"	132–138	135–145	142–156
5' 5"	134–140	137–148	144–160
5' 6"	136–142	139–151	146–164
5' 7"	138–145	142–154	149–168
5' 8"	140–148	145–157	152–172
5' 9"	142–151	148–160	155–176
5' 10"	144–154	151–163	158–180
5' 11"	146–157	154–166	161–184
6' 0"	149–160	157–170	164–188
6' 1"	152–164	160–174	168–192
6' 2"	155–168	164–178	172–197
6' 3"	158–172	167–182	176–202
6' 4"	162–176	171–187	181–207

self feeling drowsy or tired after adding carbs (in phase 2) or dairy (in phase 3)? Are you experiencing sugar or caffeine withdrawal? Did you slip off the Fat Flush wagon?

✓ HEALTH AND WELLNESS NOTES. Are your menses more regular? Is your skin clearing up and looking more radiant? Are your bowel movements regular? How are you feeling—more calm, less anxious, more energetic? Have your mood swings evened out?

✓ EXERCISE ROUTINE. How many minutes did you walk, or do the suggested trampoline workout, or spend on strength training (required in phase 3)? How did you feel during and after your exercise session? Is it getting easier each time?

✓ SLEEP TIME. Are you making it to bed by 10 p.m. and getting your eight hours of sleep?

✓ REFLECTIONS. This is the place to go when you feel like venting or talking something through, whether it's about work, your family, your weight loss, a desire to snack, etc. Use this area to jot it all down, thinking of it as your own personal sounding board—a place you can go to that is safe. No one is going to criticize you here. Then look back on it a few days later. It's a good way to learn more about who you are and what makes you tick, and what ticks you off!

✓ DAILY ACKNOWLEDGMENT. Even if you didn't do 100 percent today, reflect on what you did do, and acknowledge something good about yourself. Bolster your self-esteem and keep your momentum going by patting yourself on the back for whatever positive thing you discovered. Write down, "Today I did this well: ____," and fill in the blank. Recognize it as a good step, however small. After all, it's the little steps that lead us to those great accomplishments.

✓ GRATITUDE. Gratitude is a very powerful concept, so make it a positive habit. As Melody Beattie put it, "Gratitude unlocks the fullness of life. It turns what we have into enough and more. It turns denial into acceptance, chaos to order, confusion to clarity. It can turn a meal into a feast, a house into a home, a stranger into a friend. Gratitude makes sense of our past, brings peace for today, and creates vision for tomorrow." Aim for at least 10 things you are grateful for. If you can't do 10 quite yet, that's okay. It can take time to build up awareness of things that really make you happy in life, big or small. Start with 2 or 3, and work up to your 10.

FAT FLUSH JOURNAL

PHASE 1

MY PHASE I GOAL: *Drop 6 pounds so I can wear my favorite jeans again.*

MY PHASE I REWARD: *Get a pedicure at the new medi-spa in town.*

TODAY'S DATE: *March 30*

Meals, Beverages, & Snacks

- UPON RISING – *Had a cup hot water and lemon.*
- BREAKFAST – *Made a Blueberry Smoothie.*
- MIDMORNING SNACK – *Hard-boiled egg.*
- BEFORE LUNCH – *Had 8 oz of cran-water.*
- LUNCH – *Brought my beef stir fry to work: 4 oz lean beef with bok choy, mushrooms, and bean sprouts. Added ginger and a bit of cayenne for flavor. Also made a red-leaf salad with a few radishes, celery, fresh parsley, and some cukes. Used 1 tablespoon of flaxseed oil for dressing. Also drank 8 oz of cran-water.*
- MID-AFTERNOON SNACK – *Drank 2 glasses of cran-water (8 oz each).*
- 4 P.M. SNACK – *Had 1 pear.*
- BEFORE DINNER - *Had 8-oz of cran-water.*
- DINNER – *Made the cumin & cinnamon-scented Eggplant Delight with a side of yellow squash, asparagus, some fresh cilantro, and water chestnuts. Sautéed some greens in veggie broth with a bit of garlic.*
- MIDEVENING – *Had a cup of dandelion root tea.*

Supplements

Took my GLA-90 capsules (2 w/breakfast & 2 w/dinner). Had my multi and mineral supp w/breakfast and dinner. Took my Weight Loss formula at each meal and took two Bile Builders.

Weekly Measurements

- BUST/CHEST 36 inches
- WAIST 27 inches
- HIPS 38 inches
- THIGHS 22 inches

FOOD FOR THOUGHT – During my afternoon break with Sally and the gang, someone brought our usual Friday "snack" —a coconut cream Marie Callender pie! That was tough to turn down, but I actually felt satisfied once I had my Fat Flush snack.

HEALTH & WELLNESS NOTES – My skin is looking better than it ever has—even my husband noticed how good it looks. And I've got more energy today. I used to feel drowsy by mid-afternoon, but I actually whizzed through it with energy to spare!

EXERCISE – Went for my morning walk after I got up. It's getting easier and my mind feels clear and ready for the day.

SLEEP TIME – Got to bed a little after 10 pm. Now that I've got the temperature cooler, I'm finding it easier to sleep straight through my 8 hours.

REFLECTIONS — *Had an argument with a co-worker, who was trying to muscle in on my area to make herself look good.*

I got so upset and walked out of the office down to the vending machine. Felt so much like grabbing some cookies and a candy bar, but then decided to step outside and walk it off for a few minutes. Glad I did. It helped relieve the anger a bit and gave me time to regroup and not blow my diet with sugar!

DAILY ACKNOWLEDGMENT — *Today I twice avoided the temptation of eating my usual sugar snacks twice—and that is a great thing! Go me!*

GRATITUDE — *Today I am grateful that (1) my spouse surprised me with flowers, (2) the weather was nice on my walk this morning, (3) I get to wear my favorite pajamas to bed.*

THERAPEUTIC BATHS

On a few occasions throughout this chapter I have mentioned bathing, and now it is time for you learn to why. I cannot praise the benefits of therapeutic baths enough. Hot baths are an excellent way to reduce stress, soothe muscles, care for skin, and encourage detox by opening the pores and stimulating lymph flow—releasing toxins through perspiration. There are a few different types of baths I want you to luxuriate in, each with its unique healing properties.

Aromatherapy Baths

Adding essential oils to your bath starts with an already relaxing and health-promoting ritual and takes it to the next level. Essential oils are distilled from flowers, leaves, and roots of wild or organically grown plants. They are quickly absorbed into your body through the skin or are inhaled through your nose, and they send a soothing message to the brain, initiating feelings of well-being and harmony. These stress busters can reduce cortisol levels, decrease fat deposits and water retention, improve muscle soreness, and increase beneficial sleep. If Fat Flush had a smell, it would be the aroma of essential oils.

For Fat Flushers, the following oils provide the most healthy and beautifying benefits:

✓ ROSE. Rose oil acts as an antidepressant and anti-inflammatory that improves circulation and can help reduce heart palpitations, cravings, and stress.

✓ LAVENDER. Lavender can also reduce cravings, stress, and inflammation, as well as fight fungal infections, improve skin disorders (including acne, psoriasis, eczema, and wrinkles), lower blood pressure, and aid in digestion by stimulating production of bile and gastric juices.

✓ SANDALWOOD. Sandalwood oil relaxes the adrenal glands, which are so often fatigued, effectively lowering stress and encouraging deeper sleep.

✓ THYME. Thyme oil builds immunity, fights pathogenic bacteria, stimulates the lymphatics, reduces inflammation, and is antiparasitic.

✓ GERANIUM. Geranium oil supports adrenal function and works as an antibacterial, antifungal, antitumor, and anti-inflammatory agent.

✓ MARJORAM. Marjoram oil has a calming effect that reduces stress and can improve diabetes, irritable bowel syndrome, rheumatism, fatigue, and muscle tension.

✓ CEDARWOOD. Cedarwood oil fortifies and strengthens lungs and promotes quality sleep.

✓ ROSEMARY. Rosemary oil is especially regenerating, restorative, and detoxifying, relieving pain, stress, and indigestion.

✓ LEMON. Lemon oil improves clarity and disinfects your system; you can even use a few drops in water for a homemade household cleaning spray.

✓ JUNIPER. Juniper oil promotes toxic waste elimination with its laxative properties. It also reduces fluid retention and helps cleanse the emotions, calming an anxious mind.

✓ LEMONGRASS. Lemongrass oil tones and strengthens connective tissues, stimulates lymphatic tissues, and purges excess fluid from your system.

✓ GRAPEFRUIT. Grapefruit oil is an antimicrobial that helps dissolve fatty deposits and promotes toning and tightening of your body.

✓ PEPPERMINT. Peppermint oil alleviates flatulence, bloating, and upset stomach.

✓ CHAMOMILE. Chamomile is the ultimate calming oil and is often helpful in promoting sleep.

When adding oils to your hot bath, I recommend using 10 drops. Soak for 20 minutes at the end of the day. You can combine oils, as long as the total number of drops does not exceed 10.

It is important to check the label when purchasing essential oils. The label should state that oils have been analyzed by a gas chromatograph–mass spectrometer to ensure safety and effectiveness. This is really the only way to know that they are high quality and do not include any petrochemicals, fractions of cheaper oils, synthetic fragrance, or other degrading chemicals.

If you want the benefits of essential oils but do not have a bathtub to use them in, you can put a few drops of the oils on cold lightbulbs in lamps. The heat of the lightbulb when it is turned on will diffuse the scent. You can also purchase an oil diffuser or apply the oil directly to your skin. For skin application, apply at the pulse points and on the bottom of your feet, which is, surprisingly, the best location for absorption.

Epsom Salt Baths

Epsom salt baths are a trusty home remedy with fantastic restorative abilities for your skin and muscles. This super-salt soak also has detoxifying properties that provide a number of supplemental benefits to Fat Flushers on their health-seeking journey. The Epsom salt itself is actually magnesium sulfate, and soaking in an Epsom salt bath is an excellent way to increase the magnesium levels in your body. The sulfate half of the magnesium sulfate pair has perks all its own, helping in the formation of brain tissue, joint protein, and the strength of the digestive tract's walls. These baths will leave your body feeling better with firmer skin, more relaxed muscles, and a fitter frame.

For your Epsom salt baths, add 2 cups of Epsom salt to a tub full of hot water and soak for 20 minutes.

Castor Oil Packs

This is probably the least well known of the bathing methods, nor is it technically a bath, so allow me the privilege of introducing you to castor oil packs. Castor oil stimulates the liver and gallbladder, supporting the bile, and as well it draws toxins out of the body. Castor oil normalizes liver enzymes, decreases elevated cholesterol levels, and provides a sense of well-being. I include castor oil treatments with bathing rituals because, like the other bathing methods, you are using a healing liquid to infuse your body through the skin.

Using castor oil packs is an easy and rewarding experience. All you need is a pack of 100 percent pure, cold-pressed castor oil; wool (not cotton) flannel; and a heating pad. To take your detoxification to the next level, follow these simple steps:

1. Fold the wool flannel into three or four layers and soak it with castor oil.
2. Place the soaked flannel in a baking dish and heat it slowly in the oven until it is hot to your touch.
3. Lie down, gently rub three tablespoons of castor oil on your abdomen, and then place the soaked flannel across your abdomen.
4. Cover the soaked flannel with a plastic wrap or plastic garbage bag.
5. Finally, cover the soaked flannel with the heating pad for one hour to keep it comfortably hot.

When you finish, wash the oil from your abdomen. You can keep the oil-soaked flannel sealed in a plastic wrap or place it in a plastic storage bag for further use, since castor oil does not become rancid as quickly as many other oils.

As a gentle detox, I recommend that you use the castor oil pack once a day for three days in a row, then take three days off, and then use it for another three consecutive days. Continue this pattern every week or every other week, depending upon your liver enzyme levels. If you suffer from frequent colds, infections, or chronic fatigue syndrome, consider using the castor oil pack on a daily basis for two weeks out of every month.

Daily, weekly, and monthly rituals will soon become second nature to your Fat Flush lifestyle. As Sarah Ban Breathnach so wisely observed, "Start thinking of yourself as an artist and your life as a work-in-progress. Works-in-progress are never perfect. But changes can be made. . . . Art evolves. So does life. Art is never stagnant. Neither is life. The beautiful, authentic life you are creating for yourself is your art. It's the highest art."

10 The Fat Flush Plan Away from Home

We need to be willing to let our intuition guide us, and then be willing to follow that guidance directly and fearlessly.

—J Shakti Gawain

Like it or not, fast foods are here to stay. Eating away from home has become a way of life in our twenty-first century. In 2013, 80 percent of Americans reported eating at fast-food restaurants at least monthly, and a whopping 50 percent reported eating at these local establishments at least weekly. Furthermore, the Centers for Disease Control found that 34.3 percent of children and adolescents in the United States between the ages of 2 and 19 eat fast food on any given day. Think of the public health implication of a third of American children filtering in and out of processed food pushers every single day.

It's no wonder that the fast-food industry shelled out $4.6 billion on advertising in 2012, an 8 percent increase over 2009, according to the Yale Rudd Center for Food Policy and Obesity. In comparison, the "healthy" food categories that the Yale Rudd Center analyzed, including milk, bottled water, vegetables, and fruit, only spent a collective $367 million on advertisements. All the health food categories combined totaled to only 37.8 percent of what one famous fast-food company spent on advertising: McDonald's. The analysis found that McDonald's alone spent $972 million on advertisements in 2012. Overall, the 18 assessed fast-food companies spent 12.4 times as much on advertising than all the assessed health food categories. This "helps ensure that Americans are not more than a few steps from immediate sources of relatively non-nutritious food," according to the January–February 2000 issue of *Public Health Reports*.

Yet with a little bit of know-how, you can easily Fat Flush your way through the fast-food lane. You just need a basic road map to help you make the best food decisions. And the road map I'm talking about is far from complicated—it is quite simple, in fact. It is designed with the absolutely best fat-flushing foods, based on the foundational principles of the right protein, friendly carbohydrates, and slimming smart fats—the ultimate fat burner. You will enjoy meals that are built on such staples as eggs, lean red meat, fish, vegetables, salads, fruit, and even a little bit of butter. Fortunately, many of these foods can be found just about anywhere these days.

Convenience, however, carries a definite price. You can blow a whole day's worth of salt and calories in a single fast-food meal if you are not careful. Thus, there is some challenge in making the Fat Flush Plan work at a fast-food restaurant. On the other hand, many fast-food places offer healthier options these days, such as rotisserie-prepared chicken and turkey featured as home-style meals.

Because of the greater variety of foods available on the Lifestyle Eating Plan, it is much easier to eat out when in phase 3 than when in the first two Fat Flush phases. You can enjoy fat-flushing meals away from home if you avoid certain food items, make some savvy substitutions, and lighten up on the food combination rules.

ON THE ROAD WHILE FAT FLUSHING

Whether it is fast foods or fine dining, the food choices you make can either boost fat burning or create fat storage. It is really up to you.

By far one of the biggest challenges to eating out is avoiding the trans-fat traps. These fats include the liver-clogging, weight control–inhibiting hydrogenated oils, processed oils, margarine, and fried foods. These oils, as discussed previously, should be strictly avoided because of the trans-fatty acids and/or GMO-laden ingredients they contain. The more common foods that contain them—which you wouldn't even consider on the Fat Flush Plan anyway—include fast-food biscuits, Danish pastries, chocolate chip cookies, muffins, french fries, fried onion rings, processed cheese, mayonnaise, tartar sauce, and chicken nuggets. They are virtually everywhere!

You will recall that while no one knows for certain how much trans fat the body can actually tolerate, the daily intake should never exceed 2 grams—if at that. The problem is that the most popular fast foods are really top-heavy with those nasty trans fats. In fact, the *New York Times* reported that the late nutrition expert Mary Enig, PhD, my esteemed colleague and personal friend, found an incredible "8 g of trans-fatty acids in a large order of french fries cooked in partially hydrogenated vegetable oil, 10 g in a typical serving of fast-food fried chicken or fried fish, and 8 g in 2 ounces of imitation cheese."

Just remember that the trans fats I want you to avoid may be lurking in creamy cheese sauces and dressings, which also are loaded with plenty of regular salt and sugar. This is why I encourage you to "lemonize" your salad by simply squeezing a lemon (or lime) over it instead of a restaurant dressing if you haven't brought your own dressing.

When it comes to salad dressings, do *not* rely on the common staple of balsamic vinegar and other vinaigrettes. Vinegars, with the exception of apple cider vinegar, are one of the sneakiest sources of hidden fructose.

Recall from Chapters 2 and 3 that fructose, with its delayed insulin response, goes straight to the liver, which cannot efficiently metabolize it and deposits it as fat. This can lead to elevated triglycerides, as well as the more serious nonalcoholic fatty liver disease impacting nearly 90 million people. In addition, fructose can lead to many of the same metabolic issues as the much maligned glucose due to its impact on the liver and microbiome. Instead, opt to use a healthy oil like olive oil, flaxseed oil, or macadamia nut oil and to squeeze a lemon or lime.

As a rule of thumb, if you are on phase 3 of the Fat Flush Plan (the Lifestyle Eating Plan), choose sauces that are based on wine (the alcohol burns off in cooking) or lemon or real cream ones. Or opt for a light marinara rather than a heavy-duty cheese and tomato sauce. You can even enjoy cream soups with real cream. For those who don't tolerate dairy, go for the vegetable or tomato-based ones. And remember that on the Lifestyle Eating Plan, you also can enjoy bean soup as part of your daily quality carbs—using moderation, of course.

You will want to hold back on mayonnaise because most commercially prepared mayonnaise products are made with partially hydrogenated soybean oil. So there goes ordering those tuna, egg, shrimp, and chicken salads, as well as most coleslaw and potato salad (even for Lifestyle Fat Flushers—those on the Lifestyle Eating Plan), because they all contain mayonnaise. At home, you can make your own mayo using olive or avocado oil. When out, however, think in terms of mustard or even yogurt instead of commercial mayonnaise. A side of salsa, guacamole, or hummus (chickpea pâté made with sesame paste for Lifestyle Fat Flushers) cut with lemon juice or fresh lemons can really satisfy your taste buds. And those foods don't contain the trans-fat factors that mayonnaise-based dips do.

GOING AGAINST THE GRAIN

When it comes to bread, muffins, crackers, and rolls, try to eliminate those made with gluten-containing grains like wheat, barley, rye, and spelt. This will be next to impossible in most fast-food establishments. By the way, this also goes for pasta, especially when it is the focus of your meal. No matter what the glamorous incarnation (e.g., penne, angel hair, rigatoni, ziti, spaghetti, or macaroni), pasta is almost always made from white flour—that simple carbohydrate that is rapidly absorbed into your bloodstream and sends glucose and then fat-promoting insulin levels soaring. A better bet, whenever possible, is to order gluten-free food items, such as brown rice. And do remember that like pasta, even sourdough—which may have some redeeming qualities—is still made with white refined flour.

FATS OF LIFE

Since not all fats are considered off-limits on the Fat Flush Plan, and so many are actually crucial to cultivate health, be sure to choose foods that feature healthy fats. Olive and sesame oils are two of the oils of choice for Lifestyle Fat Flush. They are often used in many higher end restaurants, especially Italian, Greek, Spanish, and Chinese establishments. Olive oil with lemon is probably the best salad dressing you can use when eating out. Just be sure it is 100% extra virgin olive oil that has that signature string to it in the back of the throat which signifies high polyphenol content. Always order it, as well as sauces, on the side. Use just one tablespoon. You can even drizzle a little bit on your entrée as well as on your salad.

Fish and other seafood, as you know by now, are a great source of omega-3 fatty acids. You may select from a wide variety. Of course, wild caught salmon (both the Atlantic and king varieties) is the "king" of the omega-3s. You can get fresh salmon most anywhere these days, but it may be farm-raised, which is not what you want. Other high–omega-3 fish you can try include mackerel, rainbow trout, halibut, cod, haddock, tuna, and, of course, anchovies.

Although a bit salty, the underrated anchovy is high in omega-3 and omega-7 fat-burning power. Salmon and other fish can be grilled, broiled, poached, or baked in wine and seasoned with lots of fresh garlic (specify fresh; otherwise, garlic salt will be used) and onions. Some Japanese and Chinese dishes use peanut oil for stir-frying. This is also acceptable, unless, of course, you have a peanut allergy.

A delicious Fat Flush smart choice in Mexican restaurants is guacamole, which contains those beneficial fats similar to those in olive oil. Guacamole can be used as a topping, in place of sour cream or heavy cheese. Just remember to lemonize whenever and wherever you can, which I believe cuts the unhealthy fats and assists in metabolism.

The Entrée

In addition to the omega-3 poultry, beef, lamb, veal, fish, and other seafood, you also can have a tempeh or tofu dish a couple of times a week. This is always best either grilled, steamed, or stir-sautéed in the right oil.

You may want to accompany your entrée with a salad, but hold those glutenous croutons. They are made with wheat, and usually with hydrogenated oil, just like the prepared salad dressings. A double portion of steamed veggies (preferably fresh) and a friendly carb for those on phase 2 Metabolic Reset or Phase 3 Lifestyle Fat Flush (such as cooked carrots, peas, a small baked potato, brown rice, or corn on the cob with a small amount of flaxseed oil blended with real butter at the table) are good choices. Be sure to ask if that's really butter on the table—not an imitation. Enjoy one pat if you so please. Side orders of roasted garlic, parsley, chives, leeks, and even chopped onions can be an added flavor booster for your meal.

For breakfast, eggs that are poached or boiled (hard or soft) are a good choice. Or ask to have an omelet prepared with lots of fresh veggies such as onions, spinach, and peppers. Although not ideal because of the high sodium and additive content in some of these selections, other breakfast foods that will work on the road are lox or smoked salmon, turkey sausage, cottage cheese, and a couple of slices of real Swiss cheese with tomatoes. If you're hankering for cereal, make sure you have enough protein and fat (such as a scoop of cottage cheese) to provide a balance so that you don't overdo the crash-and-burn carbohydrates. Otherwise, you'll wind up looking for a pick-me-up an hour later from sugar or a caffeine-laden beverage such as coffee, tea, or cola.

And speaking of caffeine and beverages, here's the lowdown. Although I know that green tea has been touted as a miracle drink, high in the phenol-based antioxidants that help to prevent certain types of cancer, I feel that caffeine is caffeine is caffeine—a theme reiterated throughout this book! There are 35 mg of caffeine in 6 ounces of green tea versus 100 mg in a 6-ounce cup of drip-brewed coffee. Besides, most teas are high in fluoride and copper, the latter mineral which seems to go hand in hand with estrogen, potentially leading to estrogen excess and water retention.

No matter what your phase, I would suggest selecting or bringing your own herbal tea bags, such as peppermint, fennel, ginger, or dandelion root tea. For Phase 3, you could bring along red tea, an antioxidant-rich tea that is also good for balancing blood sugar levels. Red tea comes from South Africa, where it has been enjoyed for over 200 years. It is high in the antioxidant-rich flavonoids. In fact, both it and dandelion tea nourish your liver.

The second-best option might be a blended herbal green tea, which cuts down on the caffeine because it also contains herbs. I would look for Tazo Om and Green Ginger, The Republic of Tea Moroccan Mint, or Celestial Seasonings Antioxidant Green.

Avoid iced teas or iced-tea mixes, because they are often presweetened with lots of sugar or aspartame. A much simpler alternative is to order hot water with lemon or lime. Just remember: when in doubt, lemonize! There is something fresh and clean about lemons and limes. I think you'll agree with me that they are quite satisfying.

FAT FLUSHING IN THE FAST-FOOD LANE

As far as takeout meals are concerned, there are some okay meals that don't exactly conform to the fat-flushing principles but are acceptable in a pinch—once you're in the Lifestyle Fat Flush eating phase, that is. Some examples are the grilled chicken sandwiches at Arby's, Dairy Queen, Hardee's, or Carl's (9 grams of fat, 28 grams of protein, and 33 grams of carbohydrate); the chicken fajita pita at Jack-in-the-Box (9 grams of fat, 28 grams of protein, and 31 grams of carbohydrate); and the chili at Wendy's (8 grams of fat, 24 grams of protein, and 29 grams of carbohydrate). Of course, try your best to eat your fast-food sandwiches as lettuce wraps.

And as mentioned previously, no matter what phase of the plan you are on, I would definitely look for places that feature rotisserie chicken or turkey, touted as a much healthier alternative to the fried version. Because rotisserie meat is not fried, the fats are not chemically altered into trans fat in the high-heat frying process, and any unhealthy fat that the meats do contain drips off during the rotisserie turning process. With a side salad and steamed vegetables, plus lots of fresh lemon, you can't beat it.

Another fantastic fast option is fish tacos. My go-to takeout taco restaurant is the fast-food restaurant Rubio's. At Rubio's, tacos contain grilled fish made from mahimahi or red snapper, and they come with a delightful yogurt-type sauce with fresh cabbage. When ordering at different establishments, make sure you order tacos with grilled fish, and ask for a corn tortilla instead of a flour tortilla or taco shell. In phase 3, a corn tortilla counts as one friendly carb, but taco shells are loaded with trans fats, and flour tortillas are, unsurprisingly, loaded with wheat flour. I usually order several fish tacos and remove the taco shells or flour tortillas. Rubio's also has lots of salsas and fresh lime for seasonings.

Speak Up

Don't be shy. Make your personal needs known to your server in a nice way. Ask a question such as, "Do you serve butter or margarine?" or "What are the ingredients in this dish?" And always ask for the butter, olive oil, and sauces on the side. I always tell my server that I'm very sensitive to certain foods from the get-go and do my best to make friends with the server. In many cases, servers have gone out of their way to accommodate my needs and have actually brought me the bottles of oil used in the making of various dressings and sauces. Sadly, canola oil is frequently used, even in the "fancier" establishments.

Also ask about methods used to prepare foods, and make it quite clear that you don't want anything that is fried (a sure bet for getting those terrible trans fats). You may want to find out what kind of fresh vegetables are available and request that they be steamed. I always look on the menu to find what veggies are served with other dishes and then politely ask if they can be included with my entrée too. This approach has been especially important for me when I can't readily get greens. For instance, I search for a dish that has sautéed spinach or escarole with garlic and then make my request.

Let your server know that you definitely don't want margarine added to your broiled or grilled entrées, which is frequently done to avoid dryness. Ditto for mayonnaise, which also is likely to have trans fats. You can add a pat of butter if you are in the Lifestyle phase.

GOING INTERNATIONAL

You can enjoy Italian, Chinese, Mexican, French, Japanese, Mediterranean, Indian, Middle Eastern, and Thai cuisine on the Fat Flush Plan. Cajun and Creole foods are not off-limits either for special occasions. Just keep in mind that highly spicy foods can cause water retention in some people.

Italian

This is the cuisine where, at least in the type of Americanized Italian food in the United States, you have to watch to not overdo carbs such as pasta, beans, and that delicious garlic bread. Thus you might want to have the server take the bread basket away as soon as you sit down. If you are really hungry, then order an appetizer right away. Grilled portobello mushrooms or an artichoke (hold the breading) is a tasty starter. You may want to indulge in a Caesar salad, which is perfectly Fat Flush legal. Just ask for it without croutons and get the dressing on the side. And if you have a taste for anchovies in the Caesar dressing, go for it! They are high in the omega-3s, although a bit on the salty side. The best news at an Italian restaurant is that you usually can get a wide variety of delicious, colorful veggies that are not as easily available elsewhere, such as zucchini, peppers, cauliflower, eggplant, and spaghetti squash. In addition, you can typically get a leafy green, such as spinach or escarole, here as well. Sautéed with onions, fresh garlic, and a little lemon in olive oil or chicken broth, these vegetables are out of this world and very Fat Flush friendly.

And oh yes, there's that cheese—the mozzarella, ricotta, and provolone. For those of you on the Lifestyle Fat Flush eating plan, keep them to a tasty minimum and use them as a condiment, please. You can even have your pesto (that sensational combination of olive oil, garlic, basil, pine nuts, and Parmesan cheese) and eat it too. Ask for it on the side so that you can enjoy a couple of tablespoons slowly and deliberately. Do not overlook the veal dishes (the Marsala, piccata, or scaloppini), which are usually quite outstanding in the finer Italian restaurants. Watch to make sure you are adhering to high-quality oils like olive oil, and learn to lemonize by ordering several lemon wedges that can help emulsify excess oil.

Chinese

Things are really simple when you go to Chinese restaurants. Just find out which dishes can be made to order and request no MSG, sugar, salt, or soy sauce. If you must, you can always add your own soy sauce at the table. If the oil is anything other than sesame or peanut oil (and there's no allergy to peanuts), then order your food steamed. I always request a stir-fry that uses chicken broth and is made from such combinations as beef, chicken, seafood, or tofu with snow peas, water chestnuts, bean sprouts, broccoli, scallions, bamboo shoots, and bok choy (Chinese cabbage).

If you are in the Lifestyle phase and want a good vegetarian meal, try Buddha's Delight, a mix of vegetables and rice cellophane noodles that can be stir-sautéed in vegetable broth. Buddha's Delight can be modified for any Fat Flush phase by omitting the noodles. You can have tofu added to the dish with a side of steamed veggies topped off with scallions, garlic, and a bit of Chinese five-spice powder, a delightful mixture of unique spices related to cinnamon. Most of the soups offered in a Chinese restaurant are made with lots of cornstarch—including egg drop soup—so it is best to skip the soup course. On the Lifestyle Fat Flush, lo mein dishes—cellophane or mung bean noodles with some chicken, beef, shrimp, or other kinds of seafood—also might be appealing. Just remember that those oyster and black bean sauces are loaded with salt, which can result in boggy, watery tissues. Try a bit of the hot mustard, minced garlic, scallions, and even some Chinese five-spice powder instead.

As for the fortune cookie—by all means have fun and open it. Read your fortune, and then leave the cookie behind. Also, try eating with chopsticks. It may help to slow you down and enhance your digestion as a result.

Mexican

You may want to select such entrées as chicken, shrimp, or beef and eat them without the tortilla unless you are on the Lifestyle Fat Flush. Look for main dishes with fish, chicken, or beef that can be prepared with onions, tomatoes, and peppers (such as Veracruz snapper), or look for dishes that can be sautéed in olive oil with a touch of garlic. If you are on the Lifestyle Fat Flush, a tasty Mexican soup (such as black bean soup) would be a great way to start your meal. If not, then how about some guacamole (loaded with the healthy monounsaturated fats) with lots of fresh lemon or lime juice? Salsa is probably your best all-over topping. Use the sour cream and cheese as condiments, with just a dollop or a few sprinkles here and there for flavor. If you are fortunate enough to locate an authentic Mexican restaurant, such foods as squash blossoms, jícama, and chayote cactus are treats for the palate. If you happen upon a restaurant on the other end of the American-Mexican food spectrum, like Tex-Mex, you can order a beef, chicken, or seafood fajita with extra vegetables, and if you are not yet in the Lifestyle Phase, eat your fajita without the corn tortilla. Be sure, as always, to watch the kind of oil that the restaurant uses to cook the fajita meat and veggies, and ask them to use as little oil as possible.

French

Ooh la la! Here you can select from a wide variety of broiled, poached, and steamed foods. Anything sautéed in a wine sauce, such as a Bordelaise sauce, is bound to be a winner. The traditional French dish fish en papillote (cooked with herbs in the fish's own juices) is highly recommended, as are such dishes as roast chicken with herbs (poulet aux fines herbes), ratatouille (a vegetable casserole), bouillabaisse, and coq au vin. Poached salmon is also a tasty choice, but go light on the butter and cream sauce in this and other selections. If you have a hankering for something outside the American mainstream, try duck, but avoid the sweet sauces it is often cooked with.

Japanese

As in Chinese cuisine, these dishes tend to feature soy sauce, which should be avoided as much as possible due to its high salt content. For the same reason, you will need to go light on the teriyaki sauce (a blend of soy sauce, rice wine, and sugar) and sukiyaki, which are used as marinades for many entrées featuring chicken and beef. Similarly, miso (the fermented soybean paste) is also high in salt. A bit of miso, however, can be used as a glaze or as a soup base with sea vegetables (hijiki and arame) and scallions.

Japanese restaurants are known for their sushi bars. I personally don't recommend eating sushi because raw fish often can be contaminated with parasites. (Please refer to my book *Guess What Came to Dinner?*) Lifestylers can go for the California rolls (avocado and cooked shrimp), and for that matter, they can also enjoy any sushi offerings that are made with smoked salmon or cooked crab, cooked shrimp, cooked egg, cooked eel, and cooked octopus. Straight vegetarian sushi (such as the kappa maki, made with cucumbers) is good too. The nori seaweed wrapping surrounding all these delights is quite nutritious in its own right—and it's loaded with trace minerals like the thyroid-boosting iodine. Of course, if brown rice is used in the sushi, then all the better.

The best strategy for eating Japanese cuisine is going for the grilled entrées of scallops, shrimp, chicken, and beef, which are prepared using the hibachi grill. Hibachi-style food preparation has become quite popular (just make sure that the food is not finished with a margarine blend, as is the custom these days). And now Mongolian-style barbecue outlets are popping up all over the country featuring the barbecue method of cooking. You can build your own meal from a variety of fresh ingredients (e.g., raw beef, chicken, shrimp, and scallops) with lots of vegetables and even sesame seeds, however you like it. As long as there is plenty of fresh garlic, parsley, and scallions, you really can't go wrong.

Mediterranean-Greek

Pita (pocket) bread is served routinely in these restaurants along with two savory vegetarian dips, hummus and baba ghanoush. Hummus is chickpea pâté; baba ghanoush is eggplant pâté. Both are made with sesame butter, garlic, and lemon. Blended with some tzatziki (yogurt and cucumbers), each can serve as a salad dressing, or just the tzatziki alone will do the honors. I would skip the pita entirely, because it is usually made from wheat flour, which, as you well know, is not recommended in any phase of the Fat Flush Plan. Instead, use celery sticks and cucumbers for the dips.

Greek salads and others that feature feta (preferably from goat) cheese are also a nutritious choice. Try a spinach pie for a satisfying taste treat and eat around the phyllo crust if you're not extremely gluten-intolerant. As a great main course for all Fat Flushers, try shish kebab (grilled meat with vegetables on the side). Souvlakis (skewered lamb, beef, chicken, and fish mixed with vegetables) are also acceptable. Sides of chopped parsley, tomatoes, and scallions with mint and lots of lemon can top off a lovely meal.

Indian

Indian cuisine featuring pilafs and biryanis (rice-based dishes) and bean-based dals is okay in moderation if you're on the Lifestyle Fat Flush, of course. Tandoori chicken and lamb, which are cooked in a clay oven to retain the moisture from the meat, are also fine for phases 1 and 2. Other tasty entrées for Lifestylers include chicken or lamb korma with coriander and yogurt sauce. Lightly curried vegetable and chicken dishes will satisfy those who like spicy foods and do not retain water from hot seasoning.

The Indian dal salad is similar to the Middle Eastern tabbouleh but is made with lentils instead of wheat. Remember that lentils are protein-rich friendly carbs—so figure them into your meals regularly. Or you can enjoy instead a couple (and only a couple) of baked pappadums (lentil wafers). The chapati and naan (kinds of flatbread) are very delicious but are also made from wheat, so it is best to stay away from them entirely.

Thai

This is a personal favorite. You can basically follow the recommendations outlined above for Indian cuisine, but you may wish to add the popular coconut milk–based soups such as tom kha. Enjoy it with some protein, such as shrimp, chicken, or beef. Coconut contains a healthful, naturally saturated fat known for its antiviral and thyroid-supporting properties. You can enjoy these soups with lemongrass and cilantro seasonings when you are on Lifestyle. The problem I find with many Thai restaurants, however, is that sugar is a prime ingredient is almost every dish. So, be proactive and ask that your dish be made from scratch without added sugar.

◆ ◆ ◆

In closing, after eating the Fat Flush way for years, I can say that the best way to eat out is to ask questions and even shop around for a restaurant that is responsive to your special requests. In Santa Fe, a Chinese restaurant used to keep a special bottle of sesame oil and cook all dishes in this oil for my family and guests. In San Diego, one of the Chinese restaurants added brown rice to the menu. The owners were more than happy to comply with my special requests, especially when I brought in huge parties of friends and publicly thanked them again for making my life so much healthier.

PARTIES, BUSINESS LUNCHEONS, AND HOLIDAY EVENTS

The holiday season? No problem, especially on Lifestyle. You just need to know the inside tips. For starters, eat a little something before you arrive. In this way, you won't be famished and tempted to eat the sugary, starchy pick-me-ups or appetizers that undoubtedly will surround you. Grab a glass of water and hold it in your hand—getting refills as needed—throughout the evening. No one will notice you're not drinking alcohol. And, of course, for those really festive times, indulge in some spirits. Light beer—maybe six ounces or so—an ounce of hard liquor, and even a half glassful of dry wine are fine for a little libation. Just don't drink on an empty stomach. Have your drinks with some vegetables and dip, with cheese, or with dinner.

Business luncheons can be a snap. First, there's usually a salad. The safest dressings are always those made from healthy oils like olive and sesame seed oil. Remember to always order them on the side. You never know about the blue cheese and ranch dressings, which may be made with trans-fat mayonnaise. You can always squeeze fresh lemon and add a little olive oil on your salad whenever in doubt. I personally order a Caesar salad because I am assured that the lettuce is really green. Romaine is higher in nutrients such as heart-healthy and bone-healthy magnesium and chlorophyll than its lackluster relatives, particularly iceberg.

If you can manage it, just ask for a double helping of the vegetables with your entrée in place of the white rice, pasta, or baked potato you can pretty much bet will be part of your meal. Remember these are the carbs that can raise your blood sugar levels quickly, especially if there's not enough protein or healthy fat to balance the surge.

If fresh fruit is for dessert (fresh berries to be exact), you're home free. I always ask for fresh berries even if they are not on the menu. Most of the time they are available, especially in finer establishments.

The important thing here is not to make a big deal about your food preferences and draw attention to yourself. If you do, people who know better but aren't following healthy principles may redirect their guilt and make you feel uncomfortable. It will be evident in their looks, facial expressions, and even their comments. I know; I have been there many times.

If a buffet is on the menu, then go out of your way to avoid the potato, pasta, and three-bean salads (which often have some added sugar to boot). Then run to the protein. Freshly carved roast beef, grilled or baked fish, chicken dishes, lamb, and the like should be your basic favorites. Check out the veggie section, choosing any green veggie you want to fill up your plate: spinach, broccoli, asparagus, and green beans. If you are a phase 2 or are a Lifestyle Fat Flush eater, then select one friendly carb (and only one) to accompany your meal based on the fat-flushing friendly carb choices.

The holidays and other special events may feel like a minefield of problems, but they don't have to be. You actually can join in the festivities, eat smart, and keep true to your Fat Flush health revolution. I know that traditionally during those special times of the year—particularly from Thanksgiving and Christmas to New Year's—many of us have let down our guard and packed on 10 to 15 pounds. Here are some ways to sidestep those holiday pounds and still have fun celebrating with your family and friends.

The first thing you'll want to do is continue taking your conjugated linoleic acid (CLA), because even with a slipup, half the weight you regain will be redeposited as muscle. Then, about an hour before you hit the holiday scene, have a salad or, if you are on Lifestyle, a bowl of soup to curb your appetite. You might want to try circulating around the room and meeting new people. Not only will it be interesting and fun, but it also will keep you from hanging out near the food. While you're making the rounds at a party, scan the food table and look for smart Fat Flush food choices. When you want to nibble on something, select raw veggies rather than the carb-rich crackers and trans-fatty chips. It's also a good idea to use a napkin, not a plate, so that you eat less. And while you're there, head on over to that dance floor and get groovin'! Dancing is a great exercise and lymph mover.

On Lifestyle, at work, where everyone seems to bring in all kinds of goodies during the holiday season, bypass the cookies and candy. Select a handful of raw nuts and fruit instead. If you are having the holiday meal at your home or if you are bringing a dish to someone else's home, cook up some mashed sweet potatoes seasoned with cinnamon instead of those candied yams. Make a Fat Flush dip, serving it with celery, cucumber, and zucchini sticks. Forget the bread stuffing and use a variety of seeds, nuts, and vegetables (such as celery, onions, and mushrooms seasoned with anise, cayenne, garlic, or parsley).

And since the holidays are an especially stressful time of year—stirring up one of those hidden weight gain factors that pile on the pounds—be sure to keep your diet nutrient-dense so that blood sugar levels remain steady, and stick to those stress-busting rituals like quality sleep, journaling, exercise, and aromatherapy baths. Keep a keen eye out for hidden sugars, and be sure to consume adequate protein and fat to balance your body's chemistry.

I also recommend getting the helpful yeast fighter Y-C Cleanse. It will help keep cravings at an all-time low. (See Chapter 15.) This is extremely important, because all those holiday cakes, cookies, and candies contain sugar, which is the favorite food of yeast. By keeping your yeast in check, you will lose your appetite for such goodies. For years I have recommended Y-C Cleanse as a preventive measure against holiday weight gain. And it really works.

Enjoy!

11 The Fat Flush Master Shopping List

*All that is necessary to break the spell of inertia and
frustration is this: Act as if it were impossible to fail. That is
the talisman, the formula, the command of right-about-face
which turns us from failure towards success.*

—Dorothea Brande

Fat Flush will really take off when you start to clean up and clear out your kitchen. The goal, of course, is to replace old habits with new ones. The first step in the process is to replace old, familiar products with newer, better ones.

To help you get started on your Fat Flush journey, here's the complete Fat Flush Plan shopping list with brand names for the tastiest and most convenient Fat Flush foods currently available. This all-in-one shopping list contains the foods you can eat in all three phases of the program, which are noted as such. The first several pages contain the approved products for phase 1, the Two-Week Fat Flush. Next you will see the products you can add for phase 2, the Metabolic Reset. The final section includes all the additional products appropriate for phase 3, the Lifestyle Eating Plan.

Keep in mind that many of these foods can be purchased at your local health food store, whereas others are available in supermarkets. The omega-3–enriched eggs listed are definitely worth the modest price increase, not to mention the superior, rich, and creamy taste of the brightly colored yolk. Naturally, organic produce (vegetables and fruit) are preferred when possible (not only are they tastier and fresher, but they do not have all those nasty pesticides, fungicides, and heavy metals your liver has to break down). For this reason, I am providing the names of some of the easier-to-obtain brands in parentheses. And, of course, if you have access to meats and dairy products rich in conjugated linoleic acid (CLA), then opt for grass-fed beef, poultry, and lamb as much as possible to maximize your body's fat loss.

Now if organic foods are not within your budget or not available in your locale, don't despair. At the end of the chapter, you'll find directions for a tried-and-true food-cleansing bath designed to return farm freshness and purity to store-bought food. Plus, do keep in mind items that are readily available throughout the country in health food stores, supermarkets, or online are listed simply by brand name. There may be many fine brand names that also meet the Fat Flush criteria. These are simply the brands that have become my personal favorites and that I find to be the most easily accessible.

You will also find more detailed descriptions about the preferred protein powders and the most suitable cuts of meat. You'll find my specific go-to frozen fruit and vegetable brands as well. You'll find lots of special occasion spice perks and treats. Now let's go shopping!

BEFORE YOU BEGIN

Beverages. Organic fair trade coffee and/or roasted dandelion root tea, which is a naturally caffeine-free herbal coffee alternative made from roasted dandelion roots. Available at health food stores, online, or through UNI KEY at 1-800-888-4353 or online at www.unikeyhealth.com.

Fennel, ginger, and peppermint tea can be found in more health food stores. This is appropriate for all phases.

INSIDER TIP	Dandelion root coffee is especially helpful as a coffee substitute and gentle but effective liver balancer for those with elevated liver enzymes or who have overdone alcohol, sugar, trans fats, and Ibuprofen and those on medications for lowering cholesterol (like Lipitor).

PHASE 1: THE TWO-WEEK FAT FLUSH

Oil. Avocado oil spray (such as Chosen Foods), coconut oil (such as Nutiva and Tropical Traditions), high-lignan and regular flaxseed oil (such as Omega and Barleans). If you do not tolerate flaxseed oil, you can use flavored fish oil (such as Carlson's) as a flaxseed oil substitute.

STORAGE TIP	Keep in fridge. An eight-ounce bottle lasts for about three weeks.

Eggs. Omega-3–enriched (The Happy Egg Co., Organic Valley, The Country Hen, and Pilgrim's Pride EggsPlus).

HEALTH TIP	These incredible eggs contain 20 times more omega-3s than their supermarket sisters. Both The Country Hen and Pilgrim's Pride Eggs-Plus contain about 200 mg of this essential fatty acid.

Protein Powders. Whey (nonvegan) powders that are hormone-free, unheated, nondenatured, lactose-free, free of added sugars or artificial sweeteners like aspartame, sucralose or Splenda, with about 20 grams of protein per serving and negligible carbohydrates from nonmutated A2 milk (Fat Flush Whey and Designs for Health Whey). Pea and rice protein powders that are low-carb, non-GMO, unsweetened, and organic, and if possible, with third-party testing for heavy metals (Fat Flush Body Protein pea and rice and Body Ecology Fermented Plant Protein).

Lean-Protein Fish. All fresh varieties, especially bass, cod, grouper, haddock, halibut, mackerel, mahimahi, orange roughy, perch, pike, pollock, salmon, sardines, sole, snapper, trout, tuna, and whitefish, and canned tuna, salmon, mackerel, sardines, and crabmeat. Canned and frozen seafood are permissible when from a reputable brand (Wild Planet, Vital Choice Seafood, Crown Prince, Skip Jack Tuna, Bar Harbor).

HEALTH TIP	If the fish is packed in oil or with added salt, drain well under running water.

Seafood. Shrimp, lobster, crab, scallops, calamari.

HEALTH TIP	If shrimp or crab is canned, then drain well under running water to remove excess salt.

Poultry. White meat of skinned turkey and chicken, either fresh, frozen, or ground (preferably free range and hormone-free, such as Tecumseh Farms Organic, Mary's Chicken, and Good Earth Farms, and local farms).

Beef. Flank, rump, round, eye of the round, chuck, brisket, sirloin, and London broil (preferably grass-fed, such as Aspen Ridge, Ayrshire Farm, Holy Cow, and local farms).

Lamb. Leg, loin, rib.

Veal. Shoulder, rib, loin.

Other Meats. Venison, ostrich, bison (or buffalo), and elk.

HEALTH TIP	These meats can be substituted for the protein in any recipe and are higher in the fat-burning omega-3s. Remember when purchasing to choose meat from organic, pasture-raised animals. If from any other nonorganic source, the meat will likely contain antibiotics, excess hormones, and other additive chemicals that are harmful to your system and cause weight gain.

Other Protein Sources. Tempeh and tofu, non-GMO soy (Mori-Nu and White Wave).

Vegetables. All fresh, in-season produce that is green, red, orange, or purple. (Fresh is always best, followed by frozen and then canned with no added salt. Bamboo shoots, water chestnuts, and artichoke hearts are Fat Flush friendly either canned or frozen. Frozen brands are Cascadian Farms and Stahlbush Island Farms.) Make sure to buy a wide variety of colors, multiple types of leaves (prioritizing bitter varieties), and sea veggies such as agar-agar, hijiki, kombu, nori, wakame, or a sea veggie–based seasoning (like Eden Seaweed Gomasio, kelp granules, or dulse flakes from Maine).

Fruits. Fresh (without mold), frozen, or canned in natural unsweetened juices and drained (frozen brands include Cascadian Farms and Stahlbush Island Farms). Remember, phase 1 only includes apples, grapefruits, oranges, plums, strawberries, large cherries, nectarines, pomegranates, peaches, pears, and berries (blueberries, blackberries, and raspberries) in certain quantities. Don't forget to pick up avocados!

Lemons. Fresh is best, although Santa Cruz Organic Pure Lemon Juice will do.

Limes. Fresh is best, although Santa Cruz Organic Pure Lime Juice will do.

HEALTH TIP	One tablespoon equals the juice of one-half lemon or lime.

Bone Broths. Beef, chicken, or fish, vegetable broth (Pacific Foods). I especially encourage purchasing ready-made bone broth, as it is heavily featured in the Fat Flush recipes (Wise Choice Market, Kettle & Fire, Pacific Foods, LonoLife, The Osso Good Co, Au Bon Broth, Bondafide Provisions).

HEALTH TIP	Herbs, spices, and accompaniments: Apple cider vinegar (Bragg), coconut vinegar (Tropical Traditions), cayenne pepper, cinnamon, cloves, coriander (dried cilantro), cumin, dill, dried mustard, garlic, turmeric, ginger, fennel, anise, salsa, and bay leaves.

Tomato Products. Mom's tomato sauces are my favorite because they contain no sugar (momspastasauce.com)! You can find more acceptable tomato products on ThriveMarket.com (such as Jovial, Bionaturae).

Flax Seeds. Organic whole brown or golden yellow flax seeds in bulk to be ground daily as needed in a coffee grinder, blender, or food processor on the fine setting. You can also purchase preground flaxseed if you do not want to buy and grind your own, but flaxseed must be ground in order to receive its full fatty acid benefits (Omega).

Chia Seeds. Whole organic or chemical-free chia seeds in bulk. Unlike flax seeds, you do not need to grind chia seeds to derive benefits (Spectrum or Uni Key chia seeds).

Hemp Seeds. You can buy hempseed in bulk to be ground daily as needed in a coffee grinder, blender, or food processor on the fine setting. You can also purchase shelled hempseed if you do not want to buy your own (Nutiva).

Cranberry Juice. Unsweetened cranberry juice (Knudsen's, Trader Joe's, Mountain Sun).

Sweeteners. Flora-Key, stevia (SweetLeaf Stevia), monk fruit and erythritol (Lankanto).

HEALTH TIP	Flora-Key does double duty as a natural sweetener and an immune booster helping to crowd out candida and other non-friendly organisms from the GI tract. The addition of the friendly bacteria–nourishing fructooligosaccharides adds even more fiber without more bulk.

Supplements. The Fat Flush Kit supplements have been formulated to my specifications in line with the requirements of the Fat Flush Plan. These include three products: The Dieters' Multi (with or without iron), GLA 90, and the Weight Loss Formula. Bile Builder is an additional detox product. It is a gentle, but effective bile cleanser and bile promoter. All of these products are available at 1-800-888-4353 or online at www.unikeyhealth.com. Autoship programs are available, and you can become entitled to a Preferred Customer discount.

You can also choose to put together your own combination of supplements from your favorite health food store.

PHASE 2: THE METABOLIC RESET

You may have these foods in addition to the ones on the phase 1 list.

Friendly Carbs. Sweet potato, frozen or fresh green peas, beets, carrots, butternut and acorn squash, quinoa, steel cut or rolled oats.

Fruit. Note that the fruit list has been expanded to include bananas and pineapple.

Supplements. Continue with the same supplements from phase 1.

PHASE 3: THE LIFESTYLE EATING PLAN

You may have these foods in addition to the ones on the phase 1 and 2 lists.

Oils and Sprays. Avocado oil (Spectrum Naturals, Primal Kitchen, La Tourangelle), extra virgin and unfiltered olive oils (California Estates, Lucini, Napa Valley Naturals, Bragg), macadamia oil (Mac Nut Oil), sesame and toasted sesame oils (Spectrum and Eden), and olive oil sprays (Spectrum Naturals, Lucini, Napa Valley Naturals).

Sweeteners. Yacon syrup (Organic Traditions, Sunfood Superfoods, Therapeutic Laboratories, Swanson Health).

Beef (Occasional). Beef jerky (Epic, B.U.L.K., New Primal, Paleo Snacks).

Turkey (Occasional). Organic, nitrate-free turkey bacon (Applegate Farms), turkey jerky (Perky Jerky, Krave Jerky, Golden Valley, New Primal).

Nuts and Seeds. Raw almonds, filberts, pecans, peanuts, walnuts, macadamia nuts, pumpkin seeds, sunflower seeds, poppy seeds, and caraway, as well as peanut, almond, and sesame butters or tahini (Living Intentions). Be sure all nut and seed butters are free of canola, sunflower, soybean, corn, and safflower oil.

STORAGE TIP: Store nuts and seeds in a cool, dry place such as the fridge or freezer. Home-toast all seeds and nuts in the oven for 15 minutes at 250 degrees Fahrenheit to help set the oil.

Fruit. Note that melon (e.g., cantaloupe, honeydew, or watermelon), kiwi, pineapple, mango, papaya, and grapes have been added in this phase.

Special-Occasion Fruit. Dried fruit (Organic Traditions, Peeled Organic).

Mayonnaise. Avocado mayo (Thrive Market).

Dairy Products. Plain Greek full-fat yogurt, cottage cheese (Friendship, Old Home), ricotta cheese (Calabro), Swiss, Cheddar, Parmesan, string cheese, Romano, mozzarella, goat cheese, sweet butter, buttermilk (prepared using milk from Horizon, Organic Valley, local farm), cream, and ghee (Organic Valley, Purity Farms, Pore Indian Foods). Make sure all dairy products are full fat and, as much as possible, from, organically raised, pasture cows.

If intolerant to dairy, use coconut or almond substitutes like coconut cream, full-fat coconut milk (Trader Joe's), coconut yogurt, and unsweetened, unflavored almond milk (Natural Directions).

HEALTH | Companies such as Nancy's and Horizon offer a wide variety
TIP | of organic dairy products.

Friendly Carbs. Gluten-free and non-GMO corn tortillas, corn on the cob, Ancient Grain lentil and quinoa pasta, tigernuts (Organic Gemini, Supreme Peeled), chestnuts, turnips, rutabaga, parsnips, pumpkin, baked potato, red potatoes, chickpeas, pinto beans, adzuki beans, black beans, kidney beans, lentils, brown rice, popcorn (Good Health Half Naked Organic Sea Salt Popcorn). Canned beans are fine if you rinse and drain them.

HEALTH | When purchasing popcorn, canned foods, chips, or any other
TIP | products that tend to be more highly processed, read the nutrition label! Only buy snack food made with olive, avocado, or coconut oil. Make sure that the sodium level does not exceed 350–400 mg per meal. I encourage you to stick to my recommended brands to avoid hidden commercial salt.

Friendly Carb Gluten-Free and Flour Alternatives (Occasional). Paleo coconut wraps (The Pure Wraps, Paleo Wraps), raw wraps (Green Leaf Foods), coconut flour, almond flour, chickpea flour, tapioca flour, tigernut flour (Organic Gemini).

Crackers. Gluten-free brown flax or rice crackers (Mary's Gone Crackers), SeaSnax Seaweed Snacks & Seaweed Chips, RW Garcia 3 Seed Crackers, organic golden flax crackers (Foods Alive), Doctor in the Kitchen Dill, Rosemary, Tomato, and Savory Flackers.

Special Occasion Snacks, Treats, and Sweets. Protein bars (Epic), baked potato chips made with virgin olive oil, coconut oil, or avocado oil (Good Health Kettle Chips, Boulder Canyon Authentic Foods), and granola made with raw, unpasteurized honey and maple syrup (Prime Island, Platte Clove Naturals).

HEALTH | If purchasing a different brand of any of the cracker or snack
TIP | products, read the labels to make sure you are not consuming too much sugar. Check out the ingredients to catch any of those hidden sources of sugar or artificial sweeteners like high-fructose corn syrup, sorbitol, mannitol, aspartame, sucralose, and xylitol. Total sugar content should stay between three to four grams per serving. Again, I encourage you to stick to my recommended brands.

Vegetable Juice. Low-sodium vegetable juices (Low Sodium V-8 Juice, Muir Glen Tomato Juice, Muir Glen 100% Vegetable Juice, and Knudsen Organic Very Veggie Juice).

Flavor Extracts. Organic vanilla, almond, and other assorted extracts (Simply Organic, Olive Nation, Nature's Flavors).

Salt. Sea salt like Selina Naturally Celtic Sea Salt. If on a sodium-restricted diet, choose Makai Pure Deep Sea Salt, which has the highest potassium level of any comparable sea salt on the market.

Herbs, Spices, and Condiments. Oregano, basil, sage, rosemary, tarragon, thyme, Chinese five-spice powder, Dijon mustard, Angostura bitters, and capers.

Special Occasion. Gluten-free tamari (San-J) and umeboshi paste (Eden).

Acceptable Teas and Coffees. Fair-trade and organic dandelion root and red tea (rooibos tea), organic coffee, fennel tea, ginger tea, and peppermint tea.

Alcohol. Organic and sulfite-free (Coturri Winery, Frey, Fetzer, Organic Wine Company, HoneyRun Winery, Hallcrest Vineyards, Marcel Lapierre, Stellar Organics, Spartico No Sulfur Added, China Bend Vineyards, Trader Joe's).

Baking Powder. Aluminum-free brands (Royal, Rumford, Price, and Schillings) and low-sodium, cereal-free brands (Cellu and Featherweight).

Thickeners. Arrowroot and kudzu.

Supplements. Continue with the same supplements from phases 1 and 2. You can also add CLA 1,000 mg to these supplements for added weight loss benefits to target tummy fat.

FOOD-CLEANSING BATHS

If organic foods are unavailable or simply too expensive, there are many new fruit and vegetable cleansers on the market that can be found in grocery and health food stores (Biokleen, Veggie Wash, Citrus Magic).

Wash fruits and veggies thoroughly to remove estrogen-mimicking pesticides, fungicides, and herbicides. I use the Chemist Formula for my fruit and veggie wash. It was created by my friend Larry Ward, a biochemist. The recipe makes 1 quart of soak that should be prepared fresh each day. The ingredients are 18 drops of grapefruit seed extract with 4 ounces of 3 percent hydrogen peroxide and 1 teaspoon of baking soda per quart. Blend and soak all produce (you can soak eggs as well) for at least 15 minutes; then rinse well, at least three times.

12 The Fat Flush Kitchen

More actual chemistry takes place in the kitchen than in any laboratory of life.

—Dr. Hazel Parcells

"Kitchen chemistry" is a term coined by Dr. Hazel Parcells. She said "When you select the pots and pans, or the equipment that you are going to use to perform the most important task of your daily regime—what you do and how you do it represents life or death, success or failure." These words ring truer today than ever before. So here's the skinny on what works and what doesn't in your Fat Flush kitchen.

First, you may want to seriously consider using heavy-duty, stainless-steel, waterless cookware, which cooks food in a vacuum seal. When food cooks in its own juices, high flavor, tenderness, and high nutritional value are guaranteed. In fact, studies have shown that cooking in vacuum-sealed cookware rather than nonsealed cookware retains more vitamins and minerals and produces less fat. At the same time, less salt and less seasoning are required for high-quality taste. Look for waterless cookware made of the highest surgical-grade stainless steel (which does not leach into your foods and cooks foods at 180 degrees Fahrenheit—the temperature that kills worrisome germs, bacteria, and parasites but doesn't destroy vitamins and minerals).

Enamel, CorningWare, glass, and Pyrex are also acceptable. For those of you who are anemic, you might consider cooking with iron-based utensils because the extra iron picked up from cooking can actually be therapeutic. When a high–acid-based food like spaghetti sauce, for example, is cooked in iron pots, it contains six times more iron than when it is made in ceramic cookware. Choose nonstick, heavy-duty tin or black steel for your baking needs.

STAY AWAY FROM ALUMINUM

Aluminum-proof the kitchen as much as possible. Aluminum inhibits the body's utilization of key minerals like magnesium, calcium, and phosphorus. Scary, right? On top of that, some researchers believe that it can neutralize pepsin, an important digestive enzyme in the stomach. Replace all aluminum steamers, measuring cups, spoons, bread pans, and cookie sheets with stainless steel or Pyrex.

You should avoid aluminum foil also. When cooking, opt for parchment paper (like Beyond Gourmet unbleached parchment paper), which the French have used for years in their "en papillote" dishes to seal in juices. This can be used for roasting veggies as well. For storing and freezing, you can first cover with wax paper then foil, which prevents the aluminum from leaching into foods.

Can't tell whether your utensils are fused with aluminum that could leach into your food? Simple: test with a magnet. A magnet will not cling to aluminum but will to tin or nickel—which is often used with stainless steel.

CURB THE COPPER

You would also be wise to replace all copper-lined cookware. This metal can upset the sensitive zinc-copper balance in your system. Excess copper has been linked to depression, insomnia, anorexia nervosa, compulsive behavior, anxiety, hyperactivity, various skin disorders, and hair loss. Need I say more?

OTHER SMART COOKWARE

Cookware
✓ Stainless steel or healthy nonstick skillets and saucepans (various sizes). Choose nonstick brands that have no PFOA (Teflon), like Ozeri, GreenPan, or GreenLife.
✓ Stainless-steel steamer.
✓ Dutch oven, six-quart slow cooker, or Crock-Pot.
✓ Air fryer (like GoWise USA).

Bakeware
✓ Ramekins
✓ Baking sheets
✓ Oven-safe baking dishes
✓ Casseroles
✓ Pizza stone

SMART WATER SYSTEM

With pure, clean water becoming extinct and with bottled water not always being reliable, a home water filter is no longer a luxury but a necessity.

I recommend the CWR Crown Ultra-Ceramic Water Filter, the most effective water filtration system available. The filter is made of ultrafine ceramic with pores so small that they trap bacteria, parasites, and particles down to 0.8 micron in size. The filtering system provides a comprehensive, three-stage process.

In the first stage the tiny pores in the ceramic remove bacteria, parasites, rust, and dirt. The second filter state is composed of high-density matrix carbon that removes chlorine, pesticides, and other chemicals like chloramines and trihalomethanes. In the third stage, a heavy metal–removing compound eliminates lead and copper.

SMART COOKING TOOLS

Knives

I would be remiss if I did not remind you how important the right knives are for chopping, paring, slicing, and carving—everything from fruits and veggies to roasts and turkeys. At the very least, you will need one high-quality utility knife and one four-inch paring knife for the majority of your cutting needs in the smart kitchen. If you are planning to purchase a new knife set and you want something durable, then I highly recommend MAC Japanese knives, which are acclaimed by chefs all over the world as the world's finest knives. The MAC knives are what I personally use because they have a razor-sharp edge, stay sharp a long time, and have thin blades for easy slicing. They are easily available online.

Thermos Cooker

A wide-mouthed thermos is helpful for taking soups, stews, and leftovers to work with you.

Flaxseed Grinder

Since ground flax seeds are such a potent source of metabolism-boosting omega-3s and fiber-rich lignans—which function as natural hormone balancers—a specially designed flaxseed grinder is a valuable smart kitchen item. The Krups F203 Electric Spice and Coffee Grinder with stainless-steel blades is an efficient, easy-to-use grinder. You can find it and similar products online.

Mortar and Pestle

Many of the recipes call for crushed dried herbs. To crush my herbs, I like to use a mortar and pestle, which is best for extracting the essence of the dried herbs and spices used in the recipes. The mortar and pestle crushes the herbs, which in turn release the volatile oils that contain the herbs' health and aromatic qualities. The aromas of the ground, dried herbs or spices are nearly four times as strong as the same herbs and spices before they are ground.

Seed Grinder

For grinding and crushing seeds (like anise, fennel, or coriander), a small hand-turned mill is very useful.

The Thrill of the Grill: Gas Versus Charcoal

Grilling is here to stay. Nothing says outdoor fun more than a cookout. Healthwise, the oxidative reaction of charcoal grilling (a combination of browning and charring) may be somewhat toxic. Food can soak up added chemicals from the charcoal briquettes, too. So if you are a charcoal fan, please be sure to cut off any charred, burned, or blackened portions of the food.

Gas grilling is another way to go, especially if there is no sensitivity to hydrocarbons, which are the by-products of gas combustion.

The safest way to protect your food from harmful substances formed during the grilling process is to marinate, marinate, marinate. Some research shows that marinades can cut down on carcinogen production by nearly 99 percent.

Fat Flush Tip: You can make easy grilling marinades by combining about 1 cup olive oil, ½ cup fresh lime or lemon juice, and ¼ cup apple cider vinegar seasoned with some of your favorite herbs—like rosemary, so rich in antioxidants. For a sweeter marinade you can also add a tablespoon of Lakanto Monk Fruit Sweetener.

Other Smart Cooking Tools and Cutlery

✓ Wooden spoons
✓ Measuring spoons
✓ Measuring cups
✓ Slotted spoon
✓ 2 chopping boards (1 for meats, 1 for veggies)
✓ Rubber spatulas
✓ Mixing bowls (various sizes)
✓ Lemon juicer
✓ Tongs
✓ Pastry brush for basting
✓ Garlic press
✓ Grater

✓ Can opener
✓ Utility knife
✓ 4-inch paring knife
✓ Scissors
✓ Ceramic sharpening rod
✓ Masher
✓ Whisk
✓ Popsicle molds
✓ Freezer-safe, airtight containers
✓ Grilling accessories (broad-headed jumbo tongs and turner tongs with one-sided spatula)
✓ Vegetable spiralizer for zucchini "zoodles"
✓ Food processor or blender for whipping up smoothies and pâtés. I like Vitamix, NutriBullet, and immersion blenders for these purposes. Blending retains more fiber and nutrients than juicing.
✓ Toaster oven

Now your kitchen is fully prepared as you embark on a new lifestyle of eating the Fat Flush way for life changing health.

13 Fat Flush Recipes

The food you eat today walks around tomorrow.

—DR. HAZEL PARCELLS

The basic Fat Flush recipes are quick and easy to prepare. Just ask the individuals who inspired them—my clients, readers, and Fat Flush Internet community members. Like most of us, these Fat Flushers juggle family and career, so they simply don't have the time or energy to fuss with meals.

But don't let the simplicity fool you. These recipes are big on flavor, especially with all the Fat Flush herbs and spices.

Just remember: buy organic when possible and read labels carefully to avoid GMOs, and the rest will follow. When it comes to produce, fresh is always best—but frozen runs a close second. Many veggies and fruits are frozen at the peak of ripeness, so they usually have a lot of flavor. If you are using canned vegetables and fruits, be sure to drain them well because the juices have added salt—usually the wrong kind. Lastly, use the oils specified in the recipes. They have been selected for specific phases and cooking qualities.

For vegans, vegetarians, and those with food allergies, I have included a list of food swaps at the end of the chapter.

Here you go—proceed with a hearty appetite!

FAT FLUSH STAPLES

Fat Flush Lemon Water

1 cup hot water
Juice of ½ lemon or lime
Pinch of ginger (optional)
Pinch of cardamom (optional)

- Squeeze the lemon into the hot water.
- Add the spices.
- Sip slowly.

ALL PHASES

Fat Flush Cran-Water

This foundational fat-flushing beverage helps melt away stubborn cellulite and release fluid from waterlogged tissues while detoxifying the liver and cleansing the lymphatic system.

8 ounces 100% unsweetened cranberry juice or 3 tablespoons concentrate
56 ounces plain filtered water or 64 ounces if using cranberry concentrate

- In a 64-ounce (½-gallon) bottle, stir together the cranberry juice or concentrate with the water.

Makes 64 ounces.

FLUSH TIP	Allergic to cranberry juice? Omit the cranberry juice and add 4 tablespoons of unfiltered apple cider vinegar or coconut vinegar to 64 ounces of plain filtered water.

If you can't find ready-made chicken or beef bone broths, you can always make your own, and even more nutritiously. The key is to use bones with your homemade bone broth and add a couple of tablespoons of apple cider vinegar. This will up the calcium content because the vinegar actually helps leach calcium from the bones. And whenever possible, I would suggest using free-range, hormone- and antibiotic-free chicken or beef rather than commercially raised chicken or beef. These bone broths can be used in every phase of the Fat Flush Plan as a base for soups and for sautéing veggies, scrambling eggs, or basting any protein dish.

Fat Flush Bone Broth

What makes this recipe truly Fat Flush special is the burdock and daikon, both of which help to metabolize fat. Burdock is a truly medicinal root that is known for its purifying and blood-cleansing properties. For our purposes it also stimulates the secretion of bile, as well as contains inulin and prebiotic blood sugar–regulating benefits that help diabetics.

2 quarts water
3 pounds chicken or beef shank with bones
3 tablespoons cider vinegar
2 cups burdock, cut in 1-inch pieces
2 cups daikon, cut in 1-inch pieces

1 large onion, cut in 1-inch pieces
3 stalks celery, cut in 1-inch pieces
4 sprigs fresh parsley
2 bay leaves

- Place all ingredients in a large pot and bring to a boil.
- Reduce heat, cover, and simmer for about 45 minutes or until the chicken or beef is done.
- Strain, and discard vegetables and bones; save the chicken or beef for another recipe.
- Refrigerate and use within 3 days or freeze.

Makes 4 servings.
ALL PHASES

FLUSH TIPS	• Freeze bone broths in an ice cube tray for convenient future use. Each bone broth ice cube is approximately 1 tablespoon of bone broth.
	• To boost the thyroid, simply add 2 teaspoons of seaweed gomasio to provide thyroid-nourishing iodine. Also add 1 cup of potassium-rich zucchini.
	• To boost the adrenal, add ½ teaspoon of sea salt for added adrenal-supporting sodium and also add 2 cups of escarole and spinach for extra-rich magnesium content.
	• To help detoxify the liver, add 1 teaspoon of turmeric, which is a potent anti-inflammatory that enhances the liver's ability to filter toxins.

Fat Flush Vegetable Broth

Enhance any mealtime with this veggie broth that vegans can use to replace bone broth in any recipe.

2 quarts filtered water
2 cups burdock, cut in 1-inch pieces
2 cups daikon, cut in 1-inch pieces
1 large onion, cut in 1-inch pieces
3 stalks celery, cut in 1-inch pieces
1 bunch green onion, chopped
8 cloves garlic, minced
8 sprigs fresh parsley
8 ounces mushrooms, cut in ½-inch slices
2 bay leaves

- Place all ingredients in a large stockpot and bring to a boil.
- Lower heat and simmer uncovered for about 1 hour.

- Strain, and discard vegetables.
- Refrigerate and use within 3 days or freeze.
- Serve with toasted nori strips

Makes 4 servings.
ALL PHASES

BREAKFAST

Fat Flush Smoothie

8 ounces water or cran-water
Small handful of romaine, kale, or spinach or a scoop of green powder
1 fruit serving of your choosing
1 scoop whey or pea and rice protein powder
1 tablespoon flaxseed or coconut oil
1 tablespoon ground flax seeds, chia seeds, or hemp seeds
1 scoop powdered probiotic (like Flora-Key)
1 tablespoon non-GMO soy or sunflower lecithin
Ice cubes (optional)

- Blend the water, powder, and fruit until smooth. Then add the other ingredients.

Makes 1 serving.
ALL PHASES

FLUSH
TIPS

- If using flaxseed oil, stream it in while the blender is running. Make 2 smoothies at a time—put the extra in the refrigerator to enjoy later.
- To burn more fat, support the thyroid, and slow down carb absorption for lower insulin, try adding a dash of turmeric, Ceylon cinnamon, cream of tartar, collagen powder, or 1 tablespoon of apple cider vinegar or coconut vinegar.

Smoothie Variations

Cinnaberry Smoothie. Use 1 cup fresh or frozen mixed berries, 1 teaspoon Ceylon cinnamon (or to taste). *ALL PHASES*

Blueberry Mint Smoothie. Use 1 cup fresh or frozen blueberries, 3–4 fresh mint leaves (or to taste). *ALL PHASES*

Choco-Cherry Smoothie. Use 10 large fresh or frozen cherries, 1 scoop chocolate whey protein. *ALL PHASES*

Citrus Surprise Smoothie. Use flesh of ¼ grapefruit, flesh of ½ orange, a touch of Ceylon cinnamon. *ALL PHASES*

Classic Strawberry Smoothie. Use 6 large fresh or frozen strawberries. *ALL PHASES*

Minty Chocolate Smoothie. Use 4–5 fresh mint leaves (or to taste), 1 scoop chocolate whey protein. *ALL PHASES*

Plum Passion Smoothie. Use 1 plum, ½ cup fresh or frozen blueberries. *ALL PHASES*

Lemon-Lime Pucker Smoothie. Use juice of 1 lemon, juice of 1 lime. *ALL PHASES*

Raspberry Harmony Smoothie. Use ½ cup fresh or frozen peaches, ½ cup fresh or frozen raspberries. *ALL PHASES*

Black Forest Smoothie. Use 10 frozen cherries with chocolate whey protein. *ALL PHASES*

Anise Kiss Smoothie. Use ½ frozen pear chunks (peeled, cored), ½ cup fresh or frozen blueberries, ½ teaspoon anise seeds. *ALL PHASES*

Lime Booster Smoothie. Use ½ cucumber, ½ avocado, 1 cup spinach, ⅓ cup of lime juice, Ceylon cinnamon (to taste). *ALL PHASES*

Peary Blueberry Smoothie. Use ½ pear, ½ cup fresh or frozen blueberries. *ALL PHASES*

Ginger 'n' Apple Smoothie. Use 1 small apple, ½-inch cube fresh ginger. *ALL PHASES*

Spiced Mocha-Choca Smoothie. Use 1 cup chilled regular organic coffee, 1 scoop chocolate whey protein, ½ teaspoon Ceylon cinnamon. *ALL PHASES*

Green Apple & Kale Smoothie. Use 1 green apple, ½-inch cube fresh ginger, ¼ lemon, 1 cup kale. *ALL PHASES*

Cherry Limeade Smoothie. Use 10 large fresh or frozen cherries, ¼ lime. *ALL PHASES*

Blueberry Smoothie. Use 1 cup fresh or frozen blueberries. *ALL PHASES*

Lemon-Berry Smoothie. Use 1 cup frozen berries, 1 tablespoon lemon juice. *ALL PHASES*

Orange-Raspberry Banana Smoothie. Use ½ cup fresh or frozen raspberries, ½ small orange, ½ banana. *PHASE 2*

Green Goddess Smoothie. Use 1 pear, ½ frozen banana, 1 cup greens (kale or spinach), fresh cilantro (to taste), ¼ avocado. *PHASE 2*

Banana Split Pineapple Smoothie. Use 3 large fresh or frozen strawberries, ½ banana, ½ cup frozen pineapple, 1 teaspoon almond extract. *PHASE 2*

Piña Colada Smoothie. Use ½ cup pineapple, 1 tablespoon coconut oil. *PHASE 2*

Strawberry Banana Rhubarb Smoothie. Use 1 cup frozen strawberries, ½ banana, 1 cup fresh or frozen rhubarb chopped into small pieces. *PHASE 2*

Sweetie Peach Pie Smoothie. Use 1 cup frozen sliced peaches (or 1 medium peach), ½ cup frozen cooked sweet potato chunks, ⅛ teaspoon Ceylon cinnamon (or to taste), ½-inch cube fresh ginger. *PHASE 2*

Cherry-Vanilla Smoothie. Use 10 large fresh or frozen cherries, ½ cup plain Greek yogurt, 1 teaspoon natural vanilla extract. *PHASE 3*

Pear Gingersnap Smoothie. Use 1 pear, ½ cup plain Greek yogurt, ¼-inch cube fresh ginger. *PHASE 3*

Strawberry Peach Smoothie. Use ½ cup fresh or frozen peaches, ½ cup fresh or frozen strawberries, ½ cup plain Greek yogurt. *PHASE 3*

Almond Coconut Smoothie. Use 1 tablespoon almond butter, 1 tablespoon coconut oil. *PHASE 3*

Peanut Butter Choco Smoothie. Use 1 scoop chocolate whey protein, 1 tablespoon peanut butter. *PHASE 3*

Strawberry Colada Smoothie. Use ½ cup fresh or frozen strawberries, ½ cup frozen pineapple, 2 tablespoons raw unsweetened shredded coconut, 1 squeeze of fresh lemon or lime (optional). *PHASE 3*

Puffy Apple Flaxcake

Avocado oil spray
1 egg
1 to 2 tablespoons filtered water
2 tablespoons shredded apple
3 tablespoons flax seeds, ground or milled
1 packet SweetLeaf Stevia
⅛ to ¼ teaspoon Ceylon cinnamon

■ Whisk all ingredients besides Ceylon cinnamon together in a small bowl.

- Lightly coat an omelet pan with avocado oil spray and heat over medium setting.
- Pour mixture into pan and cook until bottom of flaxcake is solid enough to flip (about 3 to 4 minutes).
- Carefully flip flaxcake, cooking an additional minute until done.
- Sprinkle with Ceylon cinnamon and serve.

Makes 1 serving.
ALL PHASES

Spaghetti Squash Peach Pudding

Avocado oil spray
4 large eggs
1 serving vanilla or chocolate whey protein
2 packets SweetLeaf Stevia
3 cups cooked spaghetti squash, drained well
1 cup peaches

- Preheat the oven to 350°F.
- Lightly coat a glass 9-inch pie pan (or an 11- × 7-inch dish) with a few spritzes of avocado oil.
- Mix the eggs on low speed in a blender.
- Add the whey and stevia; blend well on low speed.
- Add the spaghetti squash; blend on high until pureed.
- Sprinkle the peaches into the pan.
- Pour the spaghetti squash mixture into the pan.
- Bake for 25 to 30 minutes or until set.
- Chill.

Makes 1 to 2 servings.
ALL PHASES

Raspberry Chia Pancakes

Avocado oil spray
1 large egg
2 tablespoons cran-water or plain water
1 tablespoon chia seeds
1 serving vanilla whey protein or pea and rice protein
1 cup raspberries
1 teaspoon Flora-Key

- Lightly coat a medium-size pan with a few spritzes of avocado oil.
- In a medium-size bowl, whisk together all the ingredients except the raspberries and Flora-Key.
- Gently fold ½ cup of the raspberries into the batter.

- Heat the pan over medium heat.
- Using a tablespoon, ladle the chia mixture into the pan.
- Cook until tiny bubbles form on the surface and the chia cakes are solid enough to turn.
- Carefully flip the chia cakes, cooking only until done.
- Transfer to a plate and keep warm.
- Repeat the process with the remaining batter, coating the pan with a few spritzes of avocado oil as needed.
- Garnish with the remaining ½ cup of raspberries.
- Sprinkle with Flora-Key.

Makes 1 serving.
ALL PHASES

Whey Pancakes

Olive oil spray
2 eggs
1 scoop vanilla whey protein
1 teaspoon Ceylon cinnamon
¼ teaspoon ground cloves

- Blend eggs, whey protein, Ceylon cinnamon, and cloves until smooth.
- Spritz a pan with olive oil spray and place over medium heat.
- Spoon about 3 tablespoons of batter into the pan, tilting the pan to evenly spread the batter.
- Cook for a few minutes, until the edges are golden brown; flip and cook for about 1 minute more.
- Remove from the pan and lay flat to cool. Repeat with the rest of the batter.

Makes 4 pancakes.
ALL PHASES

Breakfast Egg Fu Yung

Got 5 minutes? Whip up this tasty egg dish to start your day off right. A complete source of protein, eggs are loaded with key nutrients, such as vitamins, minerals, amino acids, and antioxidants, as well as the cholesterol-lowering phosphatidylcholine.

1 cup mushrooms, thinly sliced
1 tablespoon bone broth
½ cup mung bean sprouts
1 garlic clove, diced
2 eggs, beaten with water

- Cook mushrooms in broth over medium heat.
- Add bean sprouts and garlic and sauté briefly.

- Pour eggs over mushrooms and sprouts.
- Cook over low heat until firm.

Makes 1 serving.
ALL PHASES

Weekend Turkey-and-Egg Bake

Pamper yourself on your day off! Savory fat-flushing herbs and fibrous veggies give this dish some real pizzazz while keeping you on track with your weight loss goals. Fennel, dill, and garlic aid the digestive process, and parsley helps reduce water weight.

½ pound lean ground turkey
1 cup mushrooms
½ cup onion, chopped
½ cup red pepper, chopped
¼ teaspoon dill, chopped
¼ teaspoon fennel
1 crushed garlic clove, minced
2 eggs, beaten
¼ cup fresh parsley, minced
2 medium tomatoes, thinly sliced
Extra virgin olive oil

- Preheat oven to 350°F.
- In a large skillet, lightly coat pan with extra virgin olive oil and cook the turkey, mushrooms, onion, red pepper, dill, fennel, and garlic together on medium heat until the turkey is done.
- Drain off the liquid and place the mixture into a pie plate.
- In a medium bowl, stir together eggs and parsley and then spread them over the turkey mixture.
- Bake uncovered for 25–30 minutes or until the top is set.
- Garnish with a nice arrangement of tomato slices and enjoy!

Makes 2 servings.
ALL PHASES

Oatmeal Banana Waffle

2 cups rolled oats
2 cups water
1 banana
¼ teaspoon SweetLeaf Stevia or 1 tablespoon Lakanto Monk Fruit Sweetener
1 teaspoon vanilla
½ teaspoon sea salt

- Preheat waffle iron according to manufacturer's directions.

- Combine all ingredients in blender.
- Blend until smooth.
- Pour batter into waffle iron.
- Cook according to manufacturer's directions and enjoy with your favorite syrup or fresh fruit.

Makes 2–3 servings.
PHASE 2

Vegetable Frittata

Gourmet taste—yet so easy to do. And it's even better with delicious phytonutrient-rich vegetables.

Avocado oil spray
½ pound fresh or frozen asparagus spears, cut up
4 eggs
½ cup cottage cheese
1 teaspoon dried mustard
½ cup mushrooms, thinly sliced
¼ cup onions, chopped
½ tomato, thinly sliced

- Preheat oven to 400°F.
- Steam asparagus for about 5 minutes until tender; then set aside.
- Beat eggs in a medium bowl until foamy.
- Beat in cottage cheese and mustard; then set aside.
- Lightly spray an ovenproof skillet with avocado oil.
- Add mushrooms and onions (optional) and cook over medium heat until tender.
- Stir in asparagus pieces.
- Pour egg mixture over veggies and cook over low heat for about 5 minutes or until it bubbles slightly.
- Bake uncovered for about 10 minutes or until set.
- Garnish with tomato slices.

Makes 2 servings.
PHASE 3

Crockpot Raspberry Walnut Oatmeal

1 cup steel cut oats
4 cups boiling water
¼ teaspoon ground ginger
⅛ teaspoon cardamom
¼ cup walnuts, chopped
1 cup raspberries
2 tablespoons flaxseed oil

- Place all ingredients except for raspberries and oil in crockpot.
- Cook overnight, about 8 hours, on low.
- Stir in the raspberries and flaxseed oil 10 minutes before serving.

Makes 4 servings.
PHASE 3

Cream Cheese Pancakes

Avocado oil spray
2 ounces cream cheese
2 eggs
1 tablespoon coconut flour
1 tablespoon chia seeds

- Blend cream cheese, eggs, coconut flour, and chia seeds until smooth.
- Spray a pan with avocado oil and place over medium heat.
- Spoon about 3 tablespoons of batter into the pan, tilting the pan to evenly spread the batter.
- Cook for a few minutes, until the edges are golden brown; flip and cook for about 1 minute more.
- Remove from the pan and lay flat to cool. Repeat with the rest of the batter.

Makes 1 serving.
PHASE 3

Sweet Potato Hash

A great Fat Flush rendition of an old-time favorite. Just add 2 eggs any style to top off this delicious dish.

1 large sweet potato, peeled and cubed
1½ tablespoons sesame oil
½ cup scallions
½ clove garlic, chopped
Sea salt
2 strips turkey bacon, well cooked
2 tablespoons fresh parsley, chopped

- Add potato to 2 cups boiling water and simmer the potato until cooked.
- Drain and dry the potato.
- Heat 1 tablespoon oil in a medium skillet over medium heat.
- Add in scallions and garlic and sauté until tender, about 4 minutes.
- Season with salt.
- Add the remaining oil to the skillet, with sweet potato.
- Cook and stir on medium heat until done, increasing heat if necessary.
- Add turkey bacon and cook until desired crispness.

■ Garnish with parsley.

Makes 2 servings.
PHASE 3

LUNCH OR DINNER ENTRÉES

Easy Stuffed Avocado with Tuna Salad

1 (6-ounce) can tuna in water, rinsed and drained
1 tablespoon Fat Flush Mayo* or Macadamia Mayo*
¼ cup celery, finely chopped
2 tablespoons onion, finely minced
¼ teaspoon turmeric
½ medium avocado

■ Mix tuna, mayo, celery, onion, and turmeric together.
■ Cut an avocado in half, remove pit, and stuff with tuna salad.

Variations:

■ Replace the avocado with red bell pepper.
■ Replace tuna with salmon, sardines, shrimp, or tempeh.
■ Add a handful of toasted pumpkin seeds or chopped walnuts for crunch appeal for phase 3.

Makes 1 serving.
ALL PHASES

Basic Stir-Fry

Looking for a tasty no-fuss meal? This stir-fry is made to order. You can alternate your protein choices for a slight twist.

¼ cup bone broth
1 pound chicken, shrimp, lamb, or lean beef
2 cups mushrooms, thinly sliced
1 cup bamboo shoots
1 cup water chestnuts
1 cup snow peas
1 cup asparagus, coarsely chopped
1 carrot, thinly sliced
¼ teaspoon ginger

■ Heat broth over medium-high heat.
■ Add your protein choice and cook until almost done.
■ Add veggies and seasonings and cook until veggies are tender.

Makes 4 servings.
ALL PHASES

Slow Cooker Cuban Ropa Vieja

Avocado oil spray
2½ pounds flank steak, cut crosswise into three pieces
2 large onions, sliced thinly
2 bell peppers (any color), seeded and sliced thinly
1 garlic clove, minced
2 tablespoons apple cider vinegar
2 cups bone broth
1 (14-ounce) can diced tomatoes
2 bay leaves
2 tablespoons ground cumin
2 tablespoons tomato paste

- Lightly coat a large pot with a few sprays of avocado oil; heat over high heat.
- Add the meat and brown on all sides, approximately 5 minutes.
- Transfer the meat to a plate and set aside.
- Spray the pot again; heat over medium-high heat.
- Add the onions, peppers, and garlic; stir until they begin to brown.
- Add the vinegar; stir, scraping up any brown bits from the bottom of the pan.
- Add the broth and diced tomatoes.
- Bring to a boil.
- Add the bay leaves, cumin, and tomato paste, stirring until all the ingredients are blended.
- Return the steak to the pot.
- Bring the mixture back up to a boil and then cover; lower the heat and simmer until the meat is very tender, about 2½ hours.
- When the meat is tender, shred gently with a fork.
- Remove and discard the bay leaves before serving.

To prepare in the slow cooker:

- Lightly coat a large sauté pan with a spray of avocado oil; heat over high heat.
- Add the meat and brown on all sides, about 5 minutes; transfer the meat to the slow cooker.
- Add the remaining ingredients.
- Cook on low for about 6 hours or until the meat is tender.
- When the meat is cooked through and tender, shred gently with a fork.
- Remove and discard the bay leaves before serving.

Makes about 8 (2-cup) servings.
ALL PHASES

Slow Cooker Beef Stew

1½ pounds of stew meat, lean and trimmed of all visible fat, cut into chunks
2 scallions, thinly sliced
1 teaspoon Fat Flush Seasoning*
1 small head cauliflower, cut into florets
1 small head broccoli, cut into florets
1 carrot, grated
1 cup water

- Mix all ingredients in a 3½-quart or larger slow cooker.
- Cover and cook on low for 6 to 8 hours until beef is cooked through and vegetables are tender.

Serves 4.
ALL PHASES

Rose's Fat Flush Soup

Try this scrumptious standby for lunch or dinner. This full-bodied soup has been a lifesaver for many on-the-go Fat Flushers wanting a "meal-in-one."

1 pound ground beef or turkey
16 ounces tomato puree or bone broth
16 ounces filtered water
½ onion, chopped
1 cup spinach, chopped
1 cup green beans, chopped
1 garlic clove, minced
½ medium green pepper, chopped
½ medium red pepper, chopped
1 stalk celery, chopped
Extra virgin olive oil

- Lightly coat skillet with extra virgin olive oil and brown meat over medium heat until no longer pink
- Drain fat.
- Place the browned meat, water, garlic, tomato puree or bone broth, and raw veggies in a large pot.
- Simmer over low-medium heat for about 1 hour.

Makes 4 servings.
ALL PHASES

Eggplant Delight

An appetizing blend of flavors your whole family will love.

1 tablespoon bone broth
½ cup diced onion
1 garlic clove, minced
1 pound ground lamb
1 teaspoon cumin
1 teaspoon Ceylon cinnamon
1 (14.5-ounce) can no-salt-added diced tomatoes
1 medium eggplant, oven roasted

- Preheat oven to 375°F.
- Heat broth over medium heat.
- Add onion and garlic and sauté until soft.
- Remove mixture to a bowl and return pan to heat.
- Place lamb in the pan and cook until it just begins to brown.
- Add the cumin and Ceylon cinnamon, stir well, and sauté until meat is browned.
- Add onion-garlic mixture and tomatoes, simmering until juices evaporate.
- In a glass baking dish, arrange alternating layers of eggplant slices and lamb.
- Bake for 10 minutes.

Makes 4 servings.
ALL PHASES

Chicken Kebab

Even the kids will eat their veggies with this dish.

1 pound skinless chicken, cut into 1-inch cubes
2 cups zucchini, cubed
2 cups yellow squash, cubed
2 cups red pepper, cubed
½ pound button mushrooms
Lemon wedges, for garnish

- Preheat grill or broiler.
- Alternate chicken, vegetable cubes, and mushrooms on skewers.
- Grill for about 15–20 minutes, turning at least once, until chicken is cooked through.
- Remove from the grill onto a serving platter.
- Garnish with lemon and serve.

Makes 4 servings.
ALL PHASES

Cider Turkey with Mushrooms

Quick and zesty. A great pick-me-up on those hurried Fat Flush days.

1 pound skinless turkey, cut into 1-inch cubes
2 tablespoons bone broth
4 cups mushrooms, sliced
¼ cup red pepper, diced (optional)
¼ cup apple cider vinegar
⅛ cup fresh parsley, chopped, for garnish

- Cook turkey in broth over medium-high heat until the turkey is cooked through.
- Add mushrooms, red pepper (optional), and vinegar, cooking until soft.
- Remove from the skillet onto a plate.
- Garnish with fresh parsley.

Makes 4 servings.
ALL PHASES

Chicken Artichoke Jumble

¼ cup avocado or macadamia nut oil
3 tablespoons fresh basil, chopped
2 tablespoons apple cider vinegar
1 pound grilled or baked chicken, chopped or shredded
1 pound mushrooms, chopped
1 (14-ounce) can artichoke hearts, drained
1 small red onion, chopped
8 black olives, chopped
Sea salt (to taste)
2 tablespoons toasted flax seeds for garnish

- Whisk oil, basil, and vinegar together in a medium bowl.
- Add chicken, mushrooms, artichoke hearts, red onion, and olives and toss to blend.
- Season with sea salt (to taste).
- Sprinkle toasted flax seeds for garnish.

Makes 4 servings.
PHASE 3

Aloha Hawaiian Salad

1½ pounds cooked turkey or chicken, cubed or stripped
1 cup scallions, chopped
¾ cup celery, chopped
⅓ cup high-lignan flaxseed oil
1 cup fresh pineapple, crushed

Sea salt (to taste)
4 tablespoons organic extra virgin olive oil
2 tablespoons apple cider vinegar
6 cups spinach
12 macadamia nuts, chopped

- Mix turkey or chicken, scallions, celery, oil, and pineapple in a large bowl.
- Season with sea salt (to taste).
- In a separate bowl, make vinaigrette by whisking oil and vinegar together.
- Toss spinach and vinaigrette in a large bowl; arrange a single serving on each plate.
- Top each serving with turkey or chicken mixture and a sprinkling of chopped macadamia nuts.

Makes 6 servings.
PHASE 3

Purely Poached Salmon

Poaching liquid:

8 cups water or fish or bone broth
1 carrot, chopped
2 shallots, chopped
1 stalk celery, chopped
2 lemons, sliced
4 sprigs fresh dill
4 sprigs fresh parsley

Salmon:

1 pound wild-caught salmon fillet
½ cup Fat Flush Mayo* or Macadamia Mayo*
4 sprigs fresh dill
4 sprigs fresh parsley
1 lemon, sliced

- Place all the poaching ingredients in a large deep skillet with a lid.
- Bring the liquid to a gentle boil; reduce to a simmer.
- Add the salmon to the poaching liquid; cover.
- Maintaining a simmer, poach for 8 to 10 minutes or until the salmon is opaque and flakes easily with a fork.
- Place the salmon on a serving plate and refrigerate for about an hour.
- Before serving, carefully slice the salmon into four fillets and top each with 2 tablespoons of Fat Flush or Macadamia Mayo.
- Garnish with sprigs of fresh dill and parsley and lemon slices.

Makes 4 servings.
ALL PHASES

Crab Cake Delight

Avocado oil spray
1 pound crabmeat, picked over, rinsed, and drained
½ medium onion, chopped
2 tablespoons bell pepper, seeded and chopped
2 tablespoons celery, chopped
2 tablespoons fresh dill, chopped
2 tablespoons fresh parsley, chopped
1 clove garlic, minced
1 tablespoon fresh lemon juice (or lime juice)
1 large egg, beaten

- Preheat the oven to 350°F.
- Lightly coat a baking sheet with a spritz of avocado oil spray.
- In a large bowl, break up the crabmeat with a fork; mix in the rest of the ingredients.
- Shape the mixture into 8 patties and place on the baking sheet.
- Bake the crab cakes for about 15 minutes or until nicely browned and cooked through.

Makes 4 (2-cup) servings.
ALL PHASES

Succulent Sea Scallops

12 large fresh sea scallops
1 tablespoon broth or macadamia nut oil
1 clove garlic, minced
1 leek, white part, minced
½ teaspoon cumin
½ teaspoon cardamom
Pinch of sea salt
1 tablespoon fresh parsley, minced

- Rinse and drain scallops.
- Heat large skillet on medium heat.
- Add macadamia nut oil.
- Sauté garlic and leek just until garlic is softened, about 30 seconds.
- Set scallops in hot oil and allow to sear to a golden brown, flipping over after about 1 minute.
- Turn off heat.
- Sprinkle scallops with remaining ingredients.
- Cover and let rest for 5 minutes.

Serves 4.
ALL PHASES

Shrimp Creole

You don't have to live in New Orleans to cook up a tantalizing Fat Flush–style Creole dish. This recipe uses colorful phytonutrients and thermogenic herbs to entice your senses—and help you shed those pounds.

4 tablespoons bone broth
3 green onions, white parts, thinly sliced
½ cup celery, thinly sliced
½ green pepper, diced
½ red pepper, diced
1 garlic clove, minced
1 (14.5-ounce) can no-salt-added tomato sauce
½ cup filtered water
1 teaspoon fresh parsley, chopped
8 ounces shrimp, peeled and deveined

- Warm broth over low-medium heat.
- Add the green onions, celery, green and red pepper, and garlic and sauté until tender.
- Add the tomato sauce, water, and parsley and simmer uncovered for 20 minutes.
- Toss in shrimp and stir. Heat to boiling. Reduce heat to low and cover, letting dish simmer 15–20 minutes or until shrimp are done.

Makes 2 servings.
ALL PHASES

Pecan-Crusted Halibut

1 pound halibut, cut into 4 (4-ounce) portions
Sea salt (to taste)
Whites of 2 large eggs, well beaten
2 cups pecans, roughly chopped in a food processor
2 tablespoons macadamia nut oil

- Season each portion of fish with sea salt.
- Spread a thin layer of the egg whites on each side of the fish and then sprinkle with the chopped pecans.
- Press in nut mixture so both sides are coated.
- Preheat the oven to 400°F.
- Heat large saucepan coated with oil to medium heat.
- Place the fish in the pan and sear for 3 to 4 minutes or until the pecans are golden brown.
- Flip the fish and cook for another 3 minutes.

■ Place the fish in a baking dish and cook in the oven for another 8 to 10 minutes.

Makes 4 servings.
PHASE 3

Mushroom Tempeh Chili

2 (8-ounce) packages plain tempeh
2 (14-ounce) cans diced tomatoes
1 onion, chopped
3 stalks celery, chopped
4 garlic cloves, minced
2 teaspoons ground cumin
1 teaspoon ground coriander
⅛ teaspoon ground cloves
3 tablespoons apple cider vinegar
½ cup fresh cilantro, chopped
½ cup fresh parsley, chopped
1 cup bone broth
8 ounces mushrooms, quartered

■ In a large soup pot over medium heat, stir together all ingredients except the mushrooms.
■ Bring the mixture to a boil; lower the heat and cover.
■ Simmer, stirring occasionally, for about 45 minutes or until the veggies are fork-tender.
■ Add the mushrooms; simmer for an additional 10 minutes.

Makes 4 (2-cup) servings.
ALL PHASES

Portobello Bun

A great gluten-free alternative to the bun. Simply choose your burger of choice (turkey, beef, lamb, or a bean burger if vegan), and you are good to go on this healthy fast-food lunch or dinner.

2 large portobello mushrooms
Sea salt
⅛ cup apple cider vinegar
2 tablespoons bone broth or coconut oil
2 teaspoons dried parsley
1 garlic, finely minced

■ Cut stems off mushrooms and place smooth side up in a shallow dish.
■ Sprinkle lightly with salt.
■ Prepare the marinade with vinegar, broth or oil, parsley, and garlic.

- Preheat grill to medium.
- Place the mushrooms on the preheated grill, keeping the marinade for basting.
- Grill mushrooms 5 to 6 minutes per side, frequently basting until done.
- Fill the portobello "bun" with the burger of your choice.

2 servings.
ALL PHASES

Slow Cooker Lentil Stew

1¼ cup dried lentils, washed and drained
2 bay leaves
6 whole cloves
2 cups boiling water
1 onion, coarsely chopped
1 garlic clove, crushed
1 bell pepper, seeded and coarsely chopped
¼ cup bone broth
½ teaspoon Ceylon cinnamon
½ teaspoon ground ginger or 1 teaspoon grated fresh
1 teaspoon turmeric
1 teaspoon ground coriander
1 lime, juiced
1 cup fresh cilantro, chopped

- Place the lentils, bay leaves, and cloves in the slow cooker; cover with the boiling water.
- Stir in the remaining ingredients except the lime juice and cilantro.
- Cook on high for 2–2½ hours or until the lentils are tender and the water has been absorbed.
- Stir in the lime juice and cilantro.
- Remove and discard the bay leaves before serving.

FAT FLUSH TIPS	• Any type of lentil makes a delicious dhal—red, green, yellow, black, or brown. • If you prefer a souplike consistency, rather than stew, cook the lentils until tender with some liquid remaining.

Makes 4 (2-cup) servings.
PHASE 3

Black Bean Cakes

Avocado oil spray
½ cup chopped red onion
¼ cup chopped celery

¼ cup red bell pepper, seeded and chopped
¼ cup green bell pepper, seeded and chopped
2 cloves garlic, minced
1 jalapeno, seeded and chopped
2 teaspoons freshly squeezed lime juice
1 teaspoon ground cumin
¼ teaspoon ground coriander
1 tablespoon dried parsley
¼ teaspoon sea salt (optional)
2 (14-ounce) cans black beans, drained and lightly mashed
1 large egg
¼ cup chia seeds

- Preheat the oven to 375°F.
- Coat a sauté pan with a few sprays of avocado oil; heat over medium heat.
- Sauté the veggies until they are softened and begin to brown; spoon into a large bowl.
- Stir in the remaining ingredients, mixing well.
- Form the mixture into eight equal-size patties.
- Lightly coat a baking sheet with a few sprays of avocado oil.
- Place the patties on the baking sheet and bake for about 15 minutes or until heated through.

Makes 8 servings.
PHASE 3

Chickpeas with Sautéed Escarole

2 heads escarole, washed and chopped coarsely
Avocado oil spray
3 cloves garlic, crushed
2 cups fresh parsley, chopped
1 (14-ounce) can chickpeas (garbanzos), rinsed and drained
2 tablespoons bone broth
2 tablespoons freshly squeezed lemon juice
Pinch of sea salt (optional)

- In a large pot with a lid, lightly steam the escarole till just tender, about 6 minutes; drain.
- Lightly coat the same pot with a few spritzes of avocado oil spray; heat over medium heat.
- Sauté the garlic for about 1 minute or until softened and just beginning to turn golden. Be careful not to burn.
- Add the escarole, parsley, and chickpeas; sauté for 2 minutes.
- Stir in the broth, lemon juice, and salt (if using).

- Continue sautéing for about 5 minutes, until escarole is tender and almost all the broth has evaporated.

Makes about 4 (2-cup) servings.
PHASE 3

Bombay Curry Tofu

1 scallion
1 green cooking apple (such as Granny Smith), cored and chopped with peel
Grass-fed butter
2 teaspoons curry powder
1 teaspoon cumin
1 tablespoon arrowroot
1 cup canned full-fat coconut milk
½ teaspoon sea salt
1 pound extra-firm non-GMO silken tofu, cut into cubes
1 red bell pepper, cut julienne
1 yellow bell pepper, cut julienne
1 stalk celery, finely chopped

- Sauté scallion and apple in grass-fed butter until tender.
- Add curry powder and cumin and simmer 2 minutes, stirring frequently.
- Add arrowroot.
- Mix thoroughly.
- Add coconut milk and salt, stirring constantly until mixture starts to bubble.
- Lower heat to simmer and add tofu, red and yellow peppers, and celery stalk.
- Cook 8–10 minutes until mixture is nice and thick and tofu and vegetables are cooked through.

Makes 4 servings.
PHASE 3

EASY SOUPS

Egg Drop Cilantro Soup

East meets the Southwest. Here's a unique Fat Flush combo that also gets that slimming protein into your diet.

4 cups bone broth
2 eggs, well beaten
¼ cup cilantro, chopped, for garnish

- Place broth in a large pot and bring to a boil over medium-high heat.
- In a small bowl, beat eggs with a fork.

- Gradually stir the beaten eggs into the bone broth.
- Reduce heat, stirring continuously with a fork until the egg stands out from the stock.
- Remove from heat and pour into bowls.
- Garnish with cilantro and serve immediately.

Makes 4 servings.
ALL PHASES

Gingered Shrimp and Snow Pea Soup

Freshly made, mouth-watering soup in just 25 minutes.

4 cups bone broth
¼ cup fresh ginger, sliced
2 cups snow peas, trimmed
1 pound shrimp, peeled and deveined
1 lemon, cut into wedges
2 tablespoons fresh cilantro or parsley, chopped

- Place broth and ginger in a large pot, and cover and simmer over medium-high heat for 15 minutes.
- Strain out ginger and return broth to pan.
- Add snow peas, simmering covered for about 5 minutes.
- Add shrimp and cook until firm (about 3 minutes).
- Squeeze lemon wedges into individual soup bowls and garnish each with cilantro (or parsley).

Makes 4 servings.
ALL PHASES

Friendly Italian Wedding Soup

Enjoy this romantic specialty from the Mediterranean—Fat Flush style.

1 pound lean ground beef
2 tablespoons garlic, minced
2 teaspoons fresh parsley, chopped
¼ cup diced onion
4 cups bone broth
1 carrot, chopped
1 cup spinach, chopped, packed, and well drained
Fresh garlic, minced, for garnish

- Combine the beef, garlic, parsley, and onion.
- Shape into ½-inch meatballs.
- Brown meatballs over medium heat until cooked; set aside.
- Pour broth into a large pot, add chopped carrot, and bring to a boil.

- Reduce heat, add meatballs, and simmer covered for about 20 minutes.
- Add spinach and simmer for 15 minutes longer.
- Garnish with lots of fresh garlic.

Makes 4 servings.
ALL PHASES

Butternut Squash Soup

3 pounds butternut squash, peeled and seeded, cut into chunks
2 Granny Smith apples, peeled and cored
2 leeks, washed well and seeded
1 teaspoon ground ginger
Sea salt (to taste)
½ teaspoon ground coriander
½ teaspoon ground cumin
¼ cup apple cider vinegar
2 cups chicken bone or vegetable broth

- Steam the squash, apples, and leeks for about 8 minutes until soft.
- In food processor or blender, chop the mixture lightly, leaving chunks.
- Place mixture in soup pot and simmer over low to medium heat for around 20 minutes.
- Stir in spices, salt, vinegar, and broth.
- Simmer for about 5 minutes more.

Makes 6 (1-cup) servings.
PHASE 2

Velvety Borscht

6 large whole beets, peeled
3 large whole carrots, peeled
8 cups water
4 tablespoons flaxseed oil
2 tablespoons apple cider vinegar

- Place beets, carrots, and water in a soup pot and bring to a boil.
- Let simmer until vegetables are soft.
- Remove beets and carrots from water and cut into small pieces, reserving cooking liquid.
- Place vegetables and liquid in a blender or food processor with flaxseed oil and apple cider vinegar.
- Blend until smooth; then chill.

Makes 6 servings.
PHASE 2

VEGGIE SIDES

Zesty Coleslaw

Want a little crunch—and a whole lot of zing? Here it is.

1 cup shredded green cabbage
½ cup shredded red cabbage
½ cup jicama, peeled and grated
½ small green pepper, coarsely chopped
½ small red pepper, coarsely chopped
½ small onion, coarsely chopped
1 small celery stalk, chopped

Dressing:

½ cup apple cider vinegar
½ teaspoon garlic, minced
½ teaspoon Flora-Key, SweetLeaf Stevia, or Lakanto Monk Fruit Sweetener
(optional)

■ Combine the cabbage, jicama, pepper, onion, and celery in a large serving
   bowl.
■ In another bowl, create the dressing by stirring the vinegar, garlic, and
   Flora-Key, SweetLeaf Stevia, or Lakanto (optional) until well blended.
■ Add the dressing to the vegetable mixture and toss lightly.
■ Cover and refrigerate for at least 1 hour before serving.

Makes 4 servings.
ALL PHASES

Jicama Salad

12 ounces jicama, peeled and cut into thin strips
1 red onion, thinly sliced
1 carrot, grated
1 cucumber, cut into thin strips

Dressing:

1 cup parsley, chopped
½ cup apple cider vinegar
½ teaspoon dill
3 tablespoons flaxseed oil
3 garlic cloves, minced
Juice of 1 lemon

■ In a large bowl, place jicama, onion, carrot, and cucumber and set aside.

- In a jar, put parsley, vinegar, dill, flaxseed oil, garlic, and lemon juice; shake well.
- Pour the dressing over the jicama mix and toss lightly.

Makes 4 servings
ALL PHASES

Artichoke and Hearts of Palm Salad

1 (14-ounce) can artichoke hearts, rinsed and drained
1 (14-ounce) can hearts of palm, rinsed and drained
1 garlic clove, minced
¼ cup flaxseed oil
2 tablespoons fresh lemon juice
1 tablespoon apple cider vinegar
1 cup fresh parsley, minced

- In a medium-size bowl, toss all ingredients together.
- Refrigerate for 1 hour prior to serving.

Makes 4 servings.
ALL PHASES

Cauliflower Rice

1 small onion, chopped
½ red pepper, chopped
½ yellow pepper, chopped
¼ cup bone broth
2 cups cooked cauliflower, diced
¼ teaspoon dried dill
½ teaspoon garlic, minced

- Sauté the onion and pepper in the broth for about 5 minutes over medium heat.
- Add the cauliflower and toss until heated through.
- Add dill and garlic.
- Transfer to a food processor (or blender) and puree, adding an additional tablespoon of broth to achieve a smooth consistency.
- Serve hot.

Makes 2–3 servings.
ALL PHASES

Glorious Greens

2 pounds assorted greens, trimmed and cleaned
2 cups water
¼ cup bone broth

1 onion, sliced
1 garlic clove, minced
Juice of 1 lemon
4 tablespoons flaxseed oil

- Place the greens in a pot and add water to cover.
- Bring to a quick boil; then lower the heat, simmer, and cook greens until barely tender (about 5–8 minutes).
- Drain, chop, and set aside.
- Heat the broth in a saucepan and sauté the onion and garlic over low heat until tender.
- Quickly add the greens to the saucepan, reducing the heat to low, and cook greens until tender.
- Dish the greens into a bowl; add the lemon juice and flaxseed oil and toss.
- Serve warm or at room temperature.

Makes 4 servings.
ALL PHASES

Warm Asparagus and Mushrooms

1 pound fresh asparagus spears, cut into 1-inch pieces
1 tablespoon bone broth
4 cups mushrooms, thinly sliced
½ cup onion, chopped
1 tablespoon garlic, minced
½ cup fresh lemon juice
2–4 tablespoons flaxseed oil or olive oil

- Take an asparagus spear and gently bend it until it snaps; discard the bottom part; continue for the rest of the spears.
- Steam the asparagus for about 5–6 minutes until crisp but tender; set aside.
- Heat the broth, mushrooms, onions, and garlic, cooking until soft.
- Add the asparagus and drizzle with lemon juice; stir to combine.
- Cook over low-medium heat until the asparagus is warmed through.
- Remove from the skillet onto serving platters and allow to cool.
- Drizzle ½ tablespoon to 1 tablespoon flaxseed (or olive) oil over each serving at room temperature.

Makes 4 servings.
ALL PHASES

Savory Spaghetti Squash

Here's a delicious way to blend those fat-flushing nutrients with the thermogenic power of Ceylon cinnamon. When selecting your smooth, watermelon-shaped squash, look for one that has a hard, deep-colored rind.

1 spaghetti squash
1 large garlic clove, minced
½ teaspoon Ceylon cinnamon
1–2 tablespoons flaxseed oil

- Cut squash in half and scoop out the seeds.
- Place the squash halves on a baking sheet, cut side down.
- Bake at 375°F for 30 minutes.
- With a fork, separate the spaghetti pulp from the skin, and place the pulp in a serving dish.
- Sprinkle on garlic, Ceylon cinnamon, and oil and toss lightly.

Makes 4 servings.
ALL PHASES

Savory Spaghetti Squash Pancakes

Avocado oil spray
2 cups cooked spaghetti squash
1 large egg
1 tablespoon chia seeds
⅛ teaspoon coriander
⅛ teaspoon cumin
Sea salt (to taste)

- Lightly coat a sauté pan with a few spritzes of avocado oil and heat over medium heat.
- In a medium-size bowl, mix the cooked spaghetti squash, coriander, cumin, and salt (if desired) with the egg and chia seeds.
- Ladle about 2 tablespoons of the squash mixture into the pan; cook until small bubbles form on the surface of the pancake.
- Flip the pancake, cover, and continue cooking until almost dry.
- Repeat with the remaining batter.

Makes 2 to 4 servings.
ALL PHASES

Pâté for All Seasons

Company's coming, and I've got just the appetizer to satisfy your guests. This is a fabulous dip that my good friend John created. I first tasted it at a Fat Flush party in my home in San Francisco many years ago, where the pâté was, and still is, a great crowd pleaser. I find it perfect to pair with veggies.

2 (13-ounce) cans water-packed tuna, rinsed and drained
1 (8-ounce) can oysters, rinsed and drained
1 (2-ounce) can anchovy fillets, well rinsed and drained
1 clove garlic, minced

2 tablespoons parsley, chopped
¼ teaspoon dill
¼ teaspoon dried mustard
1 teaspoon fresh lemon juice

- Place all ingredients in a food processor or blender and blend until smooth.
- Add more liquid if needed.

Variation: For phase 3, add ¼ teaspoon dried horseradish.

Serves 8.
ALL PHASES

Fresh Cranberry Chutney

2 cups apple, peeled, cored, and chopped
4 cups fresh or frozen cranberries
¼ cup chopped onion
2 stalks celery, chopped
1 red bell pepper, seeded and chopped
½ cup apple cider vinegar
1 tablespoon grated fresh ginger or 1 teaspoon ground ginger
1 teaspoon Ceylon cinnamon
Zest from 1 orange
1 tablespoon Flora-Key

- Combine all the ingredients except Flora-Key in a 2-quart saucepan.
- Simmer for 20 to 25 minutes or until all veggies and fruits are tender, stirring often.
- Let cool; stir in the Flora-Key.
- Store the chutney in a covered container in the refrigerator until serving.

Makes 8 servings.
ALL PHASES

Roasted Veggie Medley

½ cup red bell pepper, sliced
½ cup eggplant, sliced
½ cup onion, sliced
½ cup mushrooms, sliced
2 tablespoons vegetable or bone broth

- Preheat the broiler.
- Place veggies in a baking dish.
- Add the broth and stir to coat.
- Broil for about 10 minutes or until the veggies are cooked through.

Variation: Try adding different Fat Flush vegetables like snow peas, zucchini, or yellow squash.

Makes 1 serving.
ALL PHASES

Quinoa Tabbouleh

Juice of 1 lemon
2 tablespoons flaxseed oil
Sea salt (to taste)
2 cups cooked quinoa
2 scallions, chopped
1 cup fresh tomato, chopped
1 cucumber, chopped
⅓ cup fresh mint, chopped
⅓ cup fresh parsley, chopped
¼ cup fresh basil, chopped

- Whisk together lemon juice, flaxseed oil, and salt.
- Combine all other ingredients and then dress with lemon mixture.
- Refrigerate 1 to 2 hours; then stir and serve.

Makes 4 servings.
PHASE 2

Orange-Scented Roasted Brussels Sprouts

Avocado oil spray
1 pound brussels sprouts, tough outer leaves removed
4 teaspoons macadamia nut oil
1 tablespoon grated orange zest
1 teaspoon dried basil

- Preheat oven to 425°F.
- In a medium-size bowl, toss the brussels sprouts with the macadamia nut oil, orange zest, and basil.
- Coat a rimmed baking sheet or casserole dish with a few sprays of the oil.
- Place the brussels sprouts in a single layer on the baking sheet.
- Roast for 15 or 20 minutes or until browned and tender.

Makes 4 servings.
PHASE 3

SALAD DRESSINGS

Fat Flush Vinaigrette

5 tablespoons vegetable or bone broth
1 garlic clove, minced
1 tablespoon apple cider vinegar
1 tablespoon fresh lemon juice
1 tablespoon fresh parsley, chopped
1 teaspoon dried mustard
Dash of sea salt

- Put all ingredients in a small jar, cover, and shake vigorously until mixed.
- Use immediately or store in the refrigerator.

Variations:

For phase 1, add a few drops of unsweetened cranberry juice and ¼ teaspoon stevia for a cranberry vinaigrette.

For phase 2, add 2 teaspoons of grated beets.

For phase 3, substitute 1 cup of water and ¼ cup sherry or white wine for broth and increase the vinegar to ¼ cup. (This makes a delicious marinade for chicken, fish, and beef!)

Makes about ½ cup.
ALL PHASES

Amazing Caesar Dressing

1 large egg, raw or coddled
Grated zest from 1 lemon
Juice from 1 small lemon
1 to 2 garlic cloves
¼ to ½ teaspoon dry mustard
Pinch of sea salt (optional)
2 tablespoons apple cider vinegar
½ cup flaxseed oil

- Place all ingredients except the flaxseed oil in blender or food processor.
- Drizzle in the flaxseed oil and blend until thickened and smooth.
- Store the dressing in the refrigerator.

Makes 1 cup.
ALL PHASES

Ruby Rich Dressing

1½ pounds medium beets, trimmed
2½ tablespoons apple cider vinegar

2 tablespoons finely chopped leeks
1 teaspoon Lakanto Monk Fruit Sweetener or ½ teaspoon SweetLeaf Stevia
½ teaspoon sea salt
1 tablespoon fresh parsley
4 tablespoons flaxseed oil or sesame oil
2 tablespoons Italian flat-leaf parsley, finely chopped

- Cover beets with water in a heavy saucepan and simmer until tender, about 30 to 45 minutes.
- Drain and cool until just warm.
- Peel off skins and cut into small cubes.
- While the beets are cooking, whisk together vinegar, leeks, Lakanto or stevia, and sea salt in a large bowl.
- Add oil slowly into mix, continuing to whisk until well incorporated.
- Add warm beets and parsley.
- Pour into blender and blend until smooth.
- Serve warm or at room temperature.

Makes 4 servings.
ALL PHASES

Pepita Plum Dressing

1 cup pumpkin seeds
1 cup filtered water
2–3 umeboshi plums
2 tablespoons flax oil

- Wash and dry pumpkin seeds.
- Dry-roast them in a skillet over medium heat until they puff up and pop.
- Place roasted seeds in a blender and grind to a meallike consistency.
- Add water to blender and continue mixing.
- Add plums and oil, blending until desired taste is reached. (The more plums you add, the saltier the dressing.)

Makes 1 cup.
PHASE 3

Toasted Sesame Lemon Dressing

½ cup toasted sesame oil
2 tablespoons fresh lemon juice
½ teaspoon grated fresh lemon zest
¼ teaspoon sea salt
½ teaspoon dried dill

- Combine all ingredients in a small covered jar.
- Shake well.

- Refrigerate until ready to use.

Makes 8 tablespoons.
PHASE 3

Curry Lime Dressing

4 tablespoons full-fat coconut milk
½ teaspoon curry
½ teaspoon turmeric
½ teaspoon Lakanto Monk Fruit Sweetener
½ teaspoon sea salt
Juice of 1 lime

- Use a blender to combine all ingredients and serve over salad.

Makes 6 tablespoons.
PHASE 3

CONDIMENTS, SAUCES, AND SEASONINGS

Great Guacamole

3 tablespoons green onion, chopped
2 tablespoons cilantro, coarsely chopped
1 clove garlic, finely minced
Juice of ½ lime
¼ teaspoon cumin
Sea salt (to taste)
4 ripe avocados

- Combine all the ingredients except the avocados.
- Mash the avocados.
- Fold in the other ingredients.
- Serve immediately.

Makes 4 servings.
ALL PHASES

5-Star Artichoke Dip

1 (14-ounce) can artichoke hearts, rinsed and drained
4 cups spinach, coarsely chopped
1 garlic clove, minced
1 tablespoon lemon juice, fresh squeezed
2 tablespoons fresh dill, chopped
½ cup fresh cilantro, chopped
1 (9-ounce) can water chestnuts, rinsed, drained, and chopped
¼ cup Fat Flush Mayo*

- Combine all ingredients in a medium bowl.
- Chill thoroughly.
- Serve with veggies or flax and chia crackers.

Makes 4 servings.
ALL PHASES

Fat Flush Mayo

1 garlic clove
2 egg yolks
2 tablespoons lemon juice
½ teaspoon dried mustard
2 tablespoons apple cider vinegar
1 cup flaxseed oil

- Combine the garlic, dried mustard, egg yolks, lemon juice, and vinegar in a food processor or blender.
- With the machine running, slowly drizzle in the oil until the mixture thickens into mayonnaise.
- Keep refrigerated.

For Fresh Herbed Mayonnaise: Before blending, mix in ½ cup minced fresh green herbs (dill, cilantro, parsley, etc.). Thin with a few drops of filtered water, if desired.

Makes 4 servings.
ALL PHASES

Macadamia Mayo

1 egg
1 tablespoon freshly squeezed lemon juice
¼ teaspoon ground mustard seed
1 cup macadamia nut oil
Sea salt (to taste)

- In a blender or food processor, blend egg, lemon juice, and mustard seed.
- Slowly add in oil, 1 tablespoon at a time, continuing to blend.
- When the oil has all emulsified and you have a creamy mayonnaise, add in salt.
- Keep in a jar in the fridge. This mayo will last about a week.

Makes 4 servings.
PHASE 3

Cilantro Pesto

1½ cups packed parsley
1½ cups cilantro
2 cloves garlic
¼ cup pine nuts
¼ cup toasted pumpkin seeds
1½ cups olive oil
¼ cup lemon juice

- Place parsley, cilantro, garlic, pine nuts, toasted pumpkin seeds, and oil in a food processor or electric blender; pulse until finely chopped.
- Add lemon juice, continuing to pulse until a paste forms, scraping down the sides as needed.
- Store in a covered container in the refrigerator.

Makes about 2 cups.
PHASE 3

Fat Flush Hummus

16 ounces garbanzo beans, drained and rinsed
Juice of 1 lemon
¼ cup olive oil
3 tablespoon tahini
¼ teaspoon sea salt

- Blend all ingredients together in food processor and serve.

Makes 8 servings.
PHASE 3

Fat Flush Garam Masala

4 teaspoons ground cloves
2 tablespoons Ceylon cinnamon
4 teaspoons ground cumin
4 teaspoons ground coriander

- Combine all ingredients in a covered container.
- Store at room temperature away from the stove.

Makes 10 tablespoons.
ALL PHASES

Fat Flush Seasoning

2 tablespoons onion powder
2 tablespoons garlic powder
2 teaspoons ground coriander

¼ cup dried parsley
1 teaspoon minced lemon zest
¼ teaspoon cayenne
¼ cup ground cumin
¼ packet SweetLeaf Stevia

- Combine all the ingredients.
- Place in a covered container or shaker bottle.
- Store the seasoning at room temperature away from the stove.

Makes ½ cup.
ALL PHASES

Italian Seasoning

2 tablespoons dried basil
2 tablespoons dried oregano
2 tablespoons dried rosemary
2 tablespoons dried cilantro
2 tablespoons dried thyme

- Combine all ingredients in a food processor and blend until they are well mixed and the desired consistency is achieved.

Yields about 2 cups or 16 (1-tablespoon) servings.
PHASE 3

SNACKS

Spinach Flatbread

1 (10-ounce) package frozen chopped spinach, thawed and drained
2 large eggs
Whites of 2 large eggs
½ teaspoon minced garlic
¼ cup chopped onions
2 tablespoons flaxseed oil

- Preheat oven to 400°F.
- In a mixing bowl, stir together all the ingredients.
- Line a baking sheet with parchment paper; pour the mixture evenly onto the pan.
- Bake for 15 minutes.
- Holding the ends of the parchment paper, pick up the flatbread and lay on a cooling rack or towel.
- Cut into sandwich or wrap-size pieces and drizzle with flaxseed oil.

Makes 2 servings.
ALL PHASES

Flax Snackers

Olive or avocado oil spray
1 cup milled flax seeds
1 teaspoon SweetLeaf Stevia
2 teaspoons Ceylon cinnamon
½ teaspoon ground ginger
½ cup cran-water
1 tablespoon almond or cashew butter as topping

- Preheat oven to 275°F.
- Lightly coat a cookie sheet with oil spray.
- Mix the dry ingredients in a medium bowl.
- Add the cran-water and let stand for 5 minutes.
- Stir the mixture vigorously with a fork for about 5 minutes or until seeds stick together.
- Let mixture rest for 15 minutes.
- Spoon the flaxseed mixture onto the prepared cookie sheet.
- Cover with waxed paper and use a rolling pin to flatten the mixture out to the sides of the cookie sheet.
- When the mixture is evenly distributed, remove and discard waxed paper.
- Use a knife or pizza cutter to score the mixture into 16 sections.
- Bake for 60–90 minutes or until the crackers lift off the cookie sheet and break apart easily.
- Store crackers in an airtight container at room temperature.

Makes 8 servings, 2 crackers each.
ALL PHASES

Fabulous Chia Crax

Chia gel:
⅓ cup chia seeds
2 cups water

Rest of recipe:
¾ cup chia seeds (reserved for crackers)
½ tablespoon cumin powder
½ tablespoon garlic powder

- Prepare the chia gel by combining seeds and water. Cover, shake for 45 seconds, and let rest for 1 minute; then shake again. After 15 minutes of resting, the gel is ready.
- Preheat the oven to 275°F.
- In a medium bowl, combine the dry chia seeds and spices.
- Add the chia gel, stirring until well mixed and the seeds start to form a ball.

- Line a baking sheet with parchment paper and spoon the chia mixture over it.
- Cover with waxed paper and use a rolling pin to flatten the mixture out to the sides of the cookie sheet.
- When the mixture is evenly distributed, remove and discard the waxed paper.
- Use a knife or pizza cutter to score the mixture into 16 sections.
- Bake for 45 minutes to 1 hour or until the crackers lift off the cookie sheet and break apart easily. Store crackers in an airtight container at room temperature.

Makes 16 servings, 2 crackers each.
ALL PHASES

Fat Flush "Deviled" Eggs

There's nothing bad about these eggs! They're loaded with slimming omega-3 and dressed with fat-flushing herbs.

2 eggs, hard-boiled
½ tablespoon flaxseed oil
½ teaspoon apple cider vinegar
½ teaspoon finely minced green onion (white part)
¼ to ½ teaspoon finely minced garlic (to taste)
¼ teaspoon dried mustard
Sprigs of fresh dill and parsley, for garnish

- Cool the hard-boiled eggs under cold water.
- Peel eggs and cut in half lengthwise.
- Remove yolks and put them in a small bowl.
- Add oil, vinegar, onion, garlic, and mustard to yolks and mix thoroughly. Scoop yolk mixture with a spoon and use it to fill the egg halves.
- Top with dill and parsley.

Makes 1 to 2 servings.
ALL PHASES

Fat Flush Pickles

One of my premier Fat Flush secrets is this: when you crave something sweet, satisfy that craving with something sour. And what better than these oh-so-easy homemade pickles. These are a great snack between meals—you can actually eat all of them in one sitting if you'd like, and they can be used sliced in salads and for burgers.

8 cucumbers, cut into spears
1 cup apple cider vinegar
1 clove garlic, minced

2 teaspoons fresh dill
Dash of turmeric

- In a medium bowl, stir together cucumbers, vinegar, garlic, dill, and turmeric.
- Cover, refrigerate for at least 6 hours, and enjoy.

Serves 4.
ALL PHASES

Spinach-Stuffed Mushrooms

This is a great party food, not to mention a quick and easy snack for you to pack and have between meals.

Avocado oil spray
1 (10-ounce) package frozen spinach, thawed and drained
1 egg yolk
1 clove garlic, minced
12 large white mushrooms, cleaned and stemmed

- Heat oven to 350°F.
- Spray a small baking sheet with avocado oil.
- In a large bowl, mix spinach, egg yolk, and garlic.
- Stuff each mushroom with spinach mixture and place on baking sheet.
- Bake for 15 to 25 minutes or until mixture is firm to the touch.
- Serve hot.

Variations:

For phase 2, add ½ teaspoon basil and oregano to stuffing mix.

For phase 3, add ½ teaspoon nutmeg and ¼ cup chopped walnuts to stuffing mix.

Serves 4.
ALL PHASES

Yummy Yam or Butternut Squash Chips

2 small yams or 1 small butternut squash, thinly sliced into ⅛-inch pieces
½ teaspoon basil
½ teaspoon oregano
½ teaspoon onion powder

- Preheat oven to 425°F.
- In a self-sealing plastic bag, place yam or squash slices and herbs, shaking to coat.
- Place the yams or squash on a baking sheet sprayed with avocado cooking spray.

- Bake for about ½ hour or until slices are slightly golden, making sure to turn at least once during cooking process.

Variations:

Substitute sweet potatoes for the yams.

Change the flavor mix by substituting sweeter spices like ground anise and fennel for the Italian herbs.

For phase 3, sprinkle with a dash of sea salt or to taste.

Serves 2.
PHASE 2

Jicama Chips

1 medium jicama, cut into ¼-inch slices
Juice of 1 lime
1 tablespoon toasted sesame oil
Parchment paper or pizza stone

- Preheat oven to 325°F.
- Toss jicama slices with lime juice.
- Place on baking sheet covered with parchment paper or use a pizza stone, making sure the slices are not touching.
- Bake for about 30 minutes, turning chips about every 10 minutes.
- Be careful not to burn.
- Cover and store in refrigerator and return to warmed oven to recrisp if desired.
- Drizzle toasted sesame oil before serving.

Makes about 2 cups.
PHASE 3

Yogurt Cheese

I first learned about this idea many years ago from my clients in Southern California. This is a good healthy spread (yogurt is filled with beneficial bacteria that aid digestion and protect against pathogens), which is delightful with flax crackers or simply by itself.

2 cups plain Greek yogurt
Dash of nutmeg
Dash of Ceylon cinnamon
Dash of cardamom

- Line a colander with cheesecloth, placing a bowl underneath.
- In a bowl, mix the yogurt with the nutmeg, Ceylon cinnamon, and cardamom.

- Pour the yogurt mixture on top of the cheesecloth.
- Place in the fridge, cover, and let drain overnight.

Variation: Add ¼ teaspoon vanilla extract for an interesting flavor.

Makes 4 servings.
PHASE 3

Fat Flush Chickpea Peanuts

These are quite addictive, so careful on the quantities—a great snack for the kids, by the way.

Avocado oil spray
1 (15.5-ounce) can chickpeas, rinsed well and drained
1 tablespoon sesame oil
¼ teaspoon ground ginger
¼ teaspoon ground coriander
¼ teaspoon ground cumin

- Preheat oven to 400°F.
- In a bowl, mix the chickpeas with the sesame oil and spices.
- Place on a baking sheet sprayed with avocado cooking oil.
- Bake about ½ hour or until chickpeas are golden and crunchy.

Variation: You can substitute olive oil for the sesame oil.

Serves 4.
PHASE 3

Roasted Chestnuts

The most easily digested nuts, chestnuts are really a starchy vegetable. One of my favorite fall and winter snack treats, roasted chestnuts make me think of New York City, where street vendors sell them on wintry days.

12 chestnuts, rinsed and dried

- Preheat the oven to 425°F.
- Use a knife to score an X on the side of each chestnut where it is most flat.
- Place on a baking sheet in a single layer.
- Roast in oven for about 20 to 25 minutes or until chestnuts are tender, turning occasionally.
- Remove from oven and cool before peeling off the outer and inner shell.

Variation: You can also cook on top of the stove. Put chestnuts in a pot, cover with cold water, and bring water to a boil, cook for 30–35 minutes, lower the heat, and simmer for another 3 to 5 minutes until soft. Chestnuts go well with a dash of cloves, allspice, or nutmeg.

Makes 3 servings.
PHASE 3

TREATS

Sweety Pie Grapefruit

½ teaspoon olive oil
½ grapefruit

- Add ½ teaspoon olive oil to ½ grapefruit and let stand for ½ hour (olive oil will neutralize the acids and sweeten up the grapefruit).

This trick was taught to me years ago by Dr. Hazel Parcells.

Makes 1 serving.
ALL PHASES

Fruity Fruit Sorbet

Once you've graduated to the Lifestyle Eating Plan, treat yourself to this delightful dessert. It's allowed only in phase 3 because, unlike the blended fruits, protein powder, and flaxseed oil in the breakfast smoothies, this recipe is really pure fruit, without the balancing nutrition of the protein and oil to level out blood sugar. Pureeing breaks down the fiber in fruits, which also can affect blood sugar levels by concentrating the sugars.

½ cup strawberries, halved
½ cup raspberries
1 teaspoon fresh lemon juice (optional)
¼ to ½ teaspoon Flora-Key or SweetLeaf Stevia (optional to taste if fruit is not sweet enough)

- Place all ingredients in a food processor or blender and puree until smooth.
- Freeze until firm (about 3–4 hours only).

TIME SAVING FLUSHING TIP	Start with partially thawed frozen fruit so that you can eat your sorbet immediately.

Makes 1 serving.
PHASE 3

Fat Flush Coconut Milk Ice Cream

1 (13.5-ounce) can full-fat coconut milk
3 frozen bananas
Pinch of sea salt

- Combine ingredients in blender and blend until smooth.
- Pour mixture into ice cream maker or food processor.
- Mix for at least 20 minutes or until ice cream is formed.
- Stir in dry salt and serve.
- Best served immediately; if stored in freezer, place back into ice cream maker to make smooth and creamy again.

Makes 10 servings.
PHASE 3

Coconut Crème Brûlée

2 cups heavy cream
2 cups full-fat coconut milk (chilled overnight)
1 cup unsweetened coconut flakes
1 vanilla bean, split and scraped
¼ to ½ cup Lakanto Monk Fruit Sweetener
Yolks of 6 large eggs
2 quarts hot water

- Preheat oven to 325°F.
- Place the cream, coconut milk, coconut flakes, and vanilla bean and its pulp into a medium saucepan set over medium-high heat and bring to a boil.
- Remove from heat; cover for 15 minutes.
- Remove vanilla bean.
- In a medium bowl, whisk together ¼ cup Lakanto and the egg yolks.
- Add the cream mixture a little at a time, stirring continuously.
- Pour the liquid into 6 ramekins (7–8-ounce size).
- Place the ramekins into a large cake pan or roasting pan.
- Pour enough hot water into the pan to come halfway up the sides of the ramekins.
- Bake just until the crème brûlée is set, approximately 40–45 minutes.
- Remove the ramekins from the roasting pan and refrigerate the crème brûlée for 2 hours.
- Remove the crème brûlée from the refrigerator at least 30 minutes prior to adding the Lakanto on top.
- Divide the remaining ¼ cup Lakanto equally among the 6 dishes and spread evenly on top.

- Using a torch, melt the top to form a crispy layer. (It will not brown like table sugar, but it will harden.) Allow the crème brûlée to sit for at least 5 minutes before serving.

Makes 6 servings.
PHASE 3

Fruity Kebabs

Grilling isn't just for veggies. The phase 3 fruits are delicious when grilled, and you can get pretty creative with the combinations, but be mindful of the portions allowed when you mix and match.

Avocado cooking spray
½ banana
½ cup cantaloupe chunks
½ cup pineapple chunks
1 cup strawberries
4 skewers

- Preheat the grill to medium high, coating racks with avocado cooking spray.
- Make kebabs by alternating banana with cantaloupe, pineapple, and strawberries on the skewers.
- Place kebabs on the grill rack and cook for about 1½ minutes on each side or until golden.

Variations:

Substitute a kiwi for the strawberries.

For those special occasions, try ½ mango instead of the strawberries for a tropical twist.

If you like, splash with rum before grilling.

Serves 4.
PHASE 3

Avocado Key Lime Pie

For crust:

2 tablespoons butter
1 cup pecans, chopped
½ cup unsweetened coconut flakes
½ teaspoon vanilla extract
Pinch of sea salt

For filling:

2 ripe avocados
½ cup freshly squeezed lime juice (key limes are best, if you can get them)
⅓ cup Lakanto Monk Fruit Sweetener
1 tablespoon coconut oil
1 teaspoon lime zest

To make the crust:
- Melt the butter in a skillet over low heat.
- In a food processor, pulse the pecans and coconut flakes for 90 seconds.
- Next add the melted butter, vanilla, and sea salt and process the mixture until it sticks together but retains a crumbly texture.
- Press the crust into the bottom and side of a pie pan. Chill in the refrigerator.

To make the filling:
- Peel and pit the avocados and put them into a food processor or blender along with the lime juice, sweetener, oil, and lime zest.
- Blend until smooth and thick.
- Pour the filling into the chilled crust and freeze for 3 hours or until the center is firm.
- Transfer to the refrigerator and chill for 2 more hours before serving.

Makes 6–8 servings.
PHASE 3

Lemon Ginger Macaroons

5 cups unsweetened coconut, finely shredded
1½ cups Lakanto Monk Fruit Sweetener
Pinch of sea salt
½ teaspoon powdered ginger
Whites of 4 large eggs, lightly beaten
1 teaspoon lemon extract

- Preheat oven to 350°F.
- Line two large baking sheets with parchment paper.
- In a large mixing bowl, mix together the coconut, Lakanto, salt, and ginger.
- Add egg whites and lemon extract, mixing until well combined. Using your hands, form the mixture into small mounds and place on baking sheets as you work.
- Bake until the peaks of the cookies are a light golden brown, about 12–15 minutes.

Makes about 3 dozen macaroons.
PHASE 3

Chia Berry Parfait

¼ cup chia seeds
¼ teaspoon Lakanto Monk Fruit Sweetener
1 (13.5-ounce) can full-fat coconut milk
½ cup berries
Vanilla extract
Ceylon cinnamon

- Combine the chia seeds and Lakanto with ¼ cup liquid from canned coconut milk.
- Let set until gel forms. Layer gel in the bottom of a glass and top with fresh berries.
- Separately, use a hand mixer to whip only the solid portion of the canned coconut milk while adding a drop of vanilla extract and a dash of Ceylon cinnamon.
- Top berries with whipped coconut cream and enjoy!

Makes 1 serving.
PHASE 3

Walnutty Baked Apples

4 large Rome Beauty or Granny Smith apples
½ cup chopped walnuts
¼ cup macadamia nut oil
½ tablespoon Lakanto Monk Fruit Sweetener
1 teaspoon Ceylon cinnamon
Sprinkle of cardamom

- Preheat oven to 350°F.
- Wash and core apples, leaving a large hole for filling.
- Combine walnuts, macadamia nut oil, Ceylon cinnamon, and Lakanto.
- Fill each apple and sprinkle cardamom on top.
- Bake for 35 minutes.

Excellent topped with real whipped cream or stuffed with a tablespoon of raisins with the walnuts for a special occasion.

Serves 4.
PHASE 3

BEVERAGES

Ginger Tea

Warming ginger root tea can help digestion if taken with a meal. It helps regulate the system, aids in controlling diarrhea and stomach cramps, and tastes good as well. A bit of Stevia Plus may be used for sweetening.

1 teaspoon fresh ginger root
1 pint purified water

- Place the ginger root in the water in a small saucepan.
- Boil for about 15–20 minutes.
- Remove from heat, strain, and enjoy hot or cold.

Variation:

Try adding a cinnamon stick to the pot and boiling it along with the ginger root for a delightful and aromatic cinnamon flavor. Also add a pinch of ground anise and ground cloves!

Serves 1.
ALL PHASES

Fennel Tea

Fennel is an excellent herb for gas and indigestion. It has been used by mothers for years to control infant colic, and its licoricelike taste lends itself to teas for adults as well.

1 teaspoon whole fennel seeds
1 pint purified water

- Place the seeds in the water in a small saucepan.
- Boil for about 15–20 minutes.
- Strain and enjoy hot or cold.

Serves 1.
ALL PHASES

Parsley Tea

Parsley is a great natural diuretic, high in potassium and other alkalinizing minerals. This is very helpful for relief of painful urination.

1 teaspoon fresh parsley
1 pint purified water

- Place the parsley in the water in a small saucepan.

- Bring to a simmer for about 15 minutes.
- Strain and enjoy hot or cold.

Serves 1.
ALL PHASES

Peppermint Tea

Very refreshing, peppermint tea is cleansing and calming to the nervous system.

1 teaspoon fresh peppermint (spearmint can also be used as a substitute)
1 pint purified water

- Place the peppermint in the water in a small saucepan.
- Bring to a simmer for about 15 minutes.
- Strain and enjoy hot or cold.

Serves 1.
ALL PHASES

Cinnamon-Cranberry Tea

For this tea, simply use ¼ cup (or 2 ounces) of unsweetened cranberry juice (subtract from your daily allotment) combined with water, and add Ceylon cinnamon. The full recipe follows:

¼ cup unsweetened cranberry juice
¾ cup purified water
½ teaspoon Ceylon cinnamon

- Combine cranberry juice and water in a small saucepan.
- Bring to a quick boil.
- Reduce heat and stir in Ceylon cinnamon.
- Serve warm.

Serves 1.
ALL PHASES

FAT FLUSH SEASONING SAVVY

No doubt you have noticed that many of the menus and recipes contain the special Fat Flush culinary herbs and spices, which can turn simple dishes into exotic entrées and sides. Cayenne pepper, cumin, parsley, cilantro, dill, anise, fennel, bay leaves, ginger, cloves, coriander, Ceylon cinnamon, mustard, and apple cider vinegar are not just your everyday flavoring favorites; they are essential to the fat-flushing strategy because they rev up the metabolism, help remove excess fluid from tissues, and control cravings. Table 13.1 presents some examples of how I like to use these Fat Flush seasonings to spice up my life. Give them a try.

Table 13.1 Pairing Foods with Herbs and Spices

FOOD	HERBS AND SPICE
Fish	Dill, fennel, ginger
Beef	Cumin, garlic, cloves
Lamb	Ceylon cinnamon, garlic, cloves
Poultry	Mustard, garlic, cayenne pepper
Eggs	Parsley, cumin, mustard
Soups	Bay leaf, parsley, dill
Cabbage	Anise, ginger, apple cider vinegar
Cucumber	Dill, apple cider vinegar, parsley
Greens	Garlic, apple cider vinegar, dill
Squash	Ceylon cinnamon, cloves, ginger

For a more cosmopolitan flavor, you can rub the following dry blends directly on your beef, fish, lamb, or poultry and cook:

Asian Inspired. ⅛ cup ground ginger, 1 tablespoon dried mustard, 1 minced garlic clove, and 1 teaspoon chopped onion

Tex-Mex Inspired. 2 tablespoons cumin, 1 teaspoon coriander, ½ teaspoon cayenne pepper, and ½ teaspoon Ceylon cinnamon

Moroccan Inspired. ½ cup chopped onion, 1 minced garlic clove, 2 teaspoons cumin and coriander, and ¼ teaspoon cayenne pepper

FAT FLUSH SWAPS

Here are some tips on how to modify recipe ingredients for your old-time favorites or holiday specialties to make them Fat Flush friendly for the Lifestyle Eating Plan phase of the program. I have found many tasty ways to cut out the trans fats, sugar, salt, refined carbohydrates, and gluten from my recipes without sacrificing flavor. Table 13.2 provides some easy-to-use tips for replacing traditional recipe ingredients. I guarantee that taste will not be sacrificed by these substitutions—in fact, it is enhanced. Try them out for yourself. Even your company won't know the difference.

Table 13.2 Helpful Substitutions

WHEN THE RECIPE CALLS FOR	USE THIS FAT FLUSH INGREDIENT INSTEAD
1 tablespoon margarine or vegetable cooking oil	Use butter, coconut, avocado, or macadamia nut oil
Sugar	Use 1 teaspoon of Flora-Key for every 2 teaspoons of sugar, or use aromatic crushed seeds such as fennel, cardamom, anise, caraway, or coriander. Can also use ½ to ¼ the amount of Lakanto or ½ packet of stevia for every teaspoon of sugar. (To replace honey in recipes to lower sugar, use equal amount of yacon syrup.)
1 cup whole or skim milk	2 heaping tablespoons high-protein whey powder plus 1 cup filtered water
Hot pepper sauce	Dash of cayenne pepper
1 teaspoon dried herbs	1 tablespoon fresh herbs
1 teaspoon salt	Use sea salt. For those on lower-sodium diets, use Selina Sea Salt's Makai Pure Deep Sea Salt, which contains the lowest sodium and highest potassium levels of any comparable salt on the market
1 ounce or square of unsweetened baking chocolate	3 tablespoons cacao or carob powder plus 1 tablespoon water and 1 tablespoon coconut oil
2 tablespoons margarine mixed with 1 tablespoon flour for sauce and soup thickeners	2 tablespoons arrowroot or kudzu found in health food stores. Arrowroot adds calcium to foods, whereas kudzu is high in iron. Or use egg yolks to thicken sauces or pureed cauliflower for soups.
1 cup whole grain flour for baking	Take 2 tablespoons out of 1 cup of flour and replace it with 2 tablespoons of flax meal. This does not replace the whole cup of flour, just those 2 tablespoons. Reduce the oil in the recipe by 2 teaspoons for every 2 tablespoons of the flax meal. Bake for a shorter time or lower the heat by 25°F. Alternatively, can use tigernut flour in equal measurements.
1 egg	1 omega-3–enriched egg. (Note: If you're allergic to eggs, blend 1 tablespoon ground flax with 3 tablespoons water and let stand for a couple of minutes.)
Gelatin	Agar-agar, a seaweed gelatin available in health food stores, replaces animal-based gelatin. Agar-agar provides added fiber and lubrication in the intestinal tract by absorbing moisture.
Baking powder, regular (contains aluminum)	Equal amounts of aluminum-free baking powder, low sodium and grain-free
Breading and frying	Poach in broth, water, or wine, and then bake in a covered dish to retain moisture

OTHER COOKING HELP

Here are some quick facts on equivalent measurements to help you in following the Fat Flush recipes and in figuring out your weekly shopping list.

Dry and Liquid Equivalents

1 teaspoon or less	=	a pinch
3 teaspoons	=	1 tablespoon
4 tablespoons	=	¼ cup
5⅓ tablespoons	=	⅓ cup
8 tablespoons	=	½ cup
10⅔ tablespoons	=	⅔ cup
16 tablespoons	=	1 cup
2 cups	=	1 pint
4 cups	=	1 quart
2 pints	=	1 quart
4 quarts	=	1 gallon

1 cup chopped onion	=	1 large onion
1 cup chopped sweet pepper	=	1 large pepper
1 cup chopped tomato	=	1 large tomato
½ cup chopped tomato	=	2 plum tomatoes
½ cup diced celery	=	1 large stalk
3 tablespoons sliced scallion	=	1 large scallion
1 teaspoon chopped garlic	=	1 large clove
3 tablespoons lemon juice	=	juice of 1 medium lemon
2 tablespoons lime juice	=	juice of 1 lime
1 tablespoon fresh herb	=	1 teaspoon dried herb
1 cup sliced mushrooms	=	6 to 8 medium mushrooms

14 Because You Asked

Whether I'm consulting, online, speaking, or taping a webinar or summit, I truly love hearing from men and women around the world. In fact, getting to communicate with everybody firsthand is perhaps the most joyful and fulfilling part of what I do. I like to hear how people are inspired by the Fat Flush Plan, how commonsense diet and detox is revitalizing their lives, and how I can help them even more by answering their questions.

Since there tends to be a common thread in their concerns, I thought you might benefit from reading through some of the most frequently asked questions about the Fat Flush Plan.

AGES, STAGES, AND GENDER

Is there an age limit for Fat Flush?

Yes and no. I believe that the first two phases of the program are too stringent for children under age 12; however, phase 3 is a healthy option for most people. Regardless of their age, your children definitely can benefit from adding the right fats to their current dietary regimen whether they are on the plan or not! In fact, the most remarkable news about the omega-3–rich oils (such as flaxseed and fish oils) is their dramatic effect on children. Many clinical studies have shown how low brain chemistry levels of these essential fatty acids are connected with a multitude of neurological and psychological symptoms, including attention deficit hyperactivity disorder, depression, and violent behavior. Adding from 2 teaspoons to 1 tablespoon of flaxseed oil to your child's cereal or pancake toppings is one of the best substitutions you can make. Indeed, it is a great idea to make such changes for the whole family.

And speaking of oils, your teenage daughter can benefit from them, too. By taking black currant seed oil, which is rich in gamma-linolenic acid (GLA), for two weeks before her period, your daughter can say goodbye to PMS-related headaches, irritability, bloating, cramping, and breast tenderness. Your children will quickly experience—even faster than you—how the right fats are a friend, not a foe.

What about pregnant or breastfeeding women—can they be on the Fat Flush Plan?

There are times in a woman's life that demand optimal nutritional support and additional calories. Pregnancy and breastfeeding are definitely two such times.

A pregnant woman should be focused on gaining weight, not losing or maintaining weight—which are the primary goals of each phase of the plan. In fact, in the second and third trimesters of pregnancy, a woman needs at least 300 extra calories each day, and she needs another 500 extra calories each day while breastfeeding. For a healthy pregnancy, doctors typically recommend that most women gain between 25 and 30 pounds. If a woman is underweight, gaining 28 to 40 pounds is suggested; if overweight, adding 15 to 25 pounds is recommended.

Having said that, phase 3 can be used as a foundational eating program for pregnant or breastfeeding women, utilizing the full array of servings in every food category as a baseline—and even adding servings in each category if weight gain is not sufficient or the person is still hungry. The only dietary change, based upon the recommendation of the Food and Drug Administration, would be to limit fish intake to only 12 ounces per week and completely eliminate larger fish such as shark, swordfish, tilefish, and king mackerel while pregnant or breastfeeding. These fish are more likely to be contaminated with toxic mercury, and exposure to mercury can result in neurological problems and learning deficits in children.

The recommended weight loss supplement—with the exception of essential fatty acids and a daily multiple vitamin containing extra folate—should be omitted during pregnancy and breastfeeding.

In addition to the essential fatty acids in flaxseed oil and GLA supplements, pregnant and breastfeeding women can supplement their diet with other essential fatty acids that can be integrated into phase 3 right away. The most important is docosahexaenoic acid (DHA), which is found in algae and in the fattier fish (such as salmon and sardines) as well as in omega-3-enriched eggs. In capsule form, DHA is usually purified to remove polychlorinated biphenyls (PCBs) and heavy metals such as mercury and arsenic.

Since the human brain is composed of 60 percent fat and since the most prevalent fat is DHA, this primary building block is absolutely essential for proper cognitive and visual development. Infants depend on mother's milk for their DHA. However, the DHA level in the breast milk of American women is the lowest in the world.

I always suggest that pregnant women take a dietary supplement containing 200 mg of DHA along with their prenatal supplements. Breastfeeding women can double this amount to 400 mg, which will benefit the baby—and also benefit the mother by protecting against postpartum depression.

Mothers unable to breastfeed should consider adding 100 mg of DHA to each bottle of formula because these supplements support the development of the infant's brain and eyes. I recommend a DHA brand from Carlson called Mother's DHA—available in health food stores.

I highly recommend the initial two phases of the Fat Flush Plan after women give birth or stop breastfeeding for a safe body cleansing and weight loss regimen.

Is there anything special a woman should do at certain stages of her life, such as perimenopause or menopause?

Yes, there is. Studies comparing Asian menopausal women with Western menopausal women showed the Asian women have a much easier transition and better overall health. One of the reasons may be their daily intake (from 45 to 100 mg) of the stabilizing phytoestrogens called isoflavones. Isoflavones are highly touted for relieving such symptoms as hot flashes, sweating, etc., caused by hormonal fluctuations. They are found most prevalently in soy, red clover, kudzu root, and lignans.

These isoflavones are accepted by human cell estrogen receptors, so they satisfy the body's estrogen needs and thereby relieve perimenopausal symptoms. As weak estrogenic mimics, these isoflavones also aid in stabilizing fluctuating estrogen and progesterone levels and reduce cholesterol while helping to maintain strong bones.

For menopausal fat-flushing women, there are many elements of the daily routine that offer hormone-stabilizing benefits. Flax seeds, as well as the GLA provided by black currant seed oil, help to balance mood swings, quell hot flashes and night sweats, and provide welcome lubrication for tissue dryness. If you choose to enjoy soy-based foods in your diet, please select non-GMO organic soy that has been properly fermented, like tofu, tempeh, or miso, and limit your intake to two servings per week.

My husband wants to follow the Fat Flush Plan. What can he expect, and should men do anything differently?

Men typically lose from 8 to 16 pounds in phase 1. They have greater muscle mass than women—20 percent more. Having more lean muscle mass means that men have the ability to lose weight faster than women. Pound for pound, muscle can burn more calories than fat—giving men a built-in advantage (literally).

Men who follow the Fat Flush Plan usually make some personal adjustments to the plan. They typically jump from phase 1 to phase 3 because they need more fuel in the form of friendly carbs for their higher metabolism.

Also, some men feel that they need more than 8 ounces of protein per day, and so they increase portion sizes of meat, fish, and chicken by 2 ounces at lunch and at dinner. Many feel more comfortable if they double up on the whey protein powder in the morning.

Could my thyroid-related weight problem be tied to any other kind of hormonal imbalance?

Yes, especially if you are lacking natural progesterone and are estrogen dominant (see Chapter 3). Synthetic estrogens in the form of birth control pills or hormone replacement therapy (HRT) elevate sex hormone–binding globulin, which can depress other hormones, including thyroid hormone. The resulting symptoms range from weight gain and fatigue, to cold hands and feet as well as an inability to sweat. Estrogen and progesterone levels can be assessed through testing. You can also try using a cream with a natural form of progesterone that is identical to what your body makes. Monitor the results over a three-month period by tracking your progress in your journal, noting your energy and overall well-being. If these improve on progesterone, then your thyroid-related weight problem is tied to estrogen dominance and progesterone deficit. (See Chapter 3.) Saliva-based tests are available through Uni Key to measure sex hormone levels, so I recommend, if possible, measuring to obtain a baseline and then retesting every three to six months to monitor progress.

FAT FLUSH PROTOCOL

Do I really have to stick to the Fat Flush Plan exactly as described, or can I personalize it a bit?

You certainly can personalize the Fat Flush Plan to suit your own needs. The program is based on principles, not just on hard-and-fast dos and don'ts. Of course, I would like you to build your meals around as many fat-flushing elements as possible to get the best results—the hot water and lemon, increased water, lean protein, low-glycemic load and low-fructose fruits and vegetables, high-fiber seeds, flaxseed oil, coconut or MCT oil, and GLA supplements as well as flavorful herbs and spices. Each of these elements has specific fat-burning and diuretic properties.

Fat Flush athletes and others who maintain a high level of fitness activity—and who aren't willing to give up their heavy-duty workout routines—should consider beginning the program in phase 2. The limited carbohydrate energy that phase 1 provides is not sufficient for a highly active person, so incorporating a half cup of peas or cooked carrots, winter squash, sweet potato, or beets seems to satisfy Fat Flush fitness buffs the most.

Is there a reason why flaxseed oil is taken with food and not alone?

Yes, there is. When you blend your flaxseed oil with other foods (such as using the oil in salad dressings or topping your veggies), it helps emulsify the oil, which ensures better absorption and therefore better use of the essential fatty acids the oil contains. In fact, the famed German biochemist Dr. Johanna Budwig, who did most of the early research on flax, always combined flaxseed oil, either with vegetables or in yogurt and no-heat recipes.

Can I cook with flaxseed oil? How should I store it?

You can't cook with flaxseed oil because it is a highly unsaturated oil, which means it is very sensitive to heat, air, and light and can go rancid if not treated properly. For these reasons, you also should keep it in the fridge up to three weeks. Flaxseed oil also can be stored in the freezer for up to one year.

On the other hand, you can cook and bake with ground flax seeds. The essential fatty acids remain stable as long as the presence of fiber and water protects them from overheating.

I've heard that flax seeds can be harmful—is this true?

Lignan-rich flax seeds are safe in proper amounts. They do, however, contain a substance known as cyanogenic glycoside, as do lima beans, sweet potatoes, yams, and bamboo shoots. Cyanogenic glycosides metabolize into yet another substance known as thiocyanate—a chemical that has the potential, over time, of suppressing the thyroid's ability to take up sufficient iodine. This biochemical occurrence raises the risk of developing goiter (abnormal enlargement of the thyroid).

There are two easy ways to avoid this problem. One is to limit consumption to a maximum of three or four tablespoons of ground-up flax seeds per day. The other is to lightly bake or toast your flax seeds, which deactivates and decomposes the cyanogenic glycosides but preserves the beneficial omega-3 properties. To toast flax seeds, you spread them on a baking sheet or pan and then place the pan in a 250 degree Fahrenheit oven for 15 to 20 minutes until the seeds are crispy.

Flaxseed oil, on the other hand, is free of cyanogenic glycosides.

Why do you limit certain herbs and spices?

On the first two phases of the Fat Flush Plan, you are concentrating on dropping pounds while cleansing your system. The selected herbs and spices in these initial phases are considered either thermogenic (which means they rev up the body's metabolic fires and jump-start energy expenditure), diuretic, or helpful in carbohydrate metabolism and digestion. These spices are the ones to focus on for optimal results.

There are plenty of tasty, thermogenic choices to spice up your life, including cayenne pepper, cumin, dried mustard, ginger, and garlic. Besides providing flavor, these herbs and spices help with your weight loss and health goals. Bay leaves, cinnamon, cloves, and coriander help control insulin levels; parsley, cilantro, fennel, anise, and apple cider vinegar act as natural diuretics; dill, fennel, and anise aid digestion; and cumin helps protect against degenerative disease.

Since dairy isn't allowed in phase 1 or phase 2, how will I get enough calcium?

Not to worry. You'll get plenty with green leafy veggies, which are used liberally in the menu plans. For instance, you'll enjoy collards, kale, watercress, parsley, cilantro, escarole, salad greens, bok choy, arugula, endive, and spinach.

Just to give you an example, a cup of milk has 300 mg of calcium. A cup of collard greens has 226 mg of calcium, a cup of turnip greens has 195 mg, and a cup of dandelion greens has 147 mg. And a cup of broccoli has around 250 mg of calcium. You'll be having lots of these calcium-rich greens at lunch and dinner. And sautéed in broth with 1 to 2 teaspoons of apple cider vinegar, they are really quite tasty.

The World Health Organization recommends just 450 mg of calcium per day, which is a far cry from the 800 to 1,500 mg recommended in the United States. At levels of 250 to 400 mg of calcium per day, women in third-world countries do not have the rates of osteoporosis and hip fractures common in developed countries. In addition, on the Fat Flush plan, all the "calcium robbers," such as caffeine, sugar, alcohol, and excess fiber from grains and bran, are totally eliminated, allowing you to retain all the calcium you consume. Furthermore, additional magnesium in the plan helps your body to actually absorb all the calcium you take in.

Sea veggies are also hidden treasures from the deep, loaded with trace minerals in addition to calcium and iron. For instance, you could try some hijiki. It tastes a lot like licorice and looks like tangled black strings, yet it has 14 times the calcium of a glass of milk. You simply rinse it under cold water and soak it for approximately 20 minutes. Then you can toss it into your salad, Rose's Fat Flush Soup*, or even Fat Flush Bone Broth*! It also can be sautéed with carrots and fresh ginger.

FLUSH FLASH

Recipes for dishes marked with an asterisk can be found in Chapter 13.

Protein is an essential part of the Fat Flush Plan, but how much do I really need?

In the past, 1 gram of protein for every 2.2 pounds of body weight was the gold standard. Now this has been changed as a result of new research suggesting that certain individuals may need much more: weight lifters; individuals having a large, muscular frame; immunosuppressed individuals; and those suffering from protein deficiency (with such symptoms as prolonged water retention, sagging muscles, loss of muscle mass, expanding waistlines, fatigue, anemia, slow wound healing, hair thinning and loss). Practically doubling the previous recommendation, some authorities now recommend up to 1 to 1.5 grams of protein per pound of body weight.

So as far as exact amounts are concerned, the jury is still out. For years, I have concurred with the Food and Nutrition Board of the National Research Council, which recommends the following amounts of protein as a general rule of thumb:

Adult men	70 grams
Adult women	58 grams
Pregnant women	65 grams
Lactating women	75 grams
Girls, aged 13–15	62 grams
Girls, aged 16–20	58 grams
Boys, aged 13–15	75 grams
Boys, aged 16–20	85 grams

To me, these numbers represent the bare minimum requirements, not the amounts for optimal health. The best way to figure out what works for you is by trial and error. You can add a couple of ounces of protein to lunch and dinner or include some high-protein, lactose-free whey shakes for snacks with your daily fruit.

Here are some examples that will help you keep track of your protein grams:

1 egg = 7 grams

1 ounce of meat, fish, fowl, or cheese = 7 grams

1 or 2 scoops of whey powder = 20 grams

4 ounces of tofu = 7 grams

2 ounces of tempeh = 7 grams

1 cup of broccoli = 4 grams

1 cup of spinach = 5 grams

2 tablespoons of chia seeds = 4 grams

I'm a vegan. Is there anything special I should do—and what about using beans for my protein portions?

Vegans may be challenged to consume enough low-carb foods that provide the quality of amino acids found in meat, eggs, fish, and poultry. Vegan diets typically are lacking in 3 of the 9 essential amino acids (lysine, methionine, and tryptophan), according to biochemist Don Tyson, who ran the Aatron Medical Services Laboratory in Torrance, California for years.

Taking a well-balanced amino acid supplement containing lysine, methionine, carnitine, and taurine (tryptophan is no longer on the market) with meals would be a good first step. There is also a vegan protein powder available from Uni Key made from non-GMO brown rice and pea protein that would be appropriate for vegans because it contains the four amino acids just mentioned. In phase 2, consider choosing quinoa and oatmeal as your friendly carbs, because they offer lysine and methionine, respectively. Avocados in all phases provide healthy fat and a rich dose of methionine, too. Pumpkin seeds are a great source of tryptophan and offer essential fats along with protection from parasites, so snack on a couple of tablespoons throughout the day.

Vegetarians, of course, can increase the whey protein shake to a total of 2 per day and include a balanced amino acid supplement (as described above).

As for the beans, which are acceptable for both vegans and vegetarians, while they are a source of protein, they also contain significant amounts of carbohydrates. So these are limited to one serving per day as an alternative to animal protein.

In phase 3 of the plan, everyone is encouraged to incorporate beans back in very small amounts. (They are not part of phase 1 or phase 2.)

Is it really okay to eat egg yolks? I always thought that they were a trigger for high cholesterol.

Yes, it is perfectly okay to have two whole eggs every day in each phase of the Fat Flush Plan. Eggs contain one of the highest-quality proteins available in any food. In fact, the egg yolk contains 45 percent of the egg's protein, along with many minerals and a good deal of the egg's vitamins. Omega-3–enriched eggs are also available, which provide nearly 200 mg of cholesterol-lowering omega-3s concentrated in the yolk. The yolk is also an excellent source of the infection-fighting vitamin A and contains a nutrient called phosphatidylcholine. As part of the substance known as lecithin, phosphatidylcholine actually prevents the oxidation of cholesterol, which protects both your liver and your arteries.

In fact, numerous studies have vindicated the maligned egg yolk. The most recent studies have shown that adults can enjoy at least two eggs a day without increasing their serum cholesterol level. Two substantial Harvard studies, published in April 1999 in the *Journal of the American Medical Association*, examined the egg consumption of approximately 40,000 men and 80,000 women over an 8- to 14-year period. After taking into consideration other dietary patterns and risk factors, the researchers found that folks who ate one egg a day or more were no more likely to develop heart disease or stroke than those who consumed one egg a week or less. Researchers at Harvard Medical School actually sanction up to seven eggs per week for optimal health.

Thus, when it comes to breakfast on the Fat Flush Plan, you can count on eggs—poached, hard-cooked, soft-boiled, or scrambled. They are absolutely delicious poached or scrambled in vegetable or chicken broth. And you can enjoy them with low-glycemic vegetables, such as onions, mushrooms, or peppers, along with our special thermogenic herbs and spices, such as a dash of cayenne.

What about eating organ meats such as liver for a protein source?

Absolutely. Organ meats, such as liver and sweetbreads, are highly nutritious. In fact, liver is high in B vitamins, iron, and DHA—that important fatty acid so critical for the brain and eyes. When I was a WIC nutritionist at Bellevue Hospital in New York City many years ago, I discovered that many women suffering from anemia could increase their iron levels simply by adding 4 ounces of calf's liver twice a week to their menu plan—a step up from the iron pills that made them constipated. I still believe that liver can greatly benefit women who are menstruating and are slightly anemic. Of course, organic liver is preferred.

Why isn't pork on the food list?

Pork is not included in the program because it is a very common food intolerance among those with gallbladder issues, and also it can carry parasites if not properly cooked. The *Trichinella spiralis* organism, which causes trichinosis, lives in pigs. If you happen to eat undercooked pork, bacon, or ham, the encysted larvae can hatch in your intestines and migrate to your brain, causing seizures.

Is sushi allowed on the Fat Flush Plan when I eat out?

No, I don't recommend it. Raw fish can carry parasites such as tapeworms and microscopic invaders and even more exotic ones such as the anisakine larvae. As I write in my book *Guess What Came to Dinner: Parasites and Your Health*, when these small worms are ingested from raw or undercooked fish, they penetrate the walls of the stomach or small intestine, causing severe inflammation and pain. The symptoms can mimic appendicitis, gastric ulcer, or even stomach cancer. Surgical removal of the worms is a familiar surgery in Japan, where raw fish is a dietary staple.

Take it from me, these uninvited guests at your dinner table not only can become embedded in your intestines but also are at the source of irritable bowel syndrome, diarrhea, constipation, immune problems, and even depression in many cases. Since the Fat Flush Plan is a weight loss program that also cleanses your system, the last thing you want to do is introduce into your body such unpleasant and immunosuppressive critters that can rob you of vitality.

*I understand why sugar is out on the Fat Flush Plan, but is a sugar sub-
stitute such as aspartame really going to upset my weight loss goals
that badly?*

Not only is aspartame suspected of stimulating insulin release, and therefore
counterproductive to your weight loss goals, but it also can damage your
health.

The mere taste of such a concentrated sweetener appears to set an
instinctual insulin mechanism into place, even though aspartame contains
zero calories. A six-year study of 80,000 women shows that the higher the
artificial sweetener consumption, the more likely the women were to pack
on the pounds.

Aspartame, marketed under the Equal and Nutrasweet brand names,
also has been shown to suppress production of serotonin—the remarkable
neurotransmitter that helps control food cravings. When serotonin levels
plummet, those sugar and carb cravings skyrocket. And this increases the
likelihood of binging and added pounds.

Loading up on those diet drinks—sweetened by aspartame—can rob you
of valuable chromium, a mineral needed for proper blood sugar function.
Having an insufficient amount of chromium results in poor blood sugar regulation, which can lead to insulin resistance and increased carb intolerance.

Does that also go for Splenda and Sweet'N Low?

The only brand-name sweeteners I recommend are SweetLeaf Stevia, Lakanto
Monk Fruit Sweetener, and yacon syrup in phase 3. Stevia is far and above my
favorite. Stevia is an herb used for hundreds of years in South America by
Indian tribes in Paraguay. It is 30 times sweeter than regular sugar, is virtually
calorie-free, and does not feed yeast, nor does it trigger fat-conserving insulin
production or raise blood sugar levels like other sweeteners.

In terms of overall health, this natural herb is an antiflatulent and
reduces heartburn, hypertension, and uric acid. Even researchers have gotten on the stevia bandwagon. A study in the *Journal of Ethnopharmacology*
demonstrates how stevia dilates blood vessels, resulting in lower blood
pressure.

SweetLeaf Stevia, unlike other stevias on the market, contains no added
maltodextrin—an extremely high-glycemic substance. Instead, the natural
sweetness of SweetLeaf Stevia is enhanced with fructooligosaccharides, substances from natural grains and vegetables that provide a benefit that none
of the other sweeteners do: it nourishes the growth of friendly bacteria,
which are your best allies in keeping yeast such as candida at bay. Remember
that yeast overgrowth can make you want to overeat (see Chapter 2).

Is it all right to drink a vegetable juice such as V-8 on the Fat Flush Plan?

Yes, in phase 3 you can start drinking your veggies. However, please use only
the low-sodium brands, such as Knudsen's, available at health food stores.

Are cooking sprays allowed?

Yes. I recommend using avocado oil spray, as avocado has one of the highest smoke points of all oils—ahead of both coconut oil and olive oil. Consider investing in an oil mister to avoid potentially harmful propellants in aerosol cooking sprays.

What about eating olives on the Fat Flush Plan?

Yes, yes, yes. They are included in all three phases of the Fat Flush Plan because they are high in oleic acid, a healthy fat that aids blood sugar and keeps insulin levels low. How many? Eating three to six per day would be fine.

SUBSTITUTIONS

I don't really like the taste of flax. What about substituting flax oil capsules for the flaxseed oil?

Yes, you can certainly do that—with caution. Sometimes in the process of encapsulation, the oil's quality can be compromised. You might want to first test its quality by piercing the capsule and tasting the oil. It should have a nutty flavor. A bitter taste with an almost stinginglike aftertaste signals rancidity.

On another note, the flaxseed oil is far more economical than the capsules. However, if you travel frequently, the capsules may be more convenient. Just be certain to purchase a good-quality product. Depending upon the brand, it can take anywhere from 4 to 6 capsules of flaxseed oil to equal 1 tablespoon of the liquid oil. Just remember that with the required 2 tablespoons of flaxseed oil daily, you would be taking sometimes 12 capsules each day, staggering them throughout.

Can ground-up flax seeds be used in place of flaxseed oil?

Yes, they can. Use three tablespoons of ground-up flax seeds to one tablespoon of the flaxseed oil. In phases 1 and 2, ground flax seed can be sprinkled over your vegetables, mixed in your salad, or used in your fruit smoothies. In phase 3, you can add it to cottage cheese or yogurt.

And by using ground-up flax seeds as a substitute, you get an extra bonus of about 8 grams of additional fiber with your meals. Flax seed is also higher in lignans than the oil. Lignans, which are 800 times more concentrated in whole flax seed than in other plants, are well recognized for their antioxidant properties, phytoestrogen help in alleviating perimenopausal and menopausal discomforts, and breast cancer–fighting abilities. In fact, a study conducted at the Princess Margaret Hospital and the Toronto Hospital in Canada showed how as little as two tablespoons a day of ground flax seed markedly slowed down tumor growth in women with breast cancer. The tagline "A muffin a day could keep breast cancer at bay" hit the newswires on

December 7, 2000, after the research was presented at an international conference on breast cancer in San Antonio, Texas. Lignans are also a soluble fiber, which keeps blood sugar levels stable and lowers cholesterol.

What about taking fish oil in place of flaxseed oil? I understand that the ALA in flax must be converted to EPA and DHA to be of any benefit.

There is much misunderstanding in this area. Science confirms that the ALA content of flax oil has stand-alone benefits all its own, without having to be converted into EPA and DHA. For example, in several studies of breast cancer risk, the higher the concentration of ALA in breast tissue, the lower the risk of manifesting breast cancer. Moreover, if breast cancer arises, the higher the breast tissue concentration of ALA, the lower the risk of cancer metastasis to other parts of the body.

For most health issues, flaxseed and fish oils provide comparable benefits. In the case of male infertility and sperm cell viability, however, studies indicate that the omega-3s from flaxseed oil make it a better choice.

If you simply can't take flax for any reason, use one teaspoon of fish oil (or three capsules of Super EPA) to one tablespoon of flaxseed oil. I recommend Uni Key's Super EPA capsules, Carlson's The Very Finest Fish Oil liquid, and Carlson's The Very Finest Fish Oil chewable softgels.

May I substitute olive oil for flaxseed oil?

Sorry, no. Even though olive oil is a "heart-smart," tasty oil that's part of the Lifestyle Eating Plan, it is not a substitute for flaxseed oil. Olive oil does not contain the essential fatty acids found in flax or fish—and neither does coconut oil. Flaxseed oil not only possesses unique fat-burning power but also improves immune function, protects against heart disease, and improves male fertility. Fat Flushers who faithfully adopt the flax habit consistently remark about having glowing skin, luster-rich hair, and strong nails.

I can't find natural cranberry juice in my area. May I substitute another juice, or what would you suggest?

Please don't substitute another juice, because it negates the entire purpose of cranberry juice in the Fat Flush Plan. Cranberry juice is packed with flavonoids, enzymes, and organic acids, such as malic acid, citric acid, and quinic acid, which have an emulsifying effect on stubborn fat deposits in the lymphatic system. The lymphatic system, which has been called the "garbage collector of the body," transports all kinds of waste products not processed by the liver. With the help of the organic acid components, the cranberry juice digests stagnated lymphatic wastes, which could very well be the reason Fat Flushers claim that their cellulite disappears.

Here's what I suggest: if you can't find natural cranberry juice, there is a really simple recipe in Chapter 6 that you can use to make your own. Since it is pretty hard to find cranberries during nonholiday times, you might want to stock up when they're easily available in November and December and freeze them for future use.

I'm concerned about the carb content in the cranberry juice. What about taking concentrated cranberry capsules instead?

Concentrated cranberry capsules may be a great help in preventing or treating urinary tract infections. However, from my experience, there is no substitute for the unsweetened cranberry juice used in the cranberry juice–water mixture. Because it is liquid, the cranberry juice is absorbed immediately into the system, performing two vital jobs: helping to keep the liver's detoxification pathways open and acting as a digestive aid for the waste material stuck in the lymphatic system.

The capsules can be difficult to digest for people who have inadequate stomach acid production or insufficient digestive enzymes. If you are concerned about the carbohydrate content of the unsweetened cranberry juice, don't be. The cranberry seems to act more as a catalyst for digesting stagnated lymphatic wastes than as a food source. There are approximately 18 grams of carbohydrate in 8 ounces—the daily amount called for in the Fat Flush Plan. And since it is being diluted with water, you are not consuming it all at once to overwhelm your system.

You recommend whey or brown rice and pea protein, but can I use soy protein powders instead?

No. Although I allow fermented soy products in the form of tofu and tempeh up to twice a week, I decided long ago that less is more when it comes to soy protein powders, which are general soy protein isolates—and often incomplete proteins.

In addition, soy is a top food allergen and contains enzyme inhibitors and phytic acid, which can remove zinc and iron from the body. As a plentiful source of copper, soy can increase or exacerbate hyperactivity, panic attacks, hair loss, adrenal burnout, fatigue, and hypothyroidism. (For more information, please refer to my book *Why Am I Always So Tired?*)

Whey protein is a much better protein powder choice. It has the highest protein efficiency ratio of all the protein sources and increases production of glutathione, one of the liver's leading antioxidants in the detox process.

I do think, however, that there is a place for soy isoflavones as a natural hormone replacement therapy for perimenopausal and menopausal women (women in their early forties through middle fifties). In amounts up to 75 mg per day—the amounts Asians typically ingest on a daily basis—soy can be good medicine.

Can lime be substituted for lemon?

Certainly. You can substitute lime or mix the two, using half lemon and half lime.

SUPPLEMENTS AND MEDICATIONS

Do I have to take supplements while on the Fat Flush Plan?

You bet. Certain supplements—such as the essential fatty acids from GLA and flax as well as conjugated linoleic acid (CLA)—are really crucial to the success of the plan. These essential and critical fats are suggested throughout each phase for a specific purpose, with your weight and fat loss goals always in mind. The daily dose of 360 mg of GLA in the form of black currant seed oil helps trigger fat burning (instead of fat storage) by mobilizing brown adipose tissue, which burns off extra calories and increases energy. GLA also controls PMS symptoms and wards off rheumatoid arthritis and skin problems, such as psoriasis and eczema.

Research has proved that the one major obstacle to dieting is hunger. Taking two tablespoons daily of flaxseed oil eliminates this problem because it creates a feeling of fullness (satiety) and makes you feel fuller longer. You are happy with less food because you are less hungry. Flaxseed oil does this by revving up metabolism and eliminating the deprivation that can make you give in to temptation and cheat on your diet. In addition, the flax seeds themselves are a powerful source of antioxidants and plant sterols, responsible for a major portion of the human immune function.

In phase 3 (or sooner if you desire), you'll add 1,000 mg of CLA with each meal, which will help your body burn fat even more. CLA is your fat-proof insurance policy. Even if you somehow regain some weight, you'll redeposit that weight as 50 percent muscle. And CLA even aids in the prevention of breast cancer by acting as a powerful antioxidant in the system. It doesn't get any better than this!

What other supplements can I take on the Fat Flush Plan?

A broad-based multivitamin and mineral supplement (like the Fat Flush Dieters' Multi) would be helpful as insurance. You also could add the Fat Flush Weight Loss Formula, which supports liver cleansing as well as carbohydrate and fat metabolism. The most important ingredients in a weight loss or fat-burning product are liver-protecting milk thistle and dandelion, blood sugar–and insulin-controlling chromium, and methionine, inositol, choline, and L-carnitine for mobilizing fat.

There is, however, one other supplement that I would suggest—magnesium. Magnesium is particularly helpful on the Fat Flush Plan for the reasons already discussed in Chapter 3. But in capsule form, it is ideal to treat those occasional headaches from caffeine withdrawal as well as challenges with constipation. Since magnesium is a major muscle relaxant, it helps restore good bowel tone and normal peristalsis—that alternating muscle relaxation and contraction in the intestines.

Magnesium also helps the liver do its job more efficiently by acting as an escort for toxins being moved through the liver, including estrogens (such as those in the pill or HRT) being broken down. In addition, magnesium is key to good bone health, balancing calcium and converting vitamin D for better calcium absorption.

Magnesium deficiency is common in our twenty-first-century lifestyle, thanks to highly processed foods, birth control pills, and stress. Even though the recommended daily allowance is 400 mg daily, most of us consume less than 100 mg. And those drinks many of us may have enjoyed BFF (before Fat Flush!)—such as coffee, tea, alcohol, and colas—don't help. They wash magnesium right out of the system via the urine. Symptoms of a magnesium deficiency include nervousness, irritability, depression, fatigue, palpitations, tremors, and spasms. According to a classic study by Guy Abraham, MD, a magnesium deficiency also will reduce blood calcium, which decreases calcium availability for your bones and further disrupts estrogen metabolism.

I would suggest taking magnesium separately from calcium (if you are still taking it) because it needs to be absorbed by itself. You can take from 400 to 1,200 mg daily, depending on bowel tolerance. You can build up to these amounts slowly if you notice any bowel intolerance.

Since I started taking birth control pills, I've gained a lot of weight. What do you suggest?

There are many low-dose birth control options on the market. However, as discussed in Chapter 2, all synthetic hormones—including those from birth control pills—put undue stress on the liver and can back up the detoxification pathways. Ultimately, this impairs bile flow, which will affect your ability to burn fat.

I encourage you to fortify your liver and enhance its ability to break down estrogens and progesterins. You may also be a candidate for a bile-building supplement to help ensure thinned bile, which carries out toxic estrogens as a method of liver cleansing. Many liver-supporting nutrients are included in the Fat Flush supporting nutrients described throughout the book. You can add more of them in the following amounts for even better liver fortification:

✓ MILK THISTLE. A powerful antioxidant that protects your liver from cell damage. It also is considered a liver regenerator and helps with bile stagnation. Take 500 to 2,000 mg daily.
✓ DANDELION. Used for centuries worldwide as a liver tonic and blood purifier. Take 500 to 2,000 mg daily.
✓ GLOBE ARTICHOKE. Another excellent blood purifier, also shown to lower blood cholesterol and help restore a damaged liver. Take 300 to 500 mg daily.

I'm on Prozac—but want to get off after reading how these kinds of antidepressants interfere with weight loss. Any suggestions?

Yes, indeed. And by the way, you are not alone battling depression—nearly 20 million Americans suffer from it. If you are getting off Prozac or any similar medications (such as Zoloft), you must do this under the care of a physician. Then you may want to investigate a breakthrough product called Ultra H-3, which balances the levels of the enzyme monoamine oxidase (MAO) in the brain. If MAO builds up in the brain, it replaces other vital substances such as norepinephrine (a hormone essential to well-being and vitality) and can cause depression as well as premature aging. Based on over 500 laboratory studies of the legendary Romanian Ultra H-3 product, Ultra H-3 is a safe and effective remedy for depression when taken for a trial period of at least three months.

Should I avoid over-the-counter products such as ibuprofen or cold medicines while on the Fat Flush Plan? What about taking Celexa, Prevacid, Claritin, or the diet drug Xenical—or even antibiotics—while on the Fat Flush Plan?

It is best to avoid over-the-counter medicines while on the Fat Flush Plan, because they all need to be broken down by the liver. One of the main purposes of the Fat Flush Plan is to protect your primary fat-burning organ, the liver, through cleansing and gentle detoxification. Increasing its workload at this time wouldn't be advisable.

You need to be especially cautious with Tylenol, which has been found to be toxic to liver function.

Keep in mind also that if you come down with a cold when your sinuses start to act up or if you start to have digestive problems, these could simply be symptoms of your cleansing process. And this is a good thing, because it means that the plan is working and you're on the way to your weight loss goals. Usually, these detoxification symptoms disappear in about four days.

If you happen to become ill while on the Fat Flush Plan and you are sure it's not related to the cleansing process—such as a sore throat, the flu, or anything similar that requires medical attention—stop the plan and consult your physician. This is not the best time for you to do the Fat Flush Plan. Wait until you are well and then begin again.

Are there any drug-nutrient interactions I should be aware of while following the Fat Flush Plan?

Yes, there are. Do be aware that cran-water acts as a mild blood thinner for some sensitive individuals. The most important drug-nutrient interactions you should be aware of are as follows, especially if you decide to use a GLA-alternative oil to the recommended black currant seed oil:

✓ EVENING PRIMROSE OIL. You shouldn't take antidepressants (such as Wellbutrin) with evening primrose oil, because it can augment the risk of seizures. This also holds true for individuals having psychotic disorders or taking phenothiazine drugs such as Thorazine, Mellaril, or Stelazine.

✓ BORAGE OIL. This has been shown to increase the blood-thinning qualities of medications such as aspirin, Dalteparin, Enoxaparin, and warfarin.

EXERCISE

I am an exercise fanatic. Do I have to change my routine while on the Fat Flush Plan?

Yes, it would be best to modify your workout routine—especially for phase 1, the Two Week Fat Flush. Since this phase of the Fat Flush Plan can be a strong detox, overexertion is not recommended, so you can preserve strength and not burn out your reserves. Phase 1 will cleanse your system as it helps you drop those extra pounds, so stick with low to moderate exercises, such as those suggested in Chapter 9, during phase 1. You'll find that brisk walking for 30 minutes and a mini-trampoline workout will help keep released toxins moving out of the lymphatic system and out of the body. You may add high intense interval training when you reach phase 2 of the program.

I hate to exercise—even if it's just walking. Do I have to?

Absolutely—for the best results. As I stated earlier, the exercises on the Fat Flush Plan are easy but necessary to escort toxins out of your body and to protect your lymphatic health. And besides, you just might enjoy it. I find my power walks inspiring. They release tension and free my mind. And that in itself helps reduce stress and those urges to binge. In addition, walking conditions the heart and respiratory system, pumping oxygen to all parts of the body. It even helps your body's response to insulin (another hidden weight gain factor).

Why not grab a friend or family member? The minutes will fly by, and you'll get in some good quality time with a loved one or new acquaintance. Or you can don some headphones and listen to your favorite tunes.

COFFEE, TEA, OR . . . ?

May I at least have one cup of coffee a day?

One cup of organic coffee is A-OK on Fat Flush. Just be aware that with commercially grown coffee, over 200 pesticides are used on most coffee plants, and that regular coffee (as well as decaf) can be one of most toxic substance for your liver to metabolize. Similar to the insulin effect from aspartame, caffeine can block weight loss efforts in many people, which is why I encourage you to add a tablespoon of coconut or MCT oil to your morning joe. When it comes to caffeine, I'm not just talking about the caffeine in coffee—this also goes for black tea, green tea, iced tea, dark or milk chocolate, colas, and over-the-counter drugs such as cold medicines, pain relievers, and allergy remedies.

And keep in mind, if you will, that coffee is a heavy-duty diuretic that strips calcium, magnesium, and sodium from your body—the very minerals you need for bone building. In fact, caffeine from coffee, tea, and soft drinks doubles the rate of calcium excretion. Three cups of black coffee can result in a 45-mg calcium loss. Thus, it is no wonder that a landmark six-year study conducted by the Department of Medicine at Boston's Brigham and Women's Hospital in the early 1980s showed a remarkable connection between caffeine and hip fractures. The researchers tracked 84,484 women from the ages of 34 to 59. The women who experienced a three times higher risk of hip fractures also had a higher intake of caffeine.

I was an avid coffee drinker and finally switched to green tea. Do I really have to give that up as well?

All I can say is this: caffeine is caffeine is caffeine. Although green tea contains about a third of the caffeine of a drip-brewed cup of regular coffee—35 mg in green tea and 100 mg in regular coffee per 6 ounces to be exact—even this lesser amount can overload the liver and inhibit its fat-burning duties. This is especially true if you are already taking birth control pills or HRT, which are very hard on the liver already. Thus, you would be adding insult to injury.

Also, both black tea and green tea are naturally high in fluoride as well as copper, a mineral potentially overabundant in many unsuspecting women. Excess copper can impair the conversion of thyroid hormones, resulting in hypothyroidism. And when this occurs, your energy production slows down, you feel tired, and your weight can escalate.

In phase 3 you can enjoy a greater variety of herbal teas. Until then, you can have ginger, fennel, peppermint, and even parsley teas as well as more water or another cup of hot water with lemon.

What about alcohol—is it okay on the weekend or a special occasion?

Once you graduate to phase 3, the Lifestyle Eating Plan, anything in moderation is fine (whether wine or even vodka). However, during phases 1 and 2, when we are trying to give the liver a well-deserved vacation, I really prefer that you abstain. When you drink alcohol in any form, it not only drains magnesium but also becomes the fuel of choice for your body to burn. And if your body is busy processing alcohol, it can't burn stored fat—and this inhibits the fat-burning process altogether. In addition, alcohol feeds yeast. Yeast-related toxins are extremely disruptive to your liver (the body's premier fat-burning organ) and serve to practically shut down the fat-burning process. Also wine lovers need to consider that for every glass consumed, circulating estrogen elevates.

OTHER CONCERNS

What if I slip and chow down a hefty pasta meal with all the trimmings—am I doomed to gaining all my weight back?

No, you are just human, like the rest of us. Although one meal won't put your weight back on, you'll probably not feel too terrific afterward. In fact, you'll more than likely feel tired or bloated. This will be enough of an incentive to help you stay more on track. Remember that the beauty of the Fat Flush Plan is that you can jump back to phase 1 or even the Three-Day Ultra Fat Flush Tune-Up—whenever you get off base—say, after a major holiday celebration.

It's my third day on the Fat Flush Plan, and I have a caffeine withdrawal headache and am very tired. Is this normal?

Yes, it is a normal reaction to cleansing and the withdrawal from coffee as well as sugar, grains, and dairy foods—especially if you've been a big consumer of these items.

A caffeine deprivation (withdrawal) headache results from the normal opening (dilation) of blood vessels that are constricted by caffeine. In other words, habitual caffeine intake keeps blood vessels in the brain constricted. When caffeine is not consumed, these blood vessels return to their normal blood flow potential, and it is this increased circulation in the brain that causes the throbbing agony of a caffeine withdrawal headache. Ultimately, the brain becomes accustomed to normal blood flow, and the headache subsides. The caffeine headache connection goes well beyond withdrawal. Caffeine itself contributes to headaches, even when it is consumed moderately and consistently.

Don't fret. After the first four days, you'll find many of your symptoms vanishing, especially the headaches—if you take it easy, rest, and follow the exercise advice outlined in Chapter 9.

I'm in phase 2—the transition part of the Fat Flush Plan—and seem to have reached a plateau. What should I do?

For starters, you need to know that you're not technically on a plateau unless you've stopped dropping weight for at least three weeks. And reaching a plateau is common, regardless of the weight plan you're following.

Since phase 2 adds two portions of the friendly carbs back into the menu, you may want to look a bit closer at this issue. Are you following the plan as suggested, or have you inadvertently overshot the carb allowances? You also may want to cut back on recipes containing onions or tomatoes, which are higher-carb veggies. Although they are healthful, cleansing foods, they can be a hidden source of weight-gaining carbs for some people. For instance, ½ cup of onions has 7.4 grams of carbohydrates, and a medium-size raw tomato (2½ inches) has 5.8 grams; 1 cup of canned tomatoes has 10 grams, and 1 cup of tomato juice has 10.4 grams.

Here's where the beauty of the Fat Flush Plan can come into play. You can go back to phase 1 for a week, cutting back on all carbs to see how you do. If this causes you to lose weight, then watching your carb levels from here on out is your primary concern. So be on the lookout for hidden sugars and read labels.

To help you achieve this, I would greatly recommend sticking to the journaling ritual. It will provide you with a clear picture of what and how much you are consuming—and reveal if there are any other ways you may be secretly sabotaging your weight loss.

You also may want to add CLA to your regimen, which is really part of phase 3. As you may remember from my discussion in Chapter 2, research over the past 20 years has shown that CLA reduces the body's ability to store fat for energy by controlling the enzymes that release fat from the cells into the bloodstream. The result is a decrease in body fat and a proportional increase in lean muscle mass.

Organic foods can get pricey—especially on my limited budget. What can I do?

Each year, the Environmental Working Group publishes a list of the "Dirty Dozen" and the "Clean 15" fruits and vegetables. You can use this guide to help prioritize your purchasing.

In any case, all fruits and veggies should be washed before consumption. Check out the Chemist Formula in Chapter 11. Alternatively, you can fill your sink with pure water and add 1 cup of raw apple cider vinegar. In this mixture, submerge your produce and manually wash it, then dry.

I'm having a problem with constipation on the diet. What should I do?

I would check to make sure that you are consuming enough water. You may also want to add 400 mg of magnesium in the morning and 400 mg in the evening, because this helps to relax the intestinal walls and establish normal peristalsis. Constipation may also be related to poor bile, so make sure you are adding the daily lecithin to your smoothie. Also consider a supplement like the Bile Builder mentioned in all three phases or find a comparable formula in your local health food store.

Should I be watching my stools during the Fat Flush Plan, and what am I looking for exactly?

Believe it or not, your stools reveal telltale signs of what's going on with your body. Here are four areas to watch for:

✓ SMELL. No, they really don't have to have a foul odor. But if they do, it's a sign that putrefaction—rotting and fermentation of food—is occurring in your digestive tract. This means that your bad bacteria are more than likely outweighing your friendly bacteria. And this spells trouble, because it's your good bacteria that help digest food by creating digestive enzymes and keeping the bad bacteria under control.

✓ FREQUENCY. Actually, having two to three bowel movements a day is considered healthy. You want to keep things moving along so that stagnation and putrefaction don't occur. This is where fiber (psyllium or ground flax seeds) comes into play to help you eliminate more readily and thereby ward off disease.

✓ FORMATION. Generally speaking, a 2-foot-long stool with a diameter about the size of a half dollar is considered the best. Anything short of this could mean that you're lacking fiber, flora, or the enzymes needed to ensure complete digestion. If food particles (notably protein) are not broken down completely, they can enter the bloodstream, which leads the way to food allergies, a weakened immune system, and various diseases.

✓ FLOTATION. If your stools sink to the bottom of the toilet, it means that they are too hard and that your diet is lacking something, possibly fiber or essential fatty acids. A healthy stool floats, is not compact, and breaks into smaller pieces as it is flushed.

Will I ever be able to have my favorite white flour foods again, such as pasta, white bread, and other carbohydrates?

Of course you can. However, I hope by the time you have completed the program, you will have lost your taste for these items.

I hope you'll crave the friendly carbs instead, such as peas, carrots, and even sweet potatoes and squash. When I am in the mood for more carbs, I slice up a squash, spread the slices on a baking sheet, and bake it at 325 degrees Fahrenheit for 30 minutes. I make believe that I am having french fries. You can also use an air fryer to make them. The slices are quite delicious with some cinnamon or cloves.

Can I ever have popcorn again?

Yes, you can have all your favorite foods. Once you graduate to phase 3 and add back friendly carbs, you might even consider drizzling 1 tablespoon of flaxseed oil on your popcorn, the way I do.

15 Resources and Support

Good information is your best medicine.

—MICHAEL E. DEBAKEY, MD

ONLINE SUPPORT

Please visit www.fatflush.com and www.annlouise.com for complete support on your Fat Flush journey and new lifestyle. Visitors to my website and subscribers to my e-mail list never miss my latest blogs and are the first to know about news and upcoming events. Plus, you can stay up-to-date with my latest online webinars, articles, and radio and television appearances. Also, do join our Fat Flush community on Facebook at www.facebook.com/groups/fatflushcommunity/ for a 24/7 connection with other members, Fat Flush–friendly recipes, diet and exercise tips, testimonials, and motivation. The folks in this group are immeasurably generous in their support and advice, knowledge, and guidance!

UNI KEY HEALTH SYSTEMS

Uni Key Health Systems has been my go-to distributor for many supplements and test kits for over 25 years. It was founded in 1992 by James Templeton, a cancer survivor who used alternative medicine to heal himself and has since dedicated his life to helping others find the root causes of disease. Uni Key Health proudly provides high-quality, natural nutritional supplements, vitamins, and health information for diet and detox, weight loss, cleansing, antiaging, energy, hormonal balance, and skin care. I have been a spokesperson and formulator for Uni Key Health Systems for over 20 years.

181 West Commerce Drive
Hayden Lake, ID 83835
800.888.4353
www.unikeyhealth.com

Fat Flush–Compatible Supplements Available from Uni Key

Bile Builder
Carlson Fish Oil and Softgels
CLA-1000
Dandelion Root Tea
Fat Flush Body Protein
Fat Flush Whey Protein
GLA-90
Liver-Lovin Formula
Mag-Key
Melatonin 3 mg
Omega Nutrition Flaxseed Oil and Softgels
Omega Nutrition Cold Milled Flax Seeds
ProgestaKey
Super-GI Cleanse
SweetLeaf Stevia
Weight Loss Formula
Whole Chia Seeds
Y-C Cleanse

Also Available from Uni Key

Earthing Products. Reconnect to the earth's natural healing electrons with products designed to ground yourself for better sleep, increased endurance, enhanced energy, and overall balance.

Salivary Hormone Test. Unlike blood tests, which do not measure bioavailable hormone activity, saliva testing is considered to be the most accurate measure of free, bioavailable hormonal activity. This personal hormone evaluation can be used to profile up to six hormones: estradiol, estriol, progesterone, testosterone, DHEA, and cortisol. Your personal results and a personal letter of recommendation from my office are mailed directly to your home.

Tissue Mineral Analysis. This test uses a small sample of hair cut from the back of your head. The analysis includes a full report, up to 20 pages, which graphically shows the levels of 32 major minerals and 6 toxic metals in the body. Each mineral is fully evaluated in terms of its relationship with other minerals, which is a key to glandular function and metabolism rate. This report provides information on the effect of vitamin deficiency and excesses. There is also a complete discussion regarding environmental influences and disease tendencies based upon mineral levels and ratios. A list of recommended food choices and supplements, based upon the individual findings, is included at the end of the report.

Water Filtration. Purify your water to protect against harmful chemicals and toxins, parasites like giardia and amoeba, chloramines, and heavy metals. A free water quality consultation with a filtration expert is also available.

EDUCATIONAL RESOURCES

Price-Pottenger Nutrition Foundation

The Price-Pottenger Nutrition Foundation is a nonprofit, tax-exempt educational organization dedicated to the promotion of enhanced health through awareness of ecology, lifestyle, and health food production and sound nutrition. At its core are the landmark works of Drs. Weston A. Price and Francis M. Pottenger, Jr., pioneers in modern research.

800.366.3748
http://ppnf.org

Broda O. Barnes, M.D., Research Foundation

The Broda O. Barnes, M.D., Research Foundation, Inc., is a not-for-profit organization dedicated to education, research, and training in the field of thyroid and metabolic balance.

203.261.2101
www.brodabarnes.org

NUTRITIONAL TRAINING RESOURCES

Certified Nutrition Specialists (CNSs)

CNSs are advanced nutrition professionals. They engage in science-based advanced medical nutrition therapy, research, education, and more, in settings such as clinics, private practice, hospitals and other institutions, industry, academia, and the community. The CNS certification is held by clinical nutritionists, physicians, and other advance-degreed healthcare professionals with a specialty in nutrition.

202.903.0267
www.nutritionspecialists.org

Certified Clinical Nutritionists (CCNs)

CCNs are board-certified professionals. The primary service provided by CCNs is educational, to optimize the experience of health through enhanced nutrition. The Clinical Nutrition Certification Board is a 501(c)(3) nonprofit tax-exempt certification agency that provides professional training, examination, and certification for healthcare organizations, specialty credentialing programs, and state license and certification examinations. The Certified Clinical Nutritionist Examination establishes reputable standards of excellence.

972.250.2829
www.cncb.org

Nutritional Therapy Association (NTA)
As an education organization, NTA is dedicated to helping healthcare professionals reverse the tragic and unsuspected effects of the modern diet on their patients and clients based on their bio-individual nutritional needs. Throughout NTA's training programs and seminars, students access a wide range of educational tools and connect nationally with other practitioners in the healing arts. Let the people at NTA know I sent you by using the code "ALG."

800.918.9798
http://nutritionaltherapy.com

The Institute for Integrative Nutrition (IIN)
IIN was founded in 1992 by Joshua Rosenthal. Once a small classroom of passionate students in New York City, it is now the largest nutrition school in the world. Through its innovative online learning platform, Integrative Nutrition has provided a global learning experience for over 60,000 students and graduates in 122 countries worldwide.

877.730.5444
www.integrativenutrition.com

Bauman College Holistic Nutrition and Culinary Arts
Bauman College educates future leaders, thinkers, and creators in the holistic nutrition and culinary arts professions to support people in achieving optimal health and create a paradigm shift in the way our world thinks about food. The college's goal is to change the way people consume food from convenience to conscious eating. Bauman provides students with a comprehensive understanding of nutrition, culinary arts, and business practices to prepare them for career success.

707.795.1284
www.baumancollege.org

American College of Healthcare Sciences
Founded in New Zealand in 1978, ACHS launched in the United States in 1989 and became the first accredited completely online college offering holistic health education, with certificate, diploma, and undergraduate and graduate degree programs.

800.487.8839
www.achs.edu

University of Bridgeport
The University of Bridgeport College of Naturopathic Medicine is committed to training physicians for the twenty-first century: doctors who are leaders in the emerging paradigm of healthcare, blending research and

innovative technologies with the art of healing and natural therapeutics to provide patient-centered care.

800.392.3582

www.bridgeport.edu/academics/graduate/naturopathic-medicine-nd

Functional Diagnostic Nutrition (FDN)
FDN is a holistic discipline that employs functional laboratory assessments to identify malfunctions and underlying conditions at the root cause of the most common health complaints. FDN embraces metabolic individuality and provides a systematic approach that allows you to achieve consistent, repeatable, and successful clinical outcomes.

858.386.0075

http://functionaldiagnosticnutrition.com

The Institute for Functional Medicine
The Institute for Functional Medicine is a leader in functional medicine education. The institute offers physicians and other healthcare professionals a systems-based approach to the prevention, diagnosis, and comprehensive management of complex chronic disease.

800.228.0622

www.functionalmedicine.org

Institute for the Psychology of Eating
The Institute for the Psychology of Eating is a unique educational organization. Its mission is to forever change the way the world understands food, body, and health. The institute offers training for professionals, programs for the public, online events, live workshops, and conferences, as well as plenty of free online content and inspiration.

303.440.7642

http://psychologyofeating.com

PROFESSIONAL ORGANIZATIONS

The American College for Advancement in Medicine (ACAM)
ACAM enables members of the public to connect with physicians who take an integrative approach to patient care and empowers individuals with information about integrative medicine treatment options. For a referral to a medical doctor or osteopath who is knowledgeable in the use of natural hormone replacement, you can contact:

800.532.3688

www.acam.org

The American Association of Naturopathic Physicians (AANP)

Naturopathic physicians are licensed in the states of Alaska, Arizona, California, Colorado, Connecticut, Hawaii, Kansas, Maine, Maryland, Minnesota, Montana, New Hampshire, North Dakota, Oregon, Utah, Vermont, and Washington; in the District of Columbia; and in the U.S. territories of Puerto Rico and the U.S. Virgin Islands. For a referral to a naturopathic physician who can guide you with natural hormone therapy, you can contact:

202.237.8150
www.naturopathic.org

American Academy of Anti-Aging (A4M)

The A4M is dedicated to the advancement of technology to detect, prevent, and treat aging-related disease and to promote research into methods to retard and optimize the human aging process. The A4M is also dedicated to educating physicians, scientists, and members of the public on biomedical sciences, breaking technologies, and anti-aging issues.

561.997.0112
www.a4m.com

American Academy of Environmental Medicine

The American Academy of Environmental Medicine, founded in 1965, is an international association of physicians and other professionals interested in the clinical aspects of humans and their environment.

316.684.5500
www.aaemonline.org

TESTING AND LABS

ZRT Laboratory

Founded by David Zava, ZRT is a CLIA-certified diagnostic laboratory and the leader in hormone and wellness testing, providing accurate and meaningful test results that assist healthcare providers in making informed treatment decisions.

866.600.1636
www.zrtlab.com

Diagnos-Techs

Founded in 1987, Diagnos-Techs has been a pioneer and leader in offering salivary hormone testing and complete GI panels for parasites, bacteria, and microbiome imbalances. The organization's commitment to assisting healthcare professionals in restoring patients' health and wellness is impressive, with over 1.2 million specimens tested per year.

425.251.0596
www.diagnostechs.com

Meridian Valley Lab Food Allergy Testing
Meridian Valley Lab is a leader in allergy and hormone testing, specializing in comprehensive 24-hour urine hormone and metabolite testing. Meridian Valley was the first lab in the United States to offer this test to help doctors use bio-identical hormone replacement therapy safely and effectively.

206.209.4200
http://meridianvalleylab.com

Cyrex Labs
Cyrex Labs is an advanced clinical laboratory focusing on mucosal, cellular, and humoral immunology and specializing in offering antibody arrays for complex thyroid, gluten, and other food-associated autoimmunity testing.

877.772.9739
www.cyrexlabs.com

Trace Elements
Trace Elements is an independent testing laboratory specializing in hair tissue mineral analysis for healthcare professionals worldwide. With continued growth since its inception in 1984, Trace Elements serves thousands of health professionals of all specialties in over 46 countries.

800.824.2314
www.traceelements.com

Immuno Laboratories
Immuno Laboratories in Fort Lauderdale, Florida, is widely recognized as one of the leading food and environmental allergy testing facilities in the world. Since its inception, the company has conducted over 33 million food sensitivity tests, with 97 percent of its physicians continuing testing for 10 years or more—a clear indication of physician and patient satisfaction.

800.231.9197
www.immunolabs.com

ELISA/ACT Biotechnologies
Exclusive providers of high-sensitivity lymphocyte response assay tests—the gold standard in delayed hypersensitivity testing.

800.553.5472
www.elisaact.com

Cell Science Systems
Cell Science Systems is the provider for the Alcat test. The Alcat test may help uncover which foods and other substances trigger chronic inflammation and its related health issues, such as gastrointestinal and metabolic disorders and others. The test measures cellular reactions to over 450

substances. In medical studies where the Alcat test was used to guide diet, patients have shown significant improvement of many common symptoms.

800.872.5228

https://cellsciencesystems.com

MAGAZINES AND NEWSLETTERS

The Health Sciences Institute (HSI) Newsletter

HSI is an independent organization dedicated to uncovering and researching the most urgent advances in modern underground medicine. As a member of the professional advisory panel, I can verify that this cutting-edge newsletter is devoted to presenting extraordinary products to its members before the products hit the marketplace. HSI was the first to break the Ultra H-3 story—the extraordinary product for arthritis, depression, and antiaging. HSI provides private access to hidden cures, powerful discoveries, breakthrough treatments, and advances in modern underground medicine.

888.213.0764

http://hsionline.com

First for Women Magazine

With an understanding that women have busy lives, *First for Women* delivers helpful tips and credible information you can't get anywhere else. The magazine provides numerous motivational articles on living a well-rounded life, nurturing family, owning a pet, preparing healthy menus, and just having fun! *First for Women* is very visual, with lots of quick tips and advice that make it easy to read as your schedule allows. I am proud to be a regular contributor.

201.569.6699

www.firstforwomen.com

Nutrition News

Siri Khalsa is a wonderful veteran journalist who has been in the business of providing health education for over 25 years. Her engaging blog covers a wide variety of contemporary and current topics, and you can receive her monthly online newsletter by subscribing.

www.nutritionnews.com

Total Health Online Magazine

The mission of *Total Health Online* magazine is to advocate self-managed natural health, emphasize the importance of becoming the cocaptain of your own healthcare team, and address the imperatives to wellness. To achieve this, the magazine provides you, the reader, with the information and resources needed to establish and maintain optimum health as well as to potentiate your immune system in times of crises. I am an associate editor for this outstanding publication.

http://totalhealthmagazine.com

Taste for Life
Taste for Life in-store magazines can be found in health food stores, natural product chains, food co-ops, and supermarkets nationwide. The publication provides excellent articles on pertinent health issues and serves as an informative educational source on a variety of levels. I am proud to sit on *Taste for Life*'s editorial board. The online website also provides a one-stop natural health resource.

603.283.0034
www.tasteforlife.com

Women's Health Letter
Dr. Janet Zand, OMD, LAc, is a board-certified acupuncturist, a doctor of traditional Chinese medicine, a nationally respected author, lecturer, and natural health practitioner, and an herbal and nutraceutical products formulator who has helped thousands of people achieve better health. Dr. Zand is the editor in chief of this informative monthly newsletter.

800.791.3459
www.womenshealthletter.com

Nutrition & Healing Newsletter
As an author of nine books on everything from thyroid disorders to back pain, Dr. Glenn S. Rothfeld has helped thousands of patients find lasting solutions to even the most stubborn health problems. These latest health discoveries are now available each month by subscribing to Dr. Rothfeld's *Nutrition & Healing* newsletter.

http://nutritionandhealing.com

Total Wellness Newsletter
Dr. Sherry A. Rogers is board certified by the American Board of Environmental Medicine; is a Fellow of the American College of Allergy, Asthma and Immunology and a Fellow of the American College of Nutrition; and for over 25 years has been board certified by the American Board of Family Practice. Her monthly newsletter, *Total Wellness*, is designed to save her readers money in office visits by keeping folks abreast of the latest cutting-edge research and findings.

800.846.6687
https://prestigepublishing.com/products/total-wellness-newsletter

BOOKS FOR YOUR BOOKSHELF

Books by Ann Louise Gittleman, PhD, CNS

Here is a list and brief descriptions of my books that are noteworthy companions for your Fat Flush journey.

The Fat Flush Cookbook
ISBN 0-07-143367-8

The Fat Flush Cookbook contains more than 200 recipes using fat-flushing foods and featuring the thermogenic herbs and spices—including ginger, cayenne pepper, mustard, anise, fennel, and cinnamon—introduced in *The Fat Flush Plan*. This heart-smart volume includes tasty, timesaving, one-dish dinners, packable lunches, recipes with delicious and unique fat-burning herbs and spices, vegetarian-friendly ideas, and an extended list of name brands suitable for fat flushing.

The Fat Flush Journal and Shopping Guide
ISBN 0-07-141497-5

The Fat Flush Journal and Shopping Guide is your handy, take-anywhere companion to *The Fat Flush Plan*. The six-week journal helps you to record your progress, weight loss, and future goals; track meals, supplements, and exercise; and stay inspired with daily motivational messages. Following the journal section is a shopping list section that features checklists of fat-flushing foods organized by grocery store aisle, lists of foods you can eat in each of the three stages of the plan, and resources for locating the hard-to-find items.

The Fat Flush Foods
ISBN 0-07-144068-2

The Fat Flush Foods highlights the "super" foods, herbs, spices, and supplements that help you speed up fat loss and reap maximum health benefits. *The Fat Flush Foods* features the top 50 super foods that burn fat, boost your metabolism, and detoxify your body while controlling cholesterol and blood sugar levels. The book features herbs and spices that burn and flush fat as well as the latest research on the antiviral, antibacterial, and antifungal properties of these herbs, spices, and foods. Tips for making fat flushing easy, economical, and delicious are also included.

Fat Flush for Life
ISBN 0-73-821431-0

Fat Flush for Life is a seasonal approach to burn stubborn body fat all year long. For each season, the guidelines transition to a specifically designed diet and wellness program to take advantage of your body's natural seasonal response. This year-round super detox plan boosts metabolism and keeps the weight off.

The Fast Track Detox Diet
ISBN 0-76-792046-5

The Fast Track Detox Diet, which was featured on ABC's *20/20*, is a healthy diet wrapped around the age-old weight loss method of fasting. The 11-day program is ideal for breaking a plateau, getting rid of unhealthy, fattening toxins, and safely losing weight with a "crash" diet that not only works in the long run but is also good for you. The program consists of the Prequel—seven days of adding liver-loving and colon-caring foods to the diet; the Fast—one day of sipping a deliciously spiced unsweetened cranberry juice; and the Sequel—three days of reintroducing supportive and immune-boosting probiotic foods into the diet. The program can be used interchangeably with Fat Flush for a jump-start and cleanse.

Before the Change
ISBN 0-06-056087-8

The *New York Times* bestseller *Before the Change* is the first complete do-it-yourself program for managing perimenopause—the period of about 10 years leading up to menopause—with natural remedies. It also includes new information on the dangers of HRT, the pros and cons of soy, and insights about hypothyroidism. When I appeared on the *Dr. Phil Show* to discuss *Before the Change*, Dr. Phil's wife, Robyn, said that this was the book that made her feel like 25, at 50!

Guess What Came to Dinner?
ISBN 1-58-333096-8

Parasites are alive and well in twenty-first-century America. Learn how to protect yourself and your family from this alarming epidemic, which knows no economic or social boundaries. Parasites can masquerade as numerous illnesses, and this book masterfully covers everything you wanted to know and more about the warning signs, the water and food connection, man's best friend, diagnosis, treatment, and prevention.

The Gut Flush Plan
ISBN 1-58-333343-6

The Gut Flush Plan focuses on the new frontier in health care—the new germ warfare—designed to outsmart the hidden invaders and superbugs that are spreading into the community and threatening our health. The book offers concrete steps that protect against the undetected hitchhikers in our food and in our surroundings that take up residence in our guts, making us sick, tired, and bloated. You will learn to fortify your own compromised digestive system against pathogens and parasites, flush out any lingering invaders or toxins, and feed yourself nourishing foods that encourage and rebuild GI health.

Super Nutrition for Women
ISBN 0-55-338250-0

Super Nutrition for Women is the perfect book for women in their twenties and thirties who want to learn how to combat PMS, alleviate yeast infections, lose weight, and strengthen their immune systems. This book also includes great tips on getting out bad fats, salt, and sugar and boosting the female minerals calcium and iron in your diet. Plus, terrific recipes!

Super Nutrition for Men
ISBN 0-89-529954-2

This book is a guide to combating heart disease, cholesterol, hair loss, stress, weight gain, impotence, and substance abuse problems. Although men will, of course, benefit from the prostate chapter, this book isn't just for men. The substance abuse chapter, adapted from the most successful recovery centers in this country, is a useful resource for anyone encountering the challenges of substance abuse.

Your Body Knows Best
ISBN 0-67-187591-4

Your Body Knows Best was the first book to feature the possible blood-type connection to weight and immunity issues. You will learn how you can custom-tailor a diet that meets your body's special needs. Your customized diet is determined by your ancestry and genetic heritage, your blood type, and your metabolism.

Get the Sugar Out
ISBN 0-30-739485-9

Get the Sugar Out explains that sugar contributes not only to weight gain but also to mood swings, weakened immunity, diabetes, some cancers, and cardiovascular disease. The book offers 501 simple, resourceful, and practical tips for cutting sugar from your diet, giving you the knowledge and inspiration you need to live a healthier life. Plus, you'll find over 50 new delicious recipes and an explanation of the glycemic index.

Why Am I Always So Tired?
ISBN 0-06-251594-2

Here is a groundbreaking discovery on the overlooked connection between exhaustion and a copper-zinc imbalance in our bodies. You will be amazed to read about the copper connection to other disorders such as hyperactivity, panic attacks, depression, skin conditions, and hormonal imbalances.

Copper is found in water pipes, IUDs, and birth control pills (estrogen stock-piles copper) as well as in soy products, chocolate, and regular tea.

Here Are Some of My Personal Favorites

The 150 Healthiest Foods on Earth
Jonny Bowden, PhD, CNS. ISBN 1-59-233228-5

A complete guide to the healthiest foods you can eat—and how to cook them! Why get your nutrients from expensive supplements when you can enjoy delicious, nourishing foods instead? From almonds to yucca, readers will find out what nutrients each of the 150 featured foods contains, what form contains the most nutrients, if it's been recommended to combat any diseases, where to find it, how to prepare it, and how much to eat—plus wonderful recipes using these sometimes obscure foods.

Live Better Longer
Joseph Dispenza. ISBN 0-59-516361-0

Simple steps for getting well, staying well, and gaining vitality for a long and healthy life based on the teachings of legendary holistic healer and pioneering nutritionist Hazel Parcells. Dr. Parcells, the revered grande dame of alternative medicine, who healed herself of terminal tuberculosis when she was 42 years old, inspired several generations of nutritionists and lived to the age of 106 by following a dramatically effective set of straightforward nutritional practices.

Why Stomach Acid Is Good for You
Jonathan V. Wright, MD, and Lane Lenard, PhD. ISBN 0-87-131931-4

This groundbreaking book unleashes a brilliant new plan for permanently curing heartburn by relieving the root cause of the problem: low stomach acid. The fact is that heartburn is caused by too little stomach acid—not too much, as many doctors profess. As explained in this book, the current practice of reducing stomach acid may be a temporary fix, but this fix comes at a cost to our long-term health that is being ignored by the pharmaceutical companies, the FDA, and the thousands of physicians that prescribe antacid drugs like Prilosec, Tagamet, Zantac, Pepcid, and others.

Earthing: The Most Important Health Discovery Ever?
Clinton Ober, Stephen T. Sinatra, MD, and Martin Zucker.
ISBN 1-59-120374-0

Earthing introduces readers to the landmark discovery that living in contact with the earth's natural surface charge—being grounded—naturally reduces and prevents chronic inflammation in the body. This effect has massive health implications because of the well-established link between chronic inflammation and all chronic diseases, including the diseases of aging and the aging process itself.

Pottenger's Prophecy: How Food Resets Genes for Wellness or Illness
Gray Graham, NTP, Deborah Kesten, MPH, and Larry Scherwitz, PhD.
    ISBN 1-93-505233-0

The age of nutritional epigenetics has arrived. *Pottenger's Prophecy* identifies the foods that launch your genes on a path toward illness, as well as the diet that can activate "health" genes, often instantly, to promote a longer, healthier life. The emerging new science of epigenetics—how the foods you eat switch genes on or off that can lead to either wellness or illness—has been called a "new paradigm" and "the medicine of the future."

Living a Longer, Healthier Life:
The Companion Guide to Dr. A's Habits of Health
Dr. Wayne Scott Anderson. ISBN 0-98-191462-4

This workbook serves as the companion guide to the bestselling book *Dr. A's Habits of Health*, a comprehensive manual designed to give you control of your daily habits and behaviors in order to create a life of vibrancy and optimal health. *Living a Longer, Healthier Life* is a critical piece of self-actualization.

Dr. A's Habits of Health: The Path to Permanent Weight Control and Optimal Health
Dr. Wayne Scott Anderson. ISBN 0-98-191460-8

Go from surviving to thriving! If you've ever tried to lose weight only to gain it back, *Dr. A's Habits of Health* offers a life-changing breakthrough that shows you not only how to reach and maintain your healthy weight, but how to create a life of renewed vibrancy, health, and spirit all under the easy-to-follow guidance of one of America s most esteemed and compassionate practitioners of weight loss and optimal health.

Intuitive Eating
Evelyn Tribole, MS, RD. ISBN 1-25-000404-7

First published in 1995, *Intuitive Eating* has become the go-to book on rebuilding a healthy body image and making peace with food. We've all been there—angry with ourselves for overeating, for our lack of willpower, for failing at yet another diet. But the problem is not us; it's that dieting, with its emphasis on rules and regulations, has stopped us from listening to our bodies.

The Pantry Principle
Mira Dessy, NE. ISBN 0-98-893570-8

This book will help you take back control of your pantry and your food sources. You will discover those items that are not contributing nutritional value and perhaps detracting from your health and that of your loved ones. You will learn how to stock your pantry with the healthiest choices available.

Staying Healthy with New Medicine: Integrating Natural, Eastern and Western Approaches for Optimal Health
Elson Haas, MD. ISBN 0-69-268780-7

Staying Healthy with New Medicine provides the basis for health with a deep understanding of what creates disease in the body-mind. The integration of natural, Eastern, and Western medicines offers a clearer insight into many crucial factors that affect health and healing rather than just one particular system.

The Perfect Metabolism Plan
Sarah Vance. ISBN 1-57-324643-3

When your metabolism is out of whack, your willpower, hunger hormones, insulin, and cravings all work against you. And you not only can't lose weight; you tend to feel foggy, sluggish, or generally unwell. But worry no more. *The Perfect Metabolism Plan* will show you how to reset and reboot your metabolism through 10 keys.

The Big Fat Surprise
Nina Teicholz. ISBN 1-45-162442-5

Investigative journalist Nina Teicholz reveals the unthinkable: that everything we thought we knew about dietary fats is wrong. She documents how the past 60 years of low-fat nutrition advice has amounted to a vast uncontrolled experiment on the entire population, with disastrous consequences for our health.

Smart Fat
Steven Masley, MD, and Jonny Bowden, PhD, CNS. ISBN 0-06-239229-8

The innovative guide that reveals how eating more fat—the smart kind—is the key to health, longevity, and permanent weight loss.

The Great Cholesterol Myth
Jonny Bowden, PhD, CNS, and Stephen T. Sinatra, MD.
   ISBN 1-59-233521-7

Bestselling health authors Jonny Bowden and Stephen Sinatra give readers a four-part strategy based on the latest studies and clinical findings for effectively preventing, managing, and reversing heart disease, focusing on diet, exercise, supplements, and stress and anger management.

Iodine: Why You Need It, Why You Can't Live Without It
David Brownstein, MD. ISBN 0-96-608823-9

Iodine is a misunderstood nutrient. Learn what forms of iodine you need and why there is not enough iodine in salt. See how iodine can help breast cancer, fibrocystic breast disease, detoxification, fatigue, Graves' disease, and Hashimoto's disease. Find out why iodine deficiency may be the root cause of thyroid problems including hypothyroidism and thyroid cancer. Discover how to get iodine in your diet and improve your immune system.

The China Study
Thomas Campbell II, MD, and T. Colin Campbell, PhD.
   ISBN 1-93-210066-0

In *The China Study*, Dr. T. Colin Campbell details the connection between nutrition and heart disease, diabetes, and cancer. The report also examines the source of nutritional confusion produced by powerful lobbies, government entities, and opportunistic scientists. The *New York Times* has recognized the study as the "Grand Prix of epidemiology" and the "most comprehensive large study ever undertaken of the relationship between diet and the risk of developing disease."

Hypothyroidism Type 2: The Epidemic
Mark Starr, MD. ISBN 0-97-526240-8

This exceptional book reveals the cause and successful treatment of the plague of illnesses affecting Western civilization, including obesity, heart attacks, depression, diabetes, strokes, headaches, chronic fatigue, and many more. In Dr. Starr's description of type 2 hypothyroidism, he presents overwhelming evidence showing that a majority of Americans suffer from this illness, which is due to environmental and hereditary factors.

Rare Earths: Forbidden Cures
Joel D. Wallach, BS, DVM, ND, and Ma Lan, MD, MS. ISBN 0-97-014908-5

For the first time, Dr. Joel Wallach and Dr. Ma Lan have brought together a comprehensive look at all the physical, emotional, and social problems attributed to mineral deficiencies in our soil and food supply. The book focuses on why nutritional supplementation, especially mineral supplementation, is critical to the good health of every human being.

The Calcium Lie
Robert Thompson, MD, and Kathleen Barnes. ISBN 0-98-158185-4

Most consumers and, surprisingly, most doctors believe that bones are made of calcium. Yet any basic biochemistry textbook will tell you the truth: bones are made of at least a dozen minerals, and we need all of them in perfect proportions in order to have healthy bones and healthy bodies. If you get too much calcium, through food sources or by taking supplements, you set yourself up for an array of negative health consequences, including obesity, type 2 diabetes, type 2 hypothyroidism, hypertension, depression, problem pregnancies, and more. This book gives you all the information you need to stay healthy and to regain your health if you or your doctor has been duped by "the calcium lie."

The Sleep Revolution
Arianna Huffington. ISBN 1-10-190400-3

We are in the midst of a sleep deprivation crisis, writes Arianna Huffington, the cofounder and editor in chief of the *Huffington Post*. And this has profound consequences—on our health, our job performance, our relationships, and our happiness. What is needed, she boldly asserts, is nothing short of a sleep revolution. Only by renewing our relationship with sleep can we take back control of our lives.

The Allergy Solution
Leo Galland, MD. ISBN 1-40-194939-8

In this groundbreaking book, Dr. Leo Galland reveals the shocking rise of hidden allergies that lead to weight gain, fatigue, brain fog, depression, joint pain, headaches, ADHD, digestive problems, and much more. New research shows how each of these is linked to the immune imbalance that is at the root of allergy.

Wheat Belly
William Davis, MD. ISBN 1-60-961479-8

Over 200 million Americans consume food products made of wheat every day. As a result, over 100 million experience some form of adverse health effect, ranging from minor rashes to high blood sugar to unattractive stomach bulges that cardiologist William Davis calls "wheat bellies." According to Davis, that excess fat has nothing to do with gluttony, sloth, or too much butter: it's due to the whole grain wraps we eat for lunch. After witnessing over 2,000 patients regain health after giving up wheat, Davis reached the disturbing conclusion that wheat is the single largest contributor to the nationwide obesity epidemic—and that elimination of wheat is key to dramatic weight loss and optimal health.

Going Against GMOs: The Fast-Growing Movement to Avoid Unnatural Genetically Modified "Foods" to Take Back Our Food
Melissa Diane Smith. ISBN 0-99-081521-8

This book is a definitive consumer's guide to understanding genetically modified foods, the food issue of our time, from the unique perspective of my colleague and friend Melissa Diane Smith, a trailblazing nutritionist. In this book, you'll find the top 10 reasons to stay away from GMOs; why you have to go against the status quo to avoid GMOs; the Eat GMO-Free Challenge and non-GMO optimal health guidelines; detailed instructions for avoiding GMOs when shopping and eating out; and more than 45 easy-to-make, non-GMO (and gluten-free) recipes.

Going Against the Grain
Melissa Diane Smith. ISBN 0-65-801722-5

More than a dozen years in print, this groundbreaking book challenges conventional dietary wisdom—that grains should be the centerpiece of our diet. Author Melissa Diane Smith presents scientific information in easy-to-understand terms on both the surprising nutritional problems of grains and the grain connection to conditions such as obesity, diabetes, syndrome X, autoimmune disorders, celiac disease, gluten sensitivity, grain allergies, and digestive problems.

Gluten Free Throughout the Year
Melissa Diane Smith. ISBN 1-60-910180-4

With more than 100 tips, 30 recipes, and names of the healthiest gluten-free food brands and products, this is an easy-to-read, tip-based practical guide for living a healthy gluten-free lifestyle.

Syndrome X: The Complete Nutritional Program to Prevent and Reverse Insulin Resistance
Melissa Diane Smith. ISBN 0-47-139858-6

This national bestselling book explains, in simple terms, how the prediabetic condition syndrome X (also known as metabolic syndrome) develops and is easily reversed through a change in diet. The condition is the combination of insulin resistance with extra weight around the middle, unhealthy cholesterol ratios, high triglycerides, and high blood pressure that ages people prematurely and sets the stage for heart disease, type 2 diabetes, and other common degenerative diseases.

The Fungus Link
Doug A. Kaufmann. ISBN 0-97-034180-6

Learn why so many people have failed to achieve the health goals they've worked so hard for, all because they were not aware of the fungus link to their symptoms. Pain, heart health, allergies, digestive disorders, mental health, women's health, and respiratory challenges are all covered in this groundbreaking work.

Cooking Your Way to Good Health
Doug Kaufmann and Denni Dunham. ISBN 0-98-279841-5

This cookbook is excellent! With such creative, yet so easy, recipes, you may never need another cookbook again. Plus, Doug Kaufmann assures that every dish is absolutely guilt-free. Brand-new ideas for breakfast, main dishes, side dishes, slow-cooked meals, appetizers, marinades, soups, and, yes, even sumptuous desserts, *Cooking Your Way to Good Health* hits all the marks.

PURE FOOD AND CLEAN WATER

Meat

The Eat Well Guide site includes state-by-state lists of meat that is raised without antibiotics.

212.991.1930
www.eatwellguide.org

Eat Wild provides lists of certified organic farmers known to produce safe, wholesome raw dairy products as well as grass-fed beef and other organic produce.

253.759.2318
www.EatWild.com

Weston A. Price has local chapters in most states, and many of them are connected with buying clubs in which you can easily purchase organic foods, including grass-fed raw dairy products such as milk and butter.

202.363.4394
www.westonaprice.org

The Grassfed Exchange has a list of producers selling organic and grass-fed meats across the United States.

256.996.3142
www.grassfedexchange.com

LocalHarvest will help you find good food close to you.

www.localharvest.org

National Farmers Market Directory will help you find a farmer's market near you.

http://nfmd.org

American Grassfed provides a list of certified grass-fed farms and ranches.

877.774.7277
www.americangrassfed.org

American Farmers Network will help you find 100 percent grass-fed, USDA-certified organic steaks, burgers, chicken, and more.

800.817.6180
www.americanfarmersnetwork.com

Community Involved in Sustaining Agriculture is dedicated to sustaining agriculture and promoting the products of small farms.

413.665.7100
www.buylocalfood.org

The FoodRoutes "Find Good Food" map can help you connect with local farmers to find the freshest, tastiest food possible. On FoodRoutes' interactive map, you can find a list of local farmers, CSAs, and markets near you.

814.571.8319
http://foodroutes.org

The Cornucopia Institute maintains web-based tools rating all certified organic brands of eggs, dairy products, and other commodities, based on ethical sourcing and authentic farming practices, separating CAFO "organic" production from authentic organic practices.

608.625.2000
www.cornucopia.org

Fish

Sardines from Crown Prince and Bela are often carried in finer health food stores. But if not, here is the contact information for these two fine brands:

Crown Prince

707.766.8575
www.crownprince.com

Bela Sardines

www.amazon.com/grocery

•   •   •

The following websites carry wild salmon and albacore tuna, rich sources of omega-3 fatty acids. Some, such as tunatuna.com (Fishing Vessel St. Jude), test their fish to ensure that they are virtually mercury-free.

Copper River Seafoods

888.622.1197
www.copperriverseafood.com

EcoFish

603.430.0101
www.ecofish.com

Fishing Vessel St. Jude

425.378.0680
www.tunatuna.com

East Point Seafood Market

888.317.8459
www.eastpointseafood.com

Vital Choice Seafood

800.608.4825
www.vitalchoice.com

Wild Salmon Seafood Market

206.217.3474
http://wildsalmonseafood.com

Water

Clean Water Revival (CWR)

CWR specializes in custom-designed water filtration equipment, air purifiers, and survival and personal protection equipment. Call Uni Key at 800.888.4353 to schedule a complimentary consultation with a water quality specialist to discuss the best filtration equipment solution for your health needs.

7897 SW Jack James Drive, Suite C
Stuart, FL 34997
800.444.3563
www.cwrenviro.com

Environmental Protection Agency Safe Drinking Water Hot Line

800.424.8802

National Testing Laboratories, Inc.

800.458.3330
www.ntllabs.com

Suburban Water Testing

800.433.6595
www.suburbantestinglabs.com

Organics

You can learn about organic food and organic farming from the following nonprofit organizations.

Organic Trade Association

802.275.3800
www.ota.com

Organic Farming Research Foundation

831.426.6606
http://ofrf.org

The Land Institute

785.823.5376
https://landinstitute.org

Community Alliance with Family Farmers

530.756.8518
www.facebook.com/famfarms

One Other Resource

ASEA

Over time, due to aging, stress, and environmental toxins, our bodies lose the ability to function at optimum levels. ASEA Redox Supplement, suspended in a pristine saline solution, is composed of the same life-sustaining molecules that exist in the human body. It works at the cellular level to enhance function and assist your body's natural efforts to maximize energy and vitality.

6550 South Millrock Drive, Suite 100
Salt Lake City, UT 84121
888.438.5971
www.aseaglobal.com

Appendix

FAT FLUSH JOURNAL

PHASE _____

MY PHASE ____ GOAL
_____

MY PHASE ____ REWARD
_____

TODAY'S DATE
_____

Meals, Beverages & Snacks

- UPON RISING _____
- BEFORE BREAKFAST _____
- BREAKFAST _____
- MIDMORNING SNACK _____
- BEFORE LUNCH _____
- LUNCH _____

_____

_____

_____

_____

- MIDAFTERNOON SNACK _____
- 4 P.M. SNACK _____
- BEFORE DINNER _____

- **DINNER**

_____

_____

_____

_____

_____

- **MIDEVENING**

Supplements

_____

_____

_____

_____

Measurements

- **BUST/CHEST**

- **WAIST**

- **HIPS**

- **THIGHS**

FOOD FOR THOUGHT

_____

_____

_____

_____

HEALTH & WELLNESS NOTES

_____

_____

_____

_____

EXERCISE

_____

_____

_____

_____

SLEEP TIME

_____

_____

_____

_____

REFLECTIONS

_____

_____

_____

_____

_____

_____

DAILY ACKNOWLEDGMENT

_____

_____

_____

_____

GRATITUDE

_____

_____

_____

_____

References

THE FAT FLUSH PHENOMENON

https://news.illinois.edu/blog/view/6367/204477.
www.apa.org/topics/obesity/support.aspx.

CHAPTER 1 SOMEONE LIKE YOU . . .

Anderson, K. E., and Kappas, A. "Dietary Regulation of Cytochrome P- 450." *Annu Rev Nutr* 11(1991):141–167.

Bland, J. S. *The 20-Day Rejuvenation Diet Program*. Los Angeles: Keats, 1999.

Bland, J. S. "Food and Nutrient Effects on Detoxification." *Townsend Letter for Doctors* (December 1995).

Bland, J. S., and Bralley, J. A. "Nutritional Up-Regulation of Hepatic Detoxification Enzymes." *J Appl Nutr* 3–4(1992):2–15.

Bock, K. *The Road to Immunity: How to Survive and Thrive in a Toxic World*. New York: Pocket Books, 1997.

Breecher, M. "A Natural Aid to Weight Reduction for the Chronically Fat." *Let's Live Magazine* (August 1982):70–73.

Brush, M. G., Watson, S. J., Horrobin, D. F., and Manku, M. S. "Abnormal Essential Fatty Acid Levels in Plasma of Women with Premenstrual Syndrome." *Am J Obstet Gynecol* 150(1984):363–366.

Cabot, S. *The Liver Cleansing Diet*. Scottsdale, AZ: SCB International, 1999.

Caldwell, J., and Jakoby, W. B. *Biological Basis of Detoxification*. New York: Academic Press, 1983.

Charalambous, B. M. "Erythrocyte Sodium Pump Activity in Human Obesity." *Clin Chim Acta* 141:2–3(1984):179–187.

Galland, L. *The Four Pillars of Healing*. New York: Random House, 1997.

Gittleman, A. L. *Beyond Pritikin*. New York: Bantam, 1988.

Gittleman, A. L. *Super Nutrition for Women*. New York: Bantam, 1991.

Haas, E. *The Detox Diet*. Millbrae, CA: Celestial Arts, 1996.

Haslett, C., et al. "A Double Blind Evaluation of Evening Primrose Oil as an Anti-Obesity Agent." *Int J Obesity* 7(1983):549–553.

Heaton, J. M. "The Distribution of Brown Adipose Tissue in the Human." *J Anat* 112(1972):35.

Heleniak, E. P., and Aston, B. "Prostaglandins, Brown Fat, and Weight Loss." *Med Hypoth* 28(1989):13–33.

Henry, C. J., and Emery, B. "Effect of Spiced Food on Metabolic Rate." *Hum Nutr Clin Nutr* 40:2(1986):165–168.

Himms-Hagen, J. "Obesity May Be Due to a Malfunctioning of Brown Fat." *Can Med Assoc J* 121(1976):1361–1364.

Horrobin, D. F. "The Role of Essential Fatty Acids and Prostaglandins in the Premenstrual Syndrome." *J Reprod Med* 28(1983):465–468.

Jakoby, W. B. (ed.). *Enzymatic Basis of Detoxification*, Vol II. New York: Academic Press, 1980.

Jakoby, W. B., Bend, J. R., and Caldwell, J. (eds.). *Metabolic Basis of Detoxification: Metabolism of Functional Groups.* New York: Academic Press, 1981.

Lemole, G. M. *The Healing Diet.* New York: William Morrow, 2000.

Mercer, S. W. "Effect of High Fat Diets on Energy Balance and Thermogenesis in Brown Adipose Tissue of Lean and Genetically Obese Mice." *J Nutr* 117:12(1987):2147–2153.

Mir, M. A., et al. "Erythrocyte Sodium Potassium-ATPase Transport in Obesity." *N Engl J Med* 305(1981):1264–1268.

Sears, B. *The Zone.* New York: Regan Books, 1995.

Takada, R., Saitoh, M., and Mori, T. "Dietary Gamma-Linolenic Acid-Enriched Oil Reduces Body Fat Content and Induces Liver Enzyme Activities Relating to Fatty Acid Beta-Oxidation in Rats." *J Nutr* 124(1994):469–474.

Vadaddi, K. S., and Horrobin, D. F. "Weight Loss Produced by Evening Primrose Oil Administered in Normal and Schizophrenic Individuals." *IRCS J Med Sci* 7(1979):52–55.

"Why You Need to Protect Your Liver." *Consumer Reports on Health* 13:4(April 2001):6–9.

CHAPTER 2 TOP 10 HIDDEN WEIGHT GAIN FACTORS #1 THROUGH #5

Hidden Factor #1: Your Tired, Toxic Liver

Anderson, J. W., et al. "Effects of Psyllium on Glucose and Serum Lipid Responses in Men with Type II Diabetes and Hypercholesterolemia." *Am J Clin Nutr* 70:4(1999):466–473.

Anderson, J. W., et al. "Long-Term Cholesterol-Lowering Effects of Psyllium as an Adjunct to Diet Therapy in the Treatment of Hypercholesterolemia." *Am J Clin Nutr* 71:6(2000):1433–1438.

Arrigoni-Martelli, E., and Caso, V. "Carnitine Protects Mitochondria and Removes Toxic Acyls from Xenobiotics." *Drugs Exp Clin Res* 27:1(2001):27–49.

Asai, A., Nakagawa, K., and Miyazawa, T. "Antioxidative Effects of Turmeric, Rosemary, and Capsicum Extracts on Membrane Phospholipid Peroxidation and Liver Lipid Metabolism in Mice." *Biosci Biotechnol Biochem* 63:12(1999): 2118–2122.

Berdanier, C. D. "Inositol: An Essential Nutrient?" *Nutrition Today* 27(1992):22–26.

Brevetti, G., et al. "Changes in Skeletal Muscle Histology and Metabolism in Patients Undergoing Exercise Reconditioning: Effect of Proprionyl-L-Carnitine." *Muscle Nerve* 20(1997):1115–1120.

Cabot, S. *The Liver Cleansing Diet.* Scottsdale, AZ: SCB International, 1996.

Chen, H., Zuo, Y., and Deng, Y. "Separation and Determination of Flavonoids and Other Phenolic Compounds in Cranberry Juice by High-Performance Liquid Chromatography." *J Chromatogr A* 913:1–2(2001):387–395.

Crayhon, R. *The Carnitine Miracle.* New York: Evans and Company, 1998.

Cunnane, S. C., et al. "Nutritional Attributes of Traditional Flaxseed in Healthy Young Adults." *Am J Clin Nutr* 61:1(1995):62–68.

Dayanandan, A., Kumar, P., and Panneerselvam, C. "Protective Role of L-Carnitine on Liver and Heart Lipid Peroxidation in Atherosclerotic Rats." *J Nutr Biochem* 12:5(2001):254–257.

Delergy, H. J., et al. "Effects of Amount and Type of Dietary Fiber on Short-Term Control of Appetite." *Int J Food Sci Nutr* 48:1(1997):67–77.

Dyck, D. J. "Dietary Fat Intake, Supplements, and Weight Loss." *Can J Appl Physiol* 25:6(2000):495–523.

Eldershaw, T. P., et al. "Pungent Principles of Ginger (*Zingiber officinale*) Are Thermogenic in the Perfused Rat Hindlimb." *Int J Obesity Related Metabol Disord* 16:10(1992):755–763.

Facchinetti, F., et al. "Oral Magnesium Successfully Relieves Premenstrual Mood Changes." *Obstet Gynecol* 78:2(1991):177–181.

Flora, K., et al. "Milk Thistle (*Silybum marianum*) for the Therapy of Liver Disease." *Am J Gastroenterol* 94:2(1999):545–546.

Gittleman, A. L. *Eat Fat, Lose Weight.* Blue Hills Publishing, Kindle Edition, 2015.

Gittleman, A. L. *The Living Beauty Detox Program.* New York: Harper San Francisco, 2000.

Hahn, P., and Skala, J. "The Role of Carnitine in Brown Adipose Tissue of Suckling Rats." *Comp Biochem Physiol* 51B(1975):507.

Hamadeh, M. J., et al. "Nutritional Aspects of Flaxseed in the Human Diet." *Proc Flax Inst* 4(1992):48–53.

Hu, F. B., et al. "A Prospective Study of Egg Consumption and Risk of Cardiovascular Disease in Men and Women." *JAMA* 281:15(1999):1387–1394.

Imparl-Radosevich, J., et al. "Regulation of PTP-1 and Insulin Receptor Kinase by Fractions from Cinnamon: Implications for Cinnamon Regulation of Insulin Signaling." *Horm Res* 50:3(1998):177–182.

Jenkins, D. J., et al. "Effect of Psyllium in Hypercholesterolemia at Two Monounsaturated Fatty Acid Intakes." *Am J Clin Nutr* 65:5(1997):1524–1533.

Lake, R. *Liver Cleansing Handbook.* Vancouver: Alive Books, 2000.

Langner, E., et al. "Ginger: History and Use." *Adv Ther* 15:1(1998):25–44.

Lebowitz, B. "Carnitine." *J Opt Nutr* 22(1993):90–109.

Mickelfied, G. H., et al. "Effects of Ginger on Gastroduodenal Motility." *Int J Clin Pharmacol Ther* 37:7(1999):341–346.

Mills, S. Y. *Out of the Earth: The Essential Book of Herbal Medicine.* London: Penguin Books, 1991, p. 282.

Murray, M. T., and Pizzorno, J. *Encyclopedia of Natural Medicine.* Rocklin, CA: Prima Publishing, 1991, pp. 51–56.

Olson, B. H., et al. "Psyllium-Enriched Cereals Lower Blood Total Cholesterol and LDL Cholesterol, but Not HDL Cholesterol, in Hypercholesterolemic Adults: Results of a Meta-Analysis." *J Nutr* 127:10(1997):1973–1980.

Park, B. K., and Kirreringham, N. R. "Assessment of Enzyme Induction and Enzyme Inhibition in Humans: Toxicological Implications." *Xenobiotica* 20:11(1990): 1339–1343.

Pepping, J. "Milk Thistle: *Silybum marianum*." *Am J Health Syst Pharm* 56:12(1999): 1196–1197.

Raczkotilla, E., et al. "The Action of *Taraxacum officinale* Extracts on the Body Weight Diuresis of Laboratory Animals." *Planta Med* 26(1974): 212–217.

Rutherford, P. P, and Deacon, A. C. "The Mode of Action of Dandelion Root Fructofuranosideases on Insulin." *Biochem J* 129:2(1972):511–512.

Salmi, H. A., et al. "Effect of Silymarin on Chemical, Functional, and Morphological Alterations of the Liver." *Scand J Gastroenterol* 17(1982): 512–517.

Shakil, A. O., et al. "Acute Liver Failure: Clinical Features, Outcome, Analysis, Applicability." *Liver Transplant* 6(2000):163–169.

Shear, N. H., et al. "Acetaminophen-Induced Toxicity to Human Epidermoid Cell Line A431 and Hepatoblastoma Cell Line: Hep G2, in Vitro, Is Diminished by Silymarin." *Skin Pharmacol* 8:6(1995):279–291.

Svilaas, A., et al. "Intakes of Antioxidants in Coffee, Wine, and Vegetables Are Correlated with Plasma Carotenoids in Humans." *J. Nutr* 134:3(2004): 562–567.

Velussi, M., et al. "Long-Term (12 Months) Treatment with an Antioxidant Drug (Silymarin) Is Effective on Hyperinsulinemia, Exogenous Insulin Need and Malondialdehyde Levels in Cirrhotic Diabetic Patients." *J Hepatol* 26:4(1997): 871–879.

"Why You Need to Protect Your Liver." *Consumer Reports on Health* (April 2001):6–9.

Zhi-Qian, H. E., et al. "Body Weight Reduction in Adolescents by a Combination of Measures Including Using L-Carnitine." *Acta Nutr Sinica* 19:2(1997):146–151.

https://cspinet.org/new/pdf/combined_infographic.pdf.

www.livestrong.com/article/390375-what-are-the-health-benefits-of-cane-syrup/.

Hidden Factor #2: False Fat

Adlercreutz, H., et al. "Inhibition of Human Aromatase by Mammalian Lignans and Isoflavonoid Phytoestrogens." *J Steroid Biochem Mol Biol* 44(1993):147–153.

Bateson-Koch, C. *Allergies: Diseases in Disguise*. Vancouver: Alive Books, 1994.

Bodel, P. T., Colran, R., and Kass, E. H. "Cranberry Juice and Antibacterial Action of Hippuric Acid." *J Lab Clin Med* 54(1959):881–888.

Braley, J. *Dr. Braley's Food Allergy and Nutrition Revolution*. New Canaan, CT: Keats Publishing, 1992.

Browder, S. E. *The Power*. New York: Wiley, 2001.

Chrohn, J. *Natural Detox: The Complete Guide to Allergy Relief and Prevention*. Point Roberts, WA: Hartley and Marks, 1996.

Crook, W. G. *Yeast Connection: A Medical Breakthrough*. Jackson, TN: Vintage Books, 1980.

Dancey, E. *The Cellulite Solution*. New York: St. Martin's Press, 1997.

De Stefani, F., et al. "Dietary Fiber and Risk of Breast Cancer: A Case-Controlled Study in Uruguay." *Nutr Cancer* 28(1997):14–19.

Espeland, M. A., et al. "Effect of Postmenopausal Hormone Therapy on Body Weight and Waist and Hip Girths: Postmenopausal Estrogen-Progestin Interventions Study Investigators." *J Clin Endocrinol Metab* 82:5(1997): 1549–1556.

Gittleman, A. L. *Before the Change*. New York: HarperOne, 2003.

Gittleman, A. L. *Beyond Pritikin*. New York: Bantam Books, 1996.

Gittleman, A. L. *Eat Fat, Lose Weight*. Blue Hills Publishing, Kindle Edition, 2015.

Gottesman, R. "How Symptoms Tell the Story of Hormone Imbalance." *John Lee Med Lett* (April 1998):5–6.

Greenwood-Robinson, M. *The Cellulite Breakthrough*. New York: Dell, 2000.

Guigliano, D., Torella, R., and Sgambat, S. "Effects of Alpha- and Beta-Adrenergic Inhibition and Somatostatin on Plasma Glucose, Free Fatty Acids, Insulin, Glucagon, and Growth Hormone Responses to Prostaglandin E1 in Man." *J Clin Endocrinol Metab* 48(1979):302.

Haas, E. M., and Stauth, C. *The False Fat Diet*. New York: Ballantine Books, 2000.

Horrobin, D. F. "The Role of Essential Fatty Acids and Prostaglandins in the Premenstrual Syndrome." *J Reprod Med* 28(1983):465–468.

Knotts, C. T., et al. "Endomesyum Antibodies in Blood Donors Predicts a High Prevalence of Celiac Disease in the United States." *J Gastroenterol* (April 1996).

Lee, Y. L., et al. "Does Cranberry Juice Have Antibacterial Activity?" *JAMA* 283:13(2000):1691.

Ofek, I., Goldhar, J., and Sharon, N. "Anti–*Escherichia coli* Adhesion Activity of Cranberry and Blueberry Juices." *Adv Exp Med Biol* 408(1996): 179–183.

Papas, P. N., Brusch, C. A., and Ceresia, G. C. "Cranberry Juice in the Treatment of Urinary Tract Infections." *Southwest Med* 47(1966):17–20.

Randolph, T. G. *An Alternative Approach to Allergies*. New York: HarperCollins, 1990.

Rigaud, D., et al. "Effect of Psyllium on Gastric Emptying, Hunger Feeling and Food Intake in Normal Volunteers: A Double-Blind Study." *Eur J Clin Nutr* 52:4(1998): 239–245.

Smith, I. K. "The Tylenol Scare." *Time* (April 9, 2001):81.

Thompson, L. U. "Flaxseed and Its Lignan and Oil Components Reduce Mammary Tumor Growth at Late Stage of Carcinogenesis." *Carcinogenesis* 17:6(1996): 1373–1376.

Walker, E. B., et al. "Cranberry Concentrate: UTI Prophylaxis." *J Fam Pract* 45:2(1997): 167–168.

Wang, C., et al. "Lignans and Flavonoids Inhibit Aromatase Enzyme in Human Preadipocytes." *J Steroid Biochem Mol Biol* 50(1994):205–212.

Whitaker, J. "Should You Use HRT?" *Health Healing* 6(2001):4–8.

Yeager, S. "Banish Cellulite in Minutes." *Prevention* (June 2001):150–157.

Zava, D. "Teenage Girls, Hormone Balance and Birth Control Pills." *John Lee Med Lett* (January 1999):5–6.

http://drhoffman.com/article/8-reasons-why-its-not-your-fault-youre-fat/#sthash .Ed0TReTa.dpbs.

http://pilladvised.com/2016/04/the-allergy-solution-q-a/.

http://thyroidpharmacist.com/articles/hormone-replacement-therapy-and-cancer.

www.sciencedaily.com/releases/2016/02/160219111219.htm.

www.wheatbellyblog.com/about/.

www.dukechronicle.com/article/2016/03/air-pollution-exposure-linked-to-obesity -risk-by-duke-researchers.

www.today.com/health/pea-protein-it-new-soy-t10501.

www.doctoroz.com/article/wheat-belly-author-william-davis-md-answers-faq ?page=1.

Hidden Factor #3: Fear of Eating Fat

American Chemical Society National Meeting News. "CLA Could Help Control Weight, Fat, Diabetes, and Muscle Loss," August 20, 2000.

Belury, M. A. "Role of Conjugated Linoleic Acid (CLA) in the Management of Type 2 Diabetes: Evidence from Zucker Diabetic Rats and Human Subjects." Presented at the American Chemical Society National Meeting, August 21, 2000.

Belury, M. A., and Vanden Heuvel, J. P. "Protection Against Cancer and Heart Disease by the Dietary Fatty Acid, Conjugated Linoleic Acid: Potential Mechanisms of Action." *Nutr Dis Update J* 1:2(1997):53–58.

Blankson, H., et al. "Conjugated Linoleic Acid Reduces Body Fat Mass in Overweight and Obese Humans." *J Nutr* 130:12(2000):2943–2948.

Clement, I. P., and Scimeca, J. A. "Conjugated Linoleic Acid and Linoleic Acid Are Distinctive Modulators of Mammary Carcinogenesis." *Nutr Cancer* 27:2(1997): 131–135.

Clement, I. P., et al. "Mammary Cancer Prevention by Conjugated Dienoic Derivative of Linoleic Acid." *Cancer Res* 51(1991):6118–6124.

Cunnane, S. C., et al. "n-3 Essential Fatty Acids Decrease Weight Gain in Genetically Obese Mice." *Br J Nutr* 56(1986):87–95.

Erling, T. "A Pilot Study with the Aim of Studying the Efficacy and Tolerability of Tonalin CLA on the Body Composition in Humans." Lillestrom, Norway: Medstat Research, Ltd., 1997.

Gittleman, A. L. *Eat Fat, Lose Weight.* Blue Hills Publishing, Kindle Edition, 2015.

Horrocks, L., and Yeo, Y. "Health Benefits of Docosahexaenoic Acid (DHA)." *Pharm Res* 40:3(1999):211–225.

Hudson, T. "The Good Fat for Women." *Health Products Bus* 29(October 2000):25–26.

Kirtland, S. J. "Prostaglandin E1: A Review." *Prostaglandins Leukotrienes Essential Fatty Acids* 32(1988):165–174.

Lands, W. E. "Biochemistry and Physiology of n-3 Fatty Acids." *FASEB J* 6(1992): 2530–2536.

Okuyama, H. "Dietary Fatty Acids: The N-6/N-3 Balance and Chronic Elderly Diseases: Excess Linoleic Acid (N-6) and Relative N-3 Deficiency Syndrome Seen in Japan." *Progr Lipid Res* 35:4(1997):409–457.

Pariza, M. W. "The Biological Activities of Conjugated Linoleic Acid." *Adv Conj Linoleic Acid Res* 1(1999):12–20.

Pariza, M. W. "Conjugated Linoleic Acid: A Newly Recognized Nutrient." *Chemistry and Industry* (June 16, 1997):464–466.

Pariza, M. W., Park, Y., and Cook, M. E. "Conjugated Linoleic Acid and the Control of Cancer and Obesity." *Toxicol Sci* 52(Suppl, 1999):107–110.

Park, Y., and Cook, M. E. "Mechanisms of Action of Conjugated Linoleic Acid: Evidence and Speculation." *Proc Soc Exp Biol Med* 233(2000):8–13.

Robinson, J. *Why Grassfed Is Best!* Vashon, WA: Island Press, 2000.

Siguel, E. N., and Lerman, R. H. "Prevalence of Essential Fatty Acid Deficiency in Patients with Chronic Gastrointestinal Disorders." *Metabolism* 45(1996):12–23.

Simopoulos, A. "Omega-3 Fatty Acids in Health and Disease and in Growth and Development." *Am J Clin Nutr* 54(1991):438–463.

Simopoulos, A. P. "Essential Fatty Acids in Health and Chronic Disease." *Am J Clin Nutr* 70(Suppl, 1999):560S–569S.

Simopoulos, A. P., and Robinson, J. *The Omega Diet.* New York: HarperCollins, 1998.

Storlien, L. H. "Not All Dietary Fats May Lead to Obesity." *Am J Clin Nutr* 51(1990): 1114.

Watkins, B. A., and Seifert, M. F. "Conjugated Linoleic Acid and Bone Biology." *J Am Coll Nutr* 19:4(2000):478–486.

Yeonhwa, P., et al. "Effect of Conjugated Linoleic Acid on Body Composition in Mice." *Lipids* 32:8(1997):853–858.

http://articles.mercola.com/sites/articles/archive/2002/08/14/con-ola1.aspx.

http://articles.mercola.com/sites/articles/archive/2014/04/16/saturated-fat-heart-health.aspx.

http://articles.mercola.com/sites/articles/archive/2011/07/18/why-do-exvegetarians-outnumber-current-vegetarians-three-to-one.aspx.

www.ncbi.nlm.nih.gov/pmc/articles/PMC3820047/.

www.wheatbellyblog.com/about/.

www.rice.edu/~jenky/sports/antiox.html.

www.uccs.edu/Documents/healthcircle/pnc/health-topics/Omega-3_6_and_9_Fats
.pdf.

www.doctoroz.com/article/wheat-belly-author-william-davis-md-answers-faq
?page=1.

Hidden Factor #4: Insulin Resistance and Inflammation

Anderson, R. A., et al. "Elevated Intakes of Supplemental Chromium Improve Glucose
and Insulin Variables in Individuals with Type II Diabetes." *Diabetes* 46(1997):
1786–1791.

Atkins, R. C., and Buff, S. *Dr. Atkins' Age-Defying Diet Revolution.* New York: St.
Martin's Press, 2000.

Borkman, M., et al. "The Relation Between Insulin Sensitivity and the Fatty-Acid
Composition of Skeletal-Muscle Phospholipids." *N Engl J Med* 328:4(1993):238–244.

Brand-Miller, J., et al. *The Glucose Revolution.* New York: Marlowe and Company,
1999.

Cefalu, W. T., et al. "The Effect of Chromium Supplementation on Carbohydrate
Metabolism and Body Fat Distribution." *Diabetes* 46(Suppl, 1997):55A.

Challem, J., et al. *Syndrome X: The Complete Nutritional Program to Prevent and
Reverse Insulin Resistance.* New York: Wiley, 2001.

Clarke, S. D., et al. "Fatty Acid Regulation of Gene Expression: Its Role in Fuel
Partitioning and Insulin Resistance." *Ann NY Acad Sci* 827(1997): 178–187.

Clarksen, P. M. "Nutritional Ergogenic Aids: Chromium, Exercise, and Muscle Mass."
Int J Sport Nutr 1(1991):289–293.

Collier, G. R., et al. "The Acute Effect of Fat on Insulin Secretion." *J Clin Endocrinol
Metab* 66(1988):323–326.

Evans, G. W. "Chromium: Insulin Cohort." *Total Health* (August 1994):42–43.

Evans, G. W. *Chromium Picolinate.* Garden City, NY: Avery, 1996.

Fanaian, M., et al. "The Effect of Modified Fat Diet on Insulin Resistance and Metabolic
Parameters in Type II Diabetes." Diabetologia 89(1996):A7.

Gittleman, A. L. *Eat Fat, Lose Weight.* Blue Hills Publishing, Kindle Edition, 2015.

Gittleman, A. L. *The 40/30/30 Phenomenon.* New Canaan, CT: Keats Publishing, 1997.

Gittleman, A. L. *Your Body Knows Best.* New York: Pocket Books, 1997.

Grant, P. "Does Bread Make You Fat?" *McCall's* (October 2000):100–103.

Holt, S. H., Brand-Miller, J. C., and Petocz, P. "Interrelationships Among Postprandial
Satiety, Glucose and Insulin Responses and Changes in Subsequent Food Intake."
Eur J Clin Nutr 50(December 1996):788–797.

Holt, S. H., Brand-Miller, J. C., Petocz, P., and Farmakalidis, E. "A Satiety Index of
Common Foods." *Eur J Clin Nutr* 49(September 1995):675–690.

Kozlovsky, A. S., et al. "Effects of Diets High in Simple Sugars on Urinary Chromium
Losses." *Metabolism* 35(1986):515–518.

Lee, B. M., and Wolever, T. M. S. "Effect of Glucose, Sucrose, and Fructose on Plasma
Glucose and Insulin Responses in Normal Humans: Comparison with White
Bread." *Eur J Clin Nutr* 52(1998):924–928.

Levi, B., and Werman, M. G. "Long-Term Fructose Consumption Accelerates
Glycation and Several Age-Related Variables in Male Rats." *J Nutr* 128:1(1998):
1442–1449.

McCarty, M. F. "The Case for Supplemental Chromium and a Survey of Clinical Studies
with Chromium Picolinate." *J Appl Nutr* 43(1991):58–66.

Opara, J. U., and Levine, J. H. "The Deadly Quartet: The Insulin Resistance Syndrome." *South Med J* 90(1997):1162–1168.

Perlmutter, David. *Brain Maker*. Boston: Little, Brown and Company, 2015.

Provonsha, S. "A Hypothesis Regarding Meat and the Insulin-Resistant State Known as Syndrome X." *Veget Nutr* 2:3(1988):119–126.

Reaven, G. M. "Hypothesis: Muscle Insulin Resistance Is the (Not So) Thrifty Genotype." *Diabetologia* 41(1998):482–484.

Reaven, G. M. "Insulin Resistance, the Key to Survival: A Rose by Any Other Name." *Diabetologia* 42(1988):384–385.

Reaven, G. M. "Pathophysiology of Insulin Resistance in Human Disease." *Physiol Rev* 75(1995):473–485.

Reaven, G. M. "Role of Insulin Resistance in Human Disease." *Diabetes* 37(1988): 1595–1607.

Rothwell, N .J., and Stock, M. J. "Insulin and Thermogenesis." *Int J Obesity* 12(1988): 93–102.

Schwarz, J. M., et al. "Thermogenesis in Obese Women: Effect of Fructose vs. Glucose Added to a Meal." *Am J Physiol* 262:4 (pt 1, 1992):E394–E401.

Spieth, L. E., et al. "A Low-Glycemic Index Diet in the Treatment of Pediatric Obesity." *Arch Pediatr Adolesc Med* 154:9(2000):947–951.

Storlien, L. H., et al. "The Type of Dietary Fat Has a Profound Influence on Development of Insulin Resistance in Rats." *Diabetes Res Clin Pract* 5(Suppl 1, 1988):S267.

Torjesen, P. A., et al. "Lifestyle Changes May Reverse Development of the Insulin Resistance Syndrome." *Diabetes Care* 30(1997):26–31.

Trent, L. K., et al. "Effects of Chromium Picolinate on Body Composition." *J Sports Med Phys Fitness* 35(1995):273–280.

Van Gaal, L., et al. "Carbohydrate-Induced Thermogenesis in Obese Women: Effect of Insulin and Catecholamines." *J Endocrinol Invest* 22:2(1999):109–114.

Williams, K. V., and Korytkowski, M. T. "Syndrome X: Pathogenesis, Clinical and Therapeutic Aspects." *Diabetes Nutr Metabol* 11(1998):140–152.

https://med.virginia.edu/ginutrition/wp-content/uploads/sites/199/2014/06/Parrish -June-15-2.pdf.

www.foodnavigator-usa.com/R-D/Americans-are-eating-10g-less-fat-per-day-than -they-did-in-the-late-1970s.

Hidden Factor #5: Stress as a Fat Maker

Bjorntorp, P. "Visceral Obesity: A Civil Syndrome." *Obesity Res* 1(1993):206–222.

Blackman, M. R. "Age-Related Alterations in Sleep Quality and Neuroendocrine Function: Interrelationships and Implications." *JAMA* 284:7(2000):861–868.

Browder, S. E. "Stress Busters That Can Save Your Life." *New Choices* (November 2000):41–44.

Epel, E. S., et al. "Stress and Body Shape: Stress-Induced Cortisol Secretion Is Consistently Greater Among Women with Central Fat." *Psychosom Med* 62:5(2000):623–632.

Epel, E. S., et al. "Stress-Induced Cortisol, Mood, and Fat Distribution in Men." *Obesity Res* 7:1(1999):9–15.

Epel, E. S., et al. "Stress May Add Bite to Appetite in Women: A Laboratory Study of Stress-Induced Cortisol and Eating Behavior." *Psychoneuroendocrinology* 26:1(2001):37–49.

Gaynor, M. L., and Hickey, J. *Dr. Gaynor's Cancer Prevention Program*. New York: Kensington Books, 1999.

Gittleman, A. L. *Eat Fat, Lose Weight*. Blue Hills Publishing, Kindle Edition, 2015.

Gray-Foltz, D. "The Relaxing Way to Lose Weight," *Health* (2001):90–95.

"Less Fun, Less Sleep, More Work: An American Portrait," National Sleep Foundation Poll, March 27, 2001.

Peeke, P. *Fight Fat After Forty*. New York: Penguin, 2000.

Peeke, P., and Chrousos, G. P. "Hypercortisolism and Obesity." *Ann NY Acad Sci* 77(1995):665–676.

Van Cauter, E., Leproult, R., and Plat, L. "Age-Related Changes in Slow Wave Sleep and REM Sleep and Relationship with Growth Hormone and Cortisol Levels in Healthy Men." *JAMA* 284:7(2000):879–881.

Wiley, T. S, and Formby, B. *Lights Out: Sleep, Sugar and Survival*. New York: Pocket Books, 2001.

Yudkin, J. *Sweet and Dangerous*. New York: Wyden Books, 1972.

http://articles.mercola.com/sites/articles/archive/2014/07/05/stress-effects.aspx.

http://brainconnection.brainhq.com/2003/03/12/why-zebras-dont-get-ulcers/.

http://news.stanford.edu/news/2007/march7/sapolskysr-030707.html.

https://sleepfoundation.org/media-center/press-release/lack-sleep-affecting -americans-finds-the-national-sleep-foundation.

www.nytimes.com/2016/05/01/realestate/arianna-huffingtons-sleep-revolution-starts -at-home.html.

www.apa.org/helpcenter/stress-body.aspx

www.apa.org/news/press/releases/stress/2014/stress-report.pdf.

CHAPTER 3 TOP 10 HIDDEN WEIGHT GAIN FACTORS #6 THROUGH #10

Hidden Factor # 6: Messy Microbiome

Gittleman, A. L. *The Gut Flush Plan*. New York: Avery, 2009.

Perlmutter, David. *Brain Maker*. Boston: Little, Brown and Company, 2015.

Vance, Sara. *The Perfect Metabolism Plan*. Newburyport, MA: Conari Press, 2015.

Hidden Factor #7: Poor Quality Bile

Gittleman, A. L. *Eat Fat, Lose Weight*. Blue Hills Publishing, Kindle Edition, 2015.

"The New Thyroid Cure." *First for Women* (May 16, 2016).

Ockenga, J., et al. "Plasma Bile Acids Are Associated with Energy Expenditure and Thyroid Function in Humans." *J Clin Endocrinol Metab* 97:2(2012):535–542.

Watanabe, M., et al. "Bile Acids Induce Energy Expenditure by Promoting Intracellular Thyroid Hormone Activation." *Nature* 439:(January 2006).

www.ncbi.nlm.nih.gov/pubmed/12487769.

www.ncbi.nlm.nih.gov/pubmed/12660641.

www.britannica.com/science/bile.

Hidden Factor #8: Tuckered-Out Thyroid

Gittleman, A. L. *Before the Change*. New York: HarperOne, 2003.

Gittleman, A. L. *Eat Fat, Lose Weight*. Blue Hills Publishing, Kindle Edition, 2015.

www.livestrong.com/article/328551-nori-nutrition-information/.
http://health.howstuffworks.com/human-body/systems/endocrine/why-thyroid
    -important.htm.
www.webmd.com/digestive-disorders/picture-of-the-gallbladder.

Hidden Factor #9: Hidden Hitchhikers—Parasites

Gittleman, A. L. *Guess What Came to Dinner?* New York: Avery, 2001.
Gittleman, A. L. *The Gut Flush Plan.* New York: Avery, 2009.
https://ods.od.nih.gov/factsheets/VitaminA-HealthProfessional/#h3.
www.foxnews.com/leisure/2015/04/15/americans-spend-more-on-dining-out-than
    -groceries-for-first-time-ever/.
www.nytimes.com/2016/01/18/us/obama-flint-michigan-water-fema-emergency
    -disaster.html?_r=0.

Hidden Factor #10: Missing Magnesium

Gittleman, A. L. *Before the Change.* New York: HarperOne, 2003.
www.psychologytoday.com/blog/evolutionary-psychiatry/201106/magnesium-and
    -the-brain-the-original-chill-pill.
www.westonaprice.org/health-topics/abcs-of-nutrition/magnificent-magnesium/
    #sthash.a2sdR0tq.dpuf.

CHAPTER 6 PHASE 1: THE TWO-WEEK FAT FLUSH

www.shape.com/lifestyle/mind-and-body/when-your-weight-fluctuates-whats
    -normal-and-whats-not.

CHAPTER 9 THE POWER OF RITUAL

Exercise

Alessio, H. M., et al. "Lipid Peroxidation and Scavenger Enzymes During Exercise:
    Adaptive Response to Training." *J Appl Physiol* 64:4(1988): 1333–1336.
Coates, G., O'Brodovich, H., and Goeree, G. "Hindlimb and Lung Lymph Flows During
    Prolonged Exercise." *J Appl Physiol* 75:2(1993):633–638.
Cooper, K. H. *The Antioxidant Revolution.* Nashville, TN: Thomas Nelson, 1994.
DeSouza, C. A. "Regular Aerobic Exercise Prevents and Restores Age-Related Declines
    in Endothelium-Dependent Vasodilation in Healthy Men." *Circulation*
    102:12(2000):1351–1357.
Fogelholm, M., et al. "Effects of Walking Training on Weight Maintenance After a Very
    Low-Energy Diet in Premenopausal Obese Women: A Randomized, Controlled
    Trial." *Arch Intern Med* 60:14(2000):2177–2184.
Gittleman, A. L. *The Fat Flush Fitness Plan.* New York: McGraw-Hill, 2003.
Gittleman, A. L. *Super Nutrition for Menopause.* Garden City, NY: Avery, 1998.
King, N. A., Tremblay, A., and Blundell, J. E. "Effects of Exercise on Appetite Control:
    Implications for Energy Balance." *Med Sci Sports Exerc* 29:8(1997):1076–1089.
Layne, J. E., and Nelson, M. E. "The Effects of Progressive Resistance Training on Bone
    Density: A Review." *Med Sci Sports Exerc* 31:1(1999):25–30.
Lemole, G. M. *The Healing Diet.* New York: William Morrow, 2001.

Murakami, M., et al. "Effects of Epinephrine and Lactate on the Increase in Oxygen Consumption of Nonexercising Skeletal Muscle After Aerobic Exercise." *J Biomed Opt* 5:4(2000):406–410.

Nelson, M. E., et al. "Analysis of Body-Composition Techniques and Models for Detecting Change in Soft Tissue with Strength Training." *Am J Clin Nutr* 63:5(1996):678–686.

Nelson, M. E., et al. "Effects of High-Intensity Strength Training on Multiple Risk Factors for Osteoporotic Fractures: A Randomized, Controlled Trial." *JAMA* 272(1994):1909–1914.

Nelson, M. E., et al. "Hormone and Bone Mineral Status in Endurance-Trained and Sedentary Postmenopausal Women." *J Clin Endocrinol Metab* 66:5(1988):927–933.

Thomas, E. L., et al. "Preferential Loss of Visceral Fat Following Aerobic Exercise, Measured by Magnetic Resonance Imaging." *Lipids* 35:7(2000): 769–776.

Van Aggel-Leijssen, D. P., Saris, W. H., Hul, G. B., and van Baak, M. A. "Short-Term Effects of Weight Loss with or without Low-Intensity Exercise Training on Fat Metabolism in Obese Men." *Am J Clin Nutr* 73:3(2001):523–531.

http://breakingmuscle.com/strength-conditioning/how-to-choose-the-proper-work-and-rest-periods-when-interval-training.

http://dailyburn.com/life/fitness/liss-cardio-low-intensity-workouts/.

http://greatist.com/fitness/complete-guide-interval-training-infographic.

www.mayoclinic.org/healthy-lifestyle/stress-management/in-depth/exercise-and-stress/art-20044469.

www.health.harvard.edu/staying-healthy/exercising-to-relax.

www.prevention.com/fitness/fitness-tips/high-intensity-interval-training-how-long-should-your-workout-be.

www.adaa.org/understanding-anxiety/related-illnesses/other-related-conditions/stress/physical-activity-reduces-st.

www.nytimes.com/well/guides/really-really-short-workouts.

www.bodybuilding.com/fun/wotw40.htm.

www.vitalchoice.com/shop/pc/articlesView.asp?id=2357.

Sleep

Redwine, L., et al. "Effects of Sleep and Sleep Deprivation on Interleukin-6, Growth Hormone, Cortisol, and Melatonin Levels in Humans." *J Clin Endocrinol Metab* 85:10(2000):3597–3603.

Van Cauter, E., Leproult, R., and Plat, L. "Age-Related Changes in Slow Wave Sleep and REM Sleep and Relationship with Growth Hormone and Cortisol Levels in Healthy Men." *JAMA* 284:7(2000):879–881.

Walsleben, J. A. "Does Being Female Affect One's Sleep?" *J Women's Health Gender-Based Med* 8:5(1999):571–572.

www.sleepfoundation.org.

http://ariannahuffington.com/wp-content/uploads/2016/04/Ariannas-12-Tips-for-Better-Sleep.pdf.

www.vogue.com/13423144/arianna-huffington-the-sleep-revolution-new-book-interview/.

www.nytimes.com/2016/05/01/realestate/arianna-huffingtons-sleep-revolution-starts-at-home.html?_r=0.

www.gallup.com/poll/166553/less-recommended-amount-sleep.aspx.

Journaling

McGee-Cooper, A. "Shifting from High Stress to High Energy." *Imprint* 40:4(1993):69–71.
McGee-Cooper, A. "Time Management: Cashing in on Both Brains." *AORN J* 44:2(1986):178–183.
Pennebaker, J. W., and Seagal, J. D. "Forming a Story: The Health Benefits of Narrative." *J Clin Psychol* 55:10(1999):1243–1254.

Therapeutic Baths

Gittleman, A. L. *Fat Flush for Life*. Boston: Da Capo Lifelong Books, 2011.
http://articles.mercola.com/herbal-oils/juniper-berry-oil.aspx.
http://articles.mercola.com/herbal-oils/lavender-oil.aspx.
http://articles.mercola.com/herbal-oils/lemon-oil.aspx.
http://articles.mercola.com/herbal-oils/rose-absolute-oil.aspx.
http://articles.mercola.com/herbal-oils/rosemary-oil.aspx.
http://articles.mercola.com/herbal-oils/sweet-marjoram-oil.aspx.
http://articles.mercola.com/herbal-oils/thyme-oil.aspx.
http://health.howstuffworks.com/skin-care/problems/treating/epsom-salt-baths4 .htm.
www.webmd.com/a-to-z-guides/epsom-salt-bath.

CHAPTER 10 THE FAT FLUSH PLAN AWAY FROM HOME

Mokdad, A. H., et al. "The Spread of the Obesity Epidemic in the United States, 1991–1998." *JAMA* 282(1999):1519–1522.
Must, A., et al. "The Disease Burden Associated with Overweight and Obesity." *JAMA* 282(1999):1523–1529.
"Now What? U.S. Study Says Margarine May Be Harmful." *New York Times* (October 1997).
"Update: Prevalence of Overweight Among Children, Adolescents, and Adults—United States, 1988–1994." *MMWR* 46(1997):199–202.

Fast-Food Marketing Stats

www.fastfoodmarketing.org/media/FastFoodFACTS_Report_Summary.pdf.

Consumption of Fast Food Stats

www.cdc.gov/nchs/data/databriefs/db213.htm.
www.gallup.com/poll/163868/fast-food-major-part-diet.aspx.
www.newsweek.com/fast-food-obesity-americans-national-center-health-statistics -373091.
www.latimes.com/science/la-sci-sn-fast-food-calories-kids-20150915-story.html.

CHAPTER 11 THE FAT FLUSH MASTER SHOPPING LIST

Flax Seed

www.bonappetit.com/test-kitchen/ingredients/article/how-to-eat-flaxseed.
www.berkeleywellness.com/healthy-eating/food/article/how-choose-and-use-flaxseed.
www.spectrumorganics.com.

Chia

www.spectrumorganics.com.

Hemp Seed

http://nutiva.com/company/certifications/.

CHAPTER 13 FAT FLUSH RECIPES

Finn, S. C. "Nutrition Communique: Helping Women Find Everyday Solutions." *J Women's Health Gender-Based Med* 9:9(2000):951–954.

U.S. Department of Agriculture, Agricultural Research Service. "Food and Nutrient Intakes by Individuals in the United States, by Sex and Age, 1994–1996." *Nationwide Food Surveys* (1998).

CHAPTER 14 BECAUSE YOU ASKED

Abraham, G. E. "The Calcium Controversy." *J Appl Nutr* 34(1982):69.

Abraham, G. E. "Nutritional Factors in the Etiology of the Premenstrual Tension Syndromes." J Reprod Med 28:7(1983):446–464.

Abraham, G. E., and Grewal, H. "A Total Dietary Program Emphasizing Magnesium Instead of Calcium: Effect on the Mineral Density of Calcaneous Bone in Postmenopausal Women on Hormonal Therapy." *J Repr Med* 35(1990):503.

Agostoni, C., et al. "Docosahexaenoic Acid Status and Developmental Quotient of Healthy Term Infants." *Lancet* 346(1995):638.

Aldercreitz, A. L., et al. "Dietary Phytoestrogen and the Menopause in Japan." *Lancet* 339(1992):1233.

Anderson, G. J., Connor, W. E., and Corliss, J. D. "Docosahexaenoic Acid Is the Preferred Dietary n-3 Fatty Acid for the Development of the Brain and Retina." *Pediatr Res* 27(1990):89–97.

Barber, M. D., et al. "The Effect of an Oral Nutritional Supplement Enriched with Fish Oil on Weight Loss in Patients with Pancreatic Cancer." *Br J Cancer* 81:1(1999):80–86.

Bariscoe, A. M., and Ragen, C. "Relation of Magnesium and Calcium Metabolism in Man." *Am J Clin Nutr* 19(1966):296.

Berth-Jones, J., and Graham-Brown, R. A. "Placebo-Controlled Trial of Essential Fatty Acid Supplementation in Atopic Dermatitis." *Lancet* 341(1993):1557–1560.

Berth-Jones, J., et al. "Evening Primrose Oil and Atopic Eczema." *Lancet* 345(1995):520.

Bhatty, R. S. "Nutrient Composition of Whole Flax Seed and Flax Seed Meal." In Cunnane S. C., and Thompson, L. U. (eds.), *Flaxseed in Human Nutrition*. Chicago: AOCS Press, 1995, pp. 22–42.

Blaylock, R. *Excitotoxins: The Taste That Kills*. Santa Fe, NM: Health Press, 1997.

Booth, S. "Flaxseed Improves Blood Glucose Levels." *J Hum Nutr Diet* 13(2000): 363–371.

Bordoni, A., et al. "Evening Primrose Oil in the Treatment of Children with Atopic Eczema." *Drugs Exp Clin Res* 14:4(1988):291–297.

Burgess, J. R., et al. "Long-Chain Polyunsaturated Fatty Acids in Children with Attention Deficit Hyperactivity Disorder." *Am J Clin Nutr* 71(2000): 327S–330S.

Butchko, H., and Kotsonis, F. "Postmarketing Surveillance in the Food Industry: The Aspartame Case Study." *Nutr Toxicol* (1994):235–249.

Callender, K., et al. "A Double-Blind Trial of Evening Primrose Oil in the Premenstrual Syndrome." *Hum Psychopharmacol* 3(1988):57–61.

Cameron, A. T. "Iodine Prophylaxis and Endemic Goiter." *Can J Public Health* 21(1930):541–548.

Carter, J. F. "Sensory Evaluation of Flaxseed of Different Varieties." *Proc Flax Inst* 56(1996):201–203.

Cassidy, A. "Biological Effects of Plant Estrogens in Premenopausal Women." (Abstract A866) *Am Soc Exp Biol* (1993).

Cave, W. T., Jr. "Dietary Omega-3 Polyunsaturated Fats and Breast Cancer." *Nutrition* 12(Suppl, 1996):S39–S42.

Cherken, L. C. "Health Alert: Herbs and Drugs That Don't Mix." *Family Circle* (September 12, 2000).

Choi, D. E. "Glutamate Neurotoxicity and Diseases of the Nervous System." *Neuron* 1(1988):623–634.

Colquhoun, I., and Bunday, S. "A Lack of Essential Fatty Acids as a Possible Cause of Hyperactivity in Children." *Med Hypoth* 7(1981):673–679.

Connor, W. E. "Diabetes, Fish Oil, and Vascular Disease." *Ann Intern Med* 123:12(1995):950–952.

Connor, W. E. "Importance of n-3 Fatty Acids in Health and Disease." *Am J Clin Nutr* 71(Suppl, 2000):171S–175S.

Connor, W. E., Lowensohn, R., and Hatcher, L. "Increased Docosahexaenoic Acid Levels in Human Newborn Infants by Administration of Sardines and Fish Oil During Pregnancy." *Lipids* 31(Suppl, 1996):S183–S187.

Coulombe, R. A., and Sharma, R. P. "Neurobiochemical Alterations Induced by the Artificial Sweetener Aspartame." *Toxicol Appl Pharmacol* 83(1986):79–85.

Dalderup, L. M. "The Role of Magnesium in Osteoporosis and Idiopathic Hypercalcaemia." *Voeding* 21(1960):424.

Davoli, E., et al. "Serum Methanol Concentrations in Rats and in Men after a Single Dose of Aspartame." *Food Chem Toxicol* 24:3 (1986):187–189.

Edwards, R., et al. "Omega-3 Polyunsaturated Fatty Acid Levels in the Diet and in Red Blood Cell Membranes of Depressed Patients." *J Affect Disord* 48(1998):149–155.

Flaten, H. "Fish-Oil Concentrate: Effects of Variables Related to Cardiovascular Disease." *Am J Clin Nutr* 52(1990):300–306.

Fotsis, T., et al. "Genistein, a Dietary Ingested Isoflavonoid, Inhibits Cell Proliferation and In Vitro Angiogenesis." *J Nutr* 125:3(Suppl, 1995): 790S–797S.

Frahm, D. "For Stool Observation." *Health Quarterly* (Winter 1997):2–4.

Frank, B., et al. "A Prospective Study of Egg Consumption and Risk of Cardiovascular Disease in Men and Women." *JAMA* 281(1999):1387.

Gittleman, A. L. *Guess What Came to Dinner?* New York: Avery, 2000.

Gittleman, A. L. *Why Am I Always So Tired?* New York: HarperSan Francisco, 1999.

Goh, Y. K., et al. "Effect of Omega-3 Fatty Acid on Plasma Lipids, Cholesterol, and Lipoprotein Fatty Acid Content in NIDDM Patients." *Diabetologia* 40(1997): 45–52.

Goss, P. E, et al. *Effects of Dietary Flaxseed in Women with Cyclical Mastalgia.* Toronto: University Health Network/Princess Margaret Hospital, University of Toronto, 2000.

Harris, W. S. "n-3 Fatty Acids and Serum Lipoproteins: Human Studies." *Am J Clin Nutr* 65(Suppl, 1997):1645S–1654S.

Hederos, C. A., et al. "Epogam Evening Primrose Oil Treatment in Atopic Dermatitis and Asthma." *Arch Dis Child* 75:6(1996):494–497.

Heroux, O., Peter, D., and Heggteveit, H. A. "Long-Term Effect of Suboptimal Dietary Magnesium." *J Nutr* 107(1977):1640.

Hibbelin, J. R. "Fish Consumption and Major Depression (Letter)." *Lancet* 351(1998): 1213.

Hibbelin, J. R., and Salem, N. "Dietary Polyunsaturated Fatty Acids and Depression: When Cholesterol Does Not Satisfy." *Am J Clin Nutr* 62(1995):1–9.

Holt, S. "Phytoestrogens for a Healthier Menopause." *Altern Complement Ther* 3:3(1997):187–193.

Horrobin, D. F. "The Effects of Gamma Linolenic Acid on Breast Pain and Diabetic Neuropathy: Possible Non-Eicosanoid Mechanisms." *Prostaglandins Leukotrienes Essential Fatty Acids* 48(1993):101–104.

Horrobin, D. F. "Gamma Linolenic Acid." *Rev Contem Pharmacol* 1(1990):1–45.

Hu, F. B. "A Prospective Study of Egg Consumption and Risk of Cardiovascular Disease in Men and Women." *JAMA* 281:15(1999):1387–1394.

Kahoo, S. K., et al. "Evening Primrose Oil and Treatment of Premenstrual Syndrome." *Med J Aust* 153(1990):192–198.

Knight, D. C., and Eden, J. A. "A Review of the Clinical Effects of Phytoestrogens." *Obstet Gynecol* 87(1996):897–904.

Kremer, J. M. "n-3 Fatty Acid Supplements in Rheumatoid Arthritis." *Am J Clin Nutr* 71(Suppl, 2000):349S–351S.

Kremer, J. M., et al. "Fish-Oil Fatty Acid Supplementation in Active Rheumatoid Arthritis: A Double-Blinded, Controlled, Crossover Study." *Ann Intern Med* 106(1987):497–503.

Levanthal, L. J., et al. "Treatment of Rheumatoid Arthritis with Gamma-Linolenic Acid." *Ann Intern Med* 1:9(1993):867–873.

Luo, J., et al. "Moderate Intake of n-3 Fatty Acids for 2 Months Has No Detrimental Effect on Glucose Metabolism and Could Ameliorate the Lipid Profile in Type 2 Diabetic Men." *Diabetes Care* 21(1998):717–724.

"Magnesium Deficiency in Alcoholism: Possible Contribution to Osteoporosis and Cardiovascular Disease in Alcoholics." *Alcoholism Clin Exp Res* 18:5(1994): 1076–1082.

Makrides, M., Neumann, M. A., and Gibson, R. A. "Is Dietary Docosahexaenoic Acid Essential for Term Infants?" *Lipids* 31(1996):115–119.

McManus, R. M., et al. "A Comparison of the Effects of n-3 Fatty Acids from Linseed Oil and Fish Oil in Well-Controlled Type II Diabetes." *Diabetes Care* 19(1996): 463–467.

Medalle, R., Waterhouse, C., and Hahn, T. J. "Vitamin D Resistance in Magnesium Deficiency." *Am J Clin Nutr* 29(1976):858.

Melis, M. S. "Stevia Dilates Vessels, Causing Lowered Blood Pressure and Increased Urine Flow When Given Over Long Periods." *J Ethnopharmacol* 47:3(1995):129–134.

Mitchell, E., et al. "Clinical Characteristics and Serum Essential Fatty Acid Levels in Hyperactive Children." *Clin Pediatr* 26(1987):406–411.

Mitchell, M. L., and O'Rourke, M. E. "Response of the Thyroid Gland to Thiocyanate and Thyrotropin." *J Clin Endocrinol* 20(1960):47–56.

Morton, M. S. "Determination of Lignans and Isoflavones in Human Female Plasma Following Dietary Supplementation." *J Endocrinol* 142(1994): 251–259.

Moser, R. H. "Aspartame and Memory Loss." *JAMA* 272:19(1994):1543.

Olney, J. W. "Brain Lesions, Obesity, and Other Disturbances in Mice Treated with Monosodium Glutamate." *Science* 165(1969):719–721.

Olney, J. W. "Excitoxins and Neurological Diseases." In *Proceedings of the International College of Neuropathologists*, Kyoto, Japan, 1990.

Oomah, B. D., Mazza, G., and Kenaschuk, E. O. "Cyanogenic Compounds in Flaxseed." *J Agri Food Chem* 40(1992):1346–1348.

Reisbick, S., et al. "Home Cage Behavior of Rhesus Monkeys with Long-Term Deficiency of Omega-3 Fatty Acids." *Physiol Behav* 55(1994):231–239.

Roberts, H. J. "Reactions Attributed to Aspartame-Containing Products: 551 Cases." *J Appl Nutr* 40(1988):85–94.

Salachas, A., et al. "Effects of Low-Dose Fish Oil Concentrate on Angina, Exercise Tolerance Time, Serum Triglycerides, and Platelet Function." *Angiology* 45(1994):1023–1031.

Sojka, J. E., and Weaver, C. M. "Magnesium Supplementation and Osteoporosis." *Nutr Rev* 53(1995):71.

Stellman, F., and Garfinkel, L. "A Short Report: Artificial Sweetener Use and Weight Changes in Women." *Prevent Med* 15(1986):195–202.

Stevens, L. J., et al. "Essential Fatty Acid Metabolism in Boys with Attention-Deficit Hyperactivity Disorder." *Am J Clin Nutr* 62:4(1995):761–768.

Stevens, L. J., et al. "Omega-3 Fatty Acids in Boys with Behavior, Learning, and Health Problems." *Physiol Behav* 59:4–5(1996):915–920.

Tate, G., et al. "Suppression of Acute and Chronic Inflammation by Dietary Gamma Linolenic Acid." *J Rheumatol* 16(1989):729–734.

Tham, D. M. "Clinical Review 97: Potential Health Benefits of Dietary Phytoestrogens: A Review of the Clinical, Epidemiological, and Mechanistic Evidence." *J Clin Endocrinol Metabol* 83(1998):2223–2235.

Toft, I., et al. "Effects of n-3 Polyunsaturated Fatty Acids on Glucose Homeostasis and Blood Pressure in Essential Hypertension." *Ann Intern Med* 123:12(1995):911–918.

"Turn Back the Clock with Nature's Fountain of Youth," *Health Sci Inst* 5:6(2000):1–5.

Uauy-Dagach, R., and Valenzuela, A. "Marine Oils: The Health Benefits of n-3 Fatty Acids." *Nutr Rev* 54(1996):S102–S108.

Von Schacky, C., et al. "The Effect of Dietary Omega-3 Fatty Acids on Coronary Atherosclerosis." *Ann Intern Med* 130(1999):554–562.

Index

About the Author

Ann Louise Gittleman, PhD, CNS, is undisputedly the First Lady of Nutrition. As a nutritional visionary and health pioneer, she has fearlessly stood on the front lines of diet and detox, the environment, and women's health. *Self* magazine describes her as one of the Top Ten Notable Nutritionists in the United States, and thousands of nutritionists, health coaches, and practitioners have benefited from her work.

Years before the Paleo, ketogenic, and vegan diet trends, in her first book, *Beyond Pritikin* (1988), Ann Louise was the very first to proclaim that obesity and diabetes were caused by a lack of the right type of fat and an excess of the wrong kind of carbohydrates, including gluten-rich grain. She was also the first nutritionist to write about the perils of gluten and discuss the blood-type theory in 1996, boldly stating, in her book *Your Body Knows Best*, that one diet may not be right for everyone.

She has also been a tireless crusader for women by offering natural solutions to menopause and perimenopausal symptoms, decades before anybody else, in her award-winning *Super Nutrition for Women*, as well as *Super Nutrition for Menopause* and her *New York Times* bestseller *Before the Change*.

She then revolutionized dieting in the first edition of *The Fat Flush Plan*—an international bestseller—by proclaiming that the liver was the body's primary fat-burning organ (and detoxifier).

Most recently, she led the charge against the hidden hazards of cell phones, iPads, smart meters, and WiFi in her groundbreaking book *Zapped*. She has appeared on *20/20, Dr. Phil, The View, Good Morning America, Extra!, FitTV,* and *The Early Show*. In addition, her work has been featured on ABC, CNN, PBS, CBS, NBC, MSNBC, CBN, Fox News, and the BBC.

She has served as a celebrity spokesperson and formula developer for many of the leading companies in the health foods and network marketing industry. Her work has been featured in a myriad of national publications including *Time, Newsweek, Glamour,* and the *New York Times*.

ENGAGING HEALTH

Today she continues to dedicate herself to carving out new landmarks in functional and integrative medicine with her latest e-book, *Eat Fat, Lose Weight*. She is a popular speaker on Internet summits and is actively involved with videos and her blog. Her expert advice often appears in *First for Women* magazine, where she was the nutrition columnist for more than 10 years.

In 2016 Ann Louise was presented with the Humanitarian Award from the Cancer Control Society. She currently sits on the Advisory Board for the

International Institute for Building-Biology & Ecology, the Nutritional Therapy Association, Inc., and Clear Passage, Inc.

Connect with Ann Louise at www.annlouise.com, www.fatflush.com, and facebook.com/annlouisegittleman.